DRUGS AFFECTING LIPID METABOLISM VIII

ADVANCES IN EXPERIMENTAL MEDICINE AND BIOLOGY

Recent Volumes in this Series

Volume 175
NEUROTRANSMITTER RECEPTORS: Mechanisms of Action and Regulation
Edited by Shozo Kito, Tomio Segawa, Kinya Kuriyama, Henry I. Yamamura, and Richard W. Olsen

Volume 176
HUMAN TROPHOBLAST NEOPLASMS
Edited by Roland A. Pattillo and Robert O. Hussa

Volume 177
NUTRITIONAL AND TOXICOLOGICAL ASPECTS OF FOOD SAFETY
Edited by Mendel Friedman

Volume 178
PHOSPHATE AND MINERAL METABOLISM
Edited by Shaul G. Massry, Giuseppe Maschio, and Eberhard Ritz

Volume 179
PROTEINS INVOLVED IN DNA REPLICATION
Edited by Ulrich Hübscher and Silvio Spadari

Volume 180
OXYGEN TRANSPORT TO TISSUE – VI
Edited by Duane Bruley, Haim I. Bicher, and Daniel Reneau

Volume 181
GENE EXPRESSION AND CELL-CELL INTERACTIONS IN THE DEVELOPING NERVOUS SYSTEM
Edited by Jean M. Lauder and Phillip G. Nelson

Volume 182
GENE EXPRESSION IN MUSCLE
Edited by Richard C. Strohman and Stewart Wolf

Volume 183
DRUGS AFFECTING LIPID METABOLISM VIII
Edited by David Kritchevsky, William L. Holmes, and Rodolfo Paoletti

---

DRUGS AFFECTING LIPID METABOLISM VIII

Edited by

David Kritchevsky
The Wistar Institute of Anatomy and Biology
Philadelphia, Pennsylvania

William L. Holmes
West Chester, Pennsylvania

and

Rodolfo Paoletti
Institute of Pharmacology and Pharmacognosy
University of Milan
Milan, Italy

PLENUM PRESS • NEW YORK AND LONDON

Library of Congress Cataloging in Publication Data

International Symposium on Drugs Affecting Lipid Metabolism (8th: 1983: Philadelphia, Pa.
Drugs affecting lipid metabolism VIII.

(Advances in experimental medicine and biology; v. 183)
"Proceedings of the Eighth International Symposium on Drugs Affecting Lipid Metabolism, held July 27-30, 1983, in Philadelphia, Pennsylvania"—T.p. verso.
Includes bibliographies and indexes.
1. Atherosclerosis—Congresses. 2. Blood lipids—Metabolism—Disorders—Congresses. 3. Antilipemic agents—Congresses. I. Kritchevsky, David, 1920- . II. Holmes, William L., 1918- . III. Paoletti, Rodolfo. IV. Title. V. Series. [DNLM: 1. Antilipemic Agents—congresses. 2. Arteriosclerosis—congresses. 3. Lipids—metabolism—congresses. 4. Lipoproteins—metabolism—congresses. 5. Metabolism—drug effects—congresses. W1 AS559 v. 183 / QU 85 I596 1983d]
RC692.I54 1983 616.1'36 84-26547

ISBN-13:978-1-4612-9493-1 e-ISBN-13:978-1-4613-2459-1
DOI:10.1007/978-1-4613-2459-1

Proceedings of the Eighth International Symposium on Drugs Affecting Lipid Metabolism, held July 27-30, 1983, in Philadelphia, Pennsylvania

Softcover reprint of the hardcover 1st 1985

A Division of Plenum Publishing Corporation
233 Spring Street, New York, N.Y. 10013

PREFACE

The Proceedings of the Eight International Symposium on Drugs Affecting Lipid Metabolism (8th D.A.L.M.) is the subject of this volume. Since the first symposium in 1960, each successive meeting has broken new ground in the field of pharmacological control of lipid levels - offering new and stimulating insights and exposing the audience to the state of the art. The field has progressed sufficiently to permit discussion of the cellular biology of atherosclerosis. The opening session was devoted to pathology, macrophages, lipoproteins and their receptors and cholesterol ester metabolism. Because of the recent emergence of new apolipoprotein technology, a workshop devoted solely to apolipoprotein methodology was introduced followed by a plenary session devoted to their metabolism and structure.

Another rapidly developing area of atherosclerosis research is non-invasive assessment of this condition. Accordingly, a session was devoted to new techniques for this research modality. The final plenary sessions were devoted to the roles of drugs and diet in atherosclerosis - cause, treatment and mechanisms of action. The meeting was summarized by Dr. O.J. Pollak, one of the "founding fathers" of this field. There were nine sessions of proffered papers whose abstracts appear in this volume. In addition, special workshops (to be reported elsewhere) were devoted to several drugs including Oryzanol, Probucol and Etofibrate.

We are grateful for the interest of the organizations whose generous support contributed to the success of the meeting. The sponsorship of the Lorenzini Foundation was especially appreciated. The success of this meeting was due, in part, to the strong support of the local organizing committee. We are deeply indebted to Mrs. Frances Murray Nigro for her efficient and cheerful handling of the duties of the secretariat. The smoothness of this critical operation was principally instrumental for the success of the symposium. We also wish to thank Mrs. Edith Basedow Pappas for her expert help in the preparation of this volume.

David Kritchevsky
William L. Holmes
Rudolfo Paoletti

ACKNOWLEDGEMENTS

We gratefully acknowledge support from the following companies:

Abbott Laboratories

American Cyanamid Company

Ayerst Laboratories

Best Foods, CPC International

Burroughs Wellcome Company

Daiichi Pure Chemicals Company, Ltd.

Johnson & Johnson

Kraft, Inc.

Eli Lilly and Company

NcNeil Pharmaceutical

Merrell-Dow Pharmaceuticals, Inc.

Merz and Company

Nu-Check-Prep, Inc.

Otsuka Pharmaceutical Company, Ltd.

Parke-Davis, Warner-Lambert Company

The Procter & Gamble Company

A.H. Robins Company

G.D. Searle and Company

Smith Kline and French Laboratories

Upjohn Company

INTERNATIONAL ADVISORY COMMITTEE:

Dr. S. Bergstrom (Sweden)
Dr. L.A. Carlson (Sweden
Dr. G. Fassina (Italy)
Dr. A.M. Gotto (U.S.A.)
Dr. S.M. Grundy (U.S.A.)
Dr. W.L. Holmes (U.S.A.)
Dr. D. Kritchevsky (U.S.A.)
Dr. R. Paoletti (Italy)
Dr. G. Schettler (Germany)
Dr. C. Sirtori (Italy)

ORGANIZING COMMITTEE:

Dr. N. DiTullio
Dr. W.L. Holmes
Dr. D.M. Klurfeld
Dr. D. Kritchevsky
Dr. J. Plostnieks
Dr. G. Reichard

SCIENTIFIC SECRETARIES:

Dr. W.L. Holmes
Dr. R. Paoletti

PROGRAM CHAIRMAN:

Dr. D. Kritchevsky

SPONSORED BY:

COUNCIL ON ARTERIOSCLEROSIS OF THE AMERICAN HEART ASSOCIATION

FONDAZIONE GIOVANNI LORENZINI

CONTENTS

CELLULAR BIOLOGY OF ATHEROSCLEROSIS

APOLIPOPROTEINS

NONINVASIVE ASSESSMENT OF ATHEROSCLEROSIS

DRUGS AND DIET

THE CELLULAR PATHOBIOLOGY OF ATHEROSCLEROSIS IN 1983

Robert W. Wissler

The Department of Pathology and The Specialized Center of Research in Atherosclerosis, The University of Chicago
Chicago, Illinois 60637

INTRODUCTION

The main components of the advanced atherosclerotic plaque are the necrotic cholesteryl ester-rich core from which the disease process gets part of its name (the Greek stem "athero" means gruel or porridge) and the fibrous (sclerotic) cap which contains predominantly smooth muscle cells which often become encased in their own synthesis products of collagen, elastin and proteoglycans. Typically, many of these cells and their surrounding intercellular matrix are associated with abundant lipids which are demonstrable both chemically and morphologically. Most of the signs and symptoms and most of the life-threatening effects of atherosclerosis are due to these major components. They result in its being the leading cause of death and morbidity in the urban-industrial countries of the world, especially in Europe and North America.

In this brief manuscript an effort will be made to summarize in more or less chronological order some of the major recent advances in atherosclerosis research. These have resulted in substantially improved understanding of the modern pathobiological principles of atherogenesis.[1-5]

THE RECENT DISCOVERIES AND THEIR IMPLICATIONS

About 25 years ago research in this field began to advance rapidly primarily because of two major discoveries. Electron microscopic studies of the plaque, along with immunohistochemical investigations, demonstrated that the main cell of the plaque is the smooth muscle cell and not the fibroblast as was generally believed prior to that

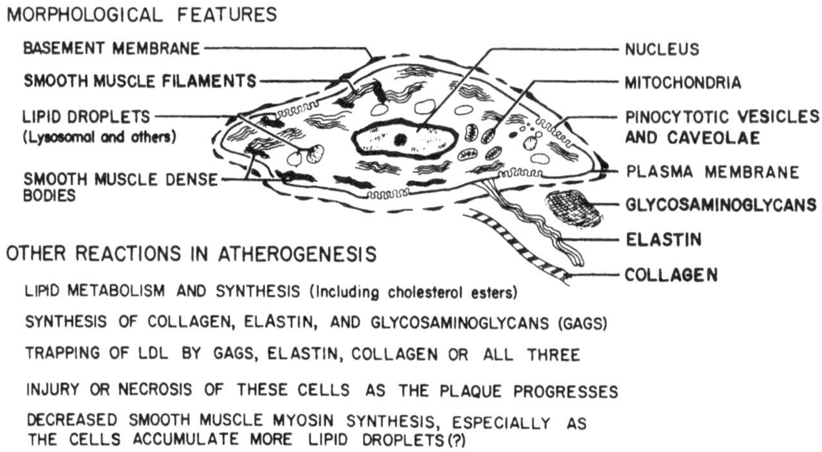

Fig. 1 The major morphological and functional features of the "multifunctional medial mesenchymal cell," the principal cell type involved in atherogenesis. This is the most prominent cell in the fibrous cap of the plaque, and probably makes most of the proteins and the other sclerotic parts of the disease process. (Modified from R. W. Wissler et al., Abnormalities of the arterial wall and its metabolism in atherogenesis, Prog. Cardiovasc. Dis. 18:5 (1976), by permission of Grune and Stratton.)

time (Fig. 1). Identification of the smooth muscle cell as the major cell of the atherosclerotic process helped to organize and unify knowledge about the plaque because this cell takes up lipid, which is an important part of the atherosclerotic process, it makes the fibrous components of the plaque, and it proliferates. It has become more and more evident that, just as in cancer, cell proliferation is an important part of the disease process in atherosclerosis.[1,2,3,6] Therefore, cell proliferation and the factors controlling the dividing of cells in the lesion are of special importance, as is the control of lipid accumulation, especially cholesteryl esters.

Additional work in the early sixties firmly established that the lipid and cholesterol in the necrotic core of the plaque come from the blood, mostly in the form of the lower density lipoproteins (LDL and VLDL). It is now well established that cholesterol-rich protein molecules, or particles, carry most of the cholesterol in the blood and supply most of the peripheral cells including the artery wall cells with cholesterol for cell membrane synthesis. The pathobiological mechanisms responsible for the buildup of cholesteryl ester deposits in and around these cells of the atherosclerotic lesion have become of increasing concern. Since almost all macromolecules in the blood get into the artery wall to some extent, it has become more and more apparent that there has to be some kind of mechanism that is trapping them or preferentially localizing these low density lipoproteins in the wall.

Many forms of lipid-protein particles circulate in the blood, and these vary greatly in their composition, with varying proportions of protein, cholesterol, cholesteryl ester, phospholipid, and triglyceride (Table 1). Low density lipoproteins, very low density lipoproteins, and broad beta very low density lipoproteins carry the highest percentage of cholesterol and cholesteryl ester in the blood. They are the ones which are most closely associated with the development of atherosclerotic plaques in animals and humans. Some of the high density lipoprotein (HDL) molecules appear to have a protective function. They can carry cholesterol out of peripheral tissues, such as arteries, and transport it back to the liver where it can be secreted into the bile and out into the feces.

As we learned more about the functions of lipid in the plasma and the interaction of lipoproteins with arterial smooth muscle cells, we found that hyperlipidemic plasma with high blood cholesterol levels, relative to the levels we consider to be normal (i.e., 150-170 mg %),[7] does several things that plasma from normal lipidemic individuals does not do. In our laboratory in the late sixties we reported that hyperlipidemic serum from rhesus monkeys fed a high fat, high cholesterol ration for several weeks stimulated proliferation of arterial medial cells whereas normal serum did not.[8] We also found that most of this excess cell division was stimulated by the LDL fraction of the hyperlipidemic serum. Whether one measures the average diameter of cultured colonies of smooth muscle cells in tissue culture flasks, or whether one uses tritiated thymidine to measure the rate of proliferation, one finds that cells that are exposed to normal monkey serum or to LDL from normal monkey serum have very low rates of cell division, and that cells which are exposed to hyperlipidemic monkey serum or LDL from hyperlipidemic monkey serum have very high rates of increase.[9,10] If HDL from normal serum is added to a system like this, one can remarkably reduce the rate of proliferation as measured by the percentage of labelled cells, as compared to the system that only has LDL from hyperlipidemic serum.[11] So there is a protective effect of high density lipoprotein in tissue culture that is consistent with what we now find epidemiologically in populations of individuals.[12] We also found that LDL molecules from hyperlipidemic plasma induce excessive ingress and storage of cholesteryl esters in these arterial smooth muscle cells.

Subcultures of these smooth muscle cells can contain abundant excess cholesterol, much more than the excess amount of cholesterol in hyperlipidemic serum,[13] and if one adds HDL to that system after the cells are loaded, the decrease in cholesteryl ester is very evident.[14] So HDL works to interrupt these cholesterol accumulating processes and will counteract the effects of low density lipoprotein from hyperlipidemic serum.[15]

In these last few years we have had the opportunity to study in vitro the interaction of smooth muscle cells of the artery wall that we have sometimes referred to as multifunctional medial mesenchymal cells because they have so many functions and take part in atherogenesis in so many ways.[16] We can study their interaction with lipoproteins in situ and have learned that the lipoproteins contribute to the fibrous cap by stimulating migration, proliferation and collagen, elastin and proteoglycan synthesis by these cells. The lipoproteins, especially the LDL from hyperlipidemic sera, can also lead to cell injury and an increase in the rate of cell death, which may be one of the major contributions to the formation of the necrotic core.[17,18]

About 1970 Dr. Russell Ross and his colleagues at the University of Washington in Seattle introduced a new concept in atherosclerosis research: injury to the endothelium, the inner lining of the artery, with subsequent platelet sticking, spreading and liberation of the platelet growth factor, may be extremely important in relation to the development of atherosclerosis, especially in certain individuals. Platelets adhere to the surface of injured endothelium, then spread out and liberate platelet derived growth factor (PDGF) from their alpha granules. This stimulates smooth muscle cells to proliferate. At this point it is a reversible process, unless something happens to make that injury or that stimulus chronic. One of the types of sustaining factors in this injury, according to Dr. Ross and his colleagues,[6] is chronic hypercholesterolemia. This hypothesis is useful in understanding the pathogenesis of the atherosclerotic process. It contributes a great deal to those of us who have been studying atherosclerosis in relation to autopsy findings and pathology. It helps to explain the occasional paradoxical or exceptional case that develops severe atherosclerosis even though the blood levels of low density lipoprotein are low, or in those where there is no history of cigarette smoking or high blood pressure--the three major risk factors that are identified with atherosclerosis. Some of those cases probably represent individuals who do have chronic endothelial injury which is severe and continuous enough so that these can develop the classical atherosclerotic process in spite of the absence of elevated levels of lipid. We believe that this is a rather unusual occurrence in most environments and is probably the exceptional way that advanced atherosclerosis develops.[19] Under usual circumstances the deposit of lipid (and apo B) in the artery wall precedes the evidence of cell proliferation. In fact, in most individuals who have low levels of low density lipoproteins, the process of cell proliferation is intermittent or relatively infrequent, and there seems to be general agreement that at least in primates those kinds of lesions will be expected to reverse completely on their own because of the rapid healing of the endothelium (Fig. 2).

According to current concepts atherosclerosis usually develops in our environment because of relatively slight but continuous elevation of low density lipoproteins in the plasma. This leads to pro-

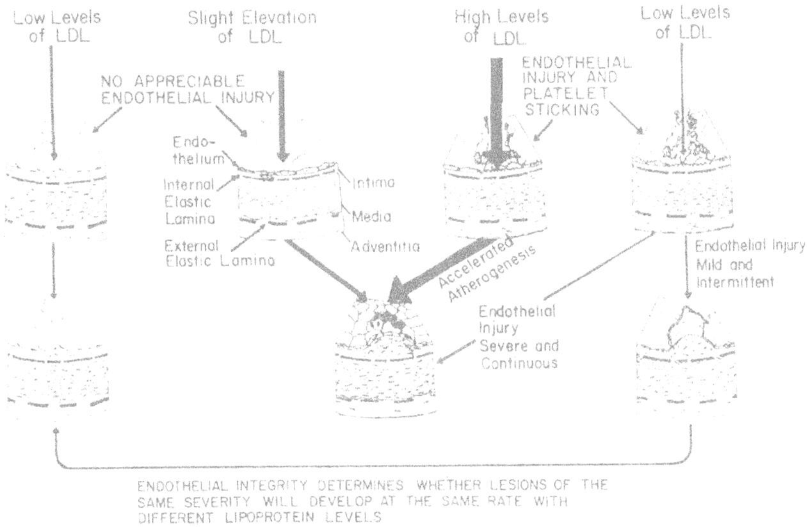

Fig. 2 Presumed pathways of interaction between elevated levels of low-density lipoprotein and arterial endothelial injury to produce a progressive atherosclerotic plaque. Although in extreme instances of continuous and severe endothelial damage, progressive plaque formation can occur even when the low-density lipoprotein levels are low (extreme right); this does not negate the protective effect of low levels of low-density lipoproteins if the endothelium is not being damaged severely (extreme left) or is damaged slightly and not very often. The accelerated atherogenesis frequently observed when familial hypercholesterolemia is present in its heterozygous or homozygous form is represented (second from right), while the usual slow pathogenesis resulting in the same kind of progressive atherosclerosis in individuals with moderate hyperlipoproteinemias over a period of decades is shown second from left. (Modified from R. Ross and J. A. Glomset, The pathogenesis of atherosclerosis, New Engl. J. Med. 295:420 (1976), reprinted by permission of the New England Journal of Medicine; see also R. W. Wissler, Principles of the pathogenesis of atherosclerosis, in: "Heart Disease: A Textbook of Cardiovascular Medicine," E. Braunwald, ed., W. B. Saunders, Philadelphia, p. 1183 (1984).)

gressive growth of the plaques due both to stimulation of smooth muscle cell proliferation and increased deposit of LDL and other low-density lipoproteins within the cells of the plaque and also between these cells.

There are also individuals with well defined genetic disorders in lipoprotein metabolism. They may account for more than 15% of the cases of advanced atherosclerosis. These unfortunate individuals often have an accelerated atherogenic process.[20] This may be augmented by nutritional hypercholesterolemia, but is primarily due to genetic abnormalities in their lipoprotein metabolism--the best known of which is the so-called familial hypercholesterolemia (FH). Some of those individiduals developed clinical complications of atherosclerosis in their teens or early twenties and many in their thirties and forties. These cases provide a strong part of the evidence that plasma lipids are very important in atherogenesis, because the components of their plaques are very similar to the plaques seen at autopsy in people in their seventies or eighties who develop atherosclerosis much more slowly.[20]

Chylomicrons and several remnant lipoprotein particles found in the plasma, particularly after a high fat meal, are large triglyceride-rich particles derived from the intestinal lymph, carry relative little cholesterol, and are often too large to gain entrance into arteries under ordinary circumstances. As a result of the work of Dr. Donald Zilversmit at Cornell,[21] and the more recent work of Dr. Robert Mahley in San Francisco,[22] we now know that there are at least two mechanisms whereby these postprandial large fat droplets may be important in atherosclerosis (Table 1). First of all, Dr. Zilversmit has demonstrated that they can furnish a good deal of cholesterol to the artery if the enzyme lipoprotein lipase acts on them close to the endothelial cells. The cholesterol released from the chylomicron in this manner can then penetrate through the artery as a much smaller remnant particle and it can become deposited. Dr. Mahley has called attention to the so-called beta very low-density lipoproteins (β-VLDL). These are probably mostly chylomicron remnant particles which are rather remarkably influenced by diets high in cholesterol, and which may be one of the most atherogenic of the particles which circulate in the blood stream.[23] It is noteworthy that Professor Scanu and his co-workers in our Specialized Center of Research,[24] and Dr. Larry Rudel and his co-workers at Bowman-Gray,[25] have found that the rhesus monkey hyperlipidemic LDL (H-LDL) has characteristics which are different from LDL of normal plasma. In this species these H-LDL particles are much larger, carry more cholesterol, and have a different kind of surface (Table 1).

Dr. Getz, the current Director of the Specialized Center of Research in Atherosclerosis at the University of Chicago, has recently studied with his co-workers a type of low-density lipoprotein usually called LDL 240, the apo B of which is largely synthesized in the gastrointestinal tract.[26] In experimental animals LDL 240 is greatly influenced by dietary factors. It is rich in apo E, and increasing evidence indicates that it is an important functional fraction of the low-density lipoproteins (Table 1).

Dr. Angelo Scanu and his co-workers at the University of Chicago have recently discovered a rather remarkable heterogeneity of rhesus monkey LDL particles.[27] They are able to identify and separate at

TABLE 1. NEW RELATIONSHIPS OF LIPOPROTEIN FRACTIONS TO ATHEROGENESIS

CURRENT LIPOPROTEIN DESIGNATIONS	PREDOMINANT APO PROTEIN(S)	FUNCTIONS AND PRESUMED FUNCTIONS IN ATHEROGENESIS
Chylomicrons	Apo B 240 Apo E	May furnish cholesterol and triglycerides for atherogenesis at the arterial cell surface due to action of lipoprotein lipase (LPL) and via other remnants
VLDL	Apo B 335 Apo E Apo C-I to C-III	Very little evidence of atherogenic effect except via LPL activity
Broad-beta VLDL	Apo B 240 Apo E	Highly atherogenic remnant particles derived from chylomicrons in subjects (especially dogs) fed a high-cholesterol, high-fat ration
H-LDL*° LDL I°	Apo B 335	Perhaps the most consistently atherogenic fraction in human species (FH) and and lipogenic and mitogenic in other primates; when altered by endothelial cells or by malondialdehyde, it is avidly taken up by macrophages in vitro
LDL II°		May support buildup of cholesterol in arterial SMC
LDL III°	Apo B 335	Little direct evidence of atherogenicity with the exception of mitogenic effect of particle after neuraminidase treatment
LDL IV°		Probably identical with LPa; epidemiological evidence supports atherogenicity
HDL_c	Apo E	Probably especially important in cholesterol excretion
HDL_1	Apo A-I Apo A-II	High-affinity receptors for hepatic apo E may help in cholesterol excretion
HDL_2	Apo E Apo A-I Apo A-II Apo C	Serum level correlated with protection against atherosclerosis in numerous species, including human Precursor to HDL_1
HDL_3	Apo A-I Apo A-II Apo C	Precursor to HDL_2, but the level is not predictive

* LDL from hyperlipidemic serum (enlarged cholesterol-rich particle)
° LDL fractions as designated by Fless and Scanu

from: R. W. Wissler, Principles of the pathogenesis of atherosclerosis, in: Heart Disease: A Textbook of Cardiovascular Medicine, 2nd Edition, E. Braunwald, ed., p 1185, W. B. Saunders Co., Philadelphia (1984).

least four fractions, LDL I, II, III, and IV, in monkey sera. Some of these may be particularly important in atherosclerosis. For example, LDL III can be converted by neuraminidase into a lipoprotein faction which stimulates smooth muscle cells to undergo proliferation even though this fraction as it circulates in the blood stream apparently has no such effect on smooth muscle cells.[28] LDL I, which is usually present in very small quantities in normal serum, also has a strong cell proliferation stimulating effect (Table 1).

Much has been learned about high density lipoproteins (HDLs) in recent years. We now know that there are at least four kinds of circulating HDLs. It is no longer sufficient to measure only the total HDL concentration, or even total HDL cholesterol in the blood, to get an accurate picture of their relative importance in atherosclerosis. The technology in the clinical chemistry laboratory needs to develop the capability of identifying the one with the apoproteins which are particularly important in relation to cholesterol modulation. Apo E, which binds most avidly to receptors in the liver, may reflect a major mechanism by which HDL protects us.[19,29]

We are now beginning to understand the pathobiology of the smooth muscle cells in the atherosclerotic plaque. We now know that many of the smooth muscle cells in the plaque, which are mostly in a synthetic state (monoclonal mutation or phenotypic modulation?), are quite different from those in the normal media of the artery.[30,31] These cells in the plaque are much more responsive to H-LDL and to the platelet derived growth factor, they are relatively noncontractile, and they are very active in connective tissue synthesis.

Furthermore, we are now beginning to think about atherosclerosis much more in terms of interaction among cells, but also interaction of cells with hyperlipidemic LDL.[1,2,5] The main target cell is the smooth muscle cell. We now know that there are numerous factors which can cause these cells to proliferate and which can lead to important changes in their biology. Endothelial cells produce a growth factor and so do macrophages, which under certain conditions get into developing lesions and produce potent mitogenic factors.[32,33] Many of these factors are now being actively investigated so that we should soon know much more about the interactions among lipoproteins, arterial smooth muscle cells, and monocytes, with endothelial cells and platelets.[2-6]

The proliferation of smooth muscle cells in the plaque may originate as a mutation from a single cell line, according to the monoclonal hypothesis developed by Dr. Earl Benditt.[30,34] Others believe that the growth is a special kind of hyperplasia of the arterial smooth muscle cells, which is probably reversible.[18] The alteration makes the cells much more sensitive to certain kinds of stimuli that accompany atherogenesis.[35]

The work of Goldstein, Brown and others on what happens to cholesterol in the form of low density lipoprotein as it comes in contact with a cell has opened up the whole new field of cell surface receptors, relevant to regulation of cholesterol uptake and cholesterol metabolism in relation to membrane formation in the cell.[36] These are highly significant new concepts with important implications for both cell metabolism and atherogenesis.

Dr. DeDuve, the great Nobel Prize winning cell biologist, has emphasized that relative deficiency in intracellular lysosomal enzyme activity may also be of importance in atherogenesis, since the lysosomal esterases probably represent one of the main ways in which cholesterol and cholesteryl esters are metabolized in the arterial cells.[37]

These concepts taken together offer striking evidence of the importance of the emerging cellular pathobiology of atherosclerosis (Fig. 3).[2] These studies as well as work in many other laboratories are now progressing rapidly into a molecular pathobiology phase which begins to offer promise of a new era of more complete understanding of the pathogenesis of atherosclerosis.

In addition to the remarkable recent growth of knowledge regarding the types and interactions of lipoprotein fractions referred to earlier in this paper (Table 1), there is rapidly expanding knowledge regarding the different cell surface receptors on the principal scavenger cell, the macrophage.[19,38] There is continued doubt and continued investigation of the macrophage as a contributor to the progression and the regression of the atherosclerotic process (Table 2). Current observations indicate that few monocyte derived macrophages are present in either human or primate plaques of young adults unless there is also damage to the artery wall by antigen-antibody (Ag-Ab) complexes [39] or if there is a severe defect in cholesterol catabolism and excretion, as characteristically observed in the rabbit model of atherosclerosis.[40]

Recent studies in this laboratory have utilized newly developed and recently validated specific histochemical procedures for identifying macrophages.[41,42] This technique has permitted us to begin to quantitate the proportion of macrophages in lesions at various stages of development and in various species to be compared with the human atherosclerotic process. Briefly, almost all human lesions show fewer than 10% of the cells to be positive for this macrophage indicator. On the other hand only one animal model thus far shows similar proportions, namely the rhesus monkey. The cynomolgus monkey, like the rabbit, usually shows a high proportion, 50% or more of its cells, as positive for this lipase reaction which presumably stains only macrophages.

Recently, a careful study of these two species of macaques, rhesus and cynomolgus, fed the same atherogenic ration for the same length of time, has revealed a number of rather consistent differences in

TABLE 2

MACROPHAGES AND ATHEROGENESIS:

ARE THEY IMPORTANT CONTRIBUTORS TO PLAQUE DEVELOPMENT?

PROS	CONS
Most "Foam Cells" are derived from macrophages (not SMC)	Virtually all models resembling the human lesion, as well as the human lesion, contain very few macrophages.
Macrophages do not require Apo B receptors to become loaded with lipid and cholesterol from broad beta VLDL or from altered (aging) LDL	The principal cell that divides, accumulates and produces collagen, elastin and proteoglycans in the plaque is the smooth muscle cell.
Macrophages may be responsible for most of the intracellular metabolism of LDL entering the artery wall and when they die they may deposit much of the intercellular lipid.	The smooth muscle cell in the lesions is a deregulated "synthetic" cell which may be coverted to a foam cell under some circumstances.
Secretion of macrophage derived growth factor provides a powerful stimulus for arterial SMC proliferation.	The macrophage rich lesions in experimental animals (rabbits, fowl, cholate fed rats) do not resemble human lesions and generally do not lead to ischemic disease or to thrombosis.
Therefore, in spite of rather small numbers, little proliferation and little matrix formation, the macrophage may exert a profound influence on lesion development.	The macrophages tend to increase during the early stages of regression of atherosclerosis and are best regarded as scavenger cells which aid in lesion healing and diminution. The lipases, collagenase and elastase they make may help in plaque regression.

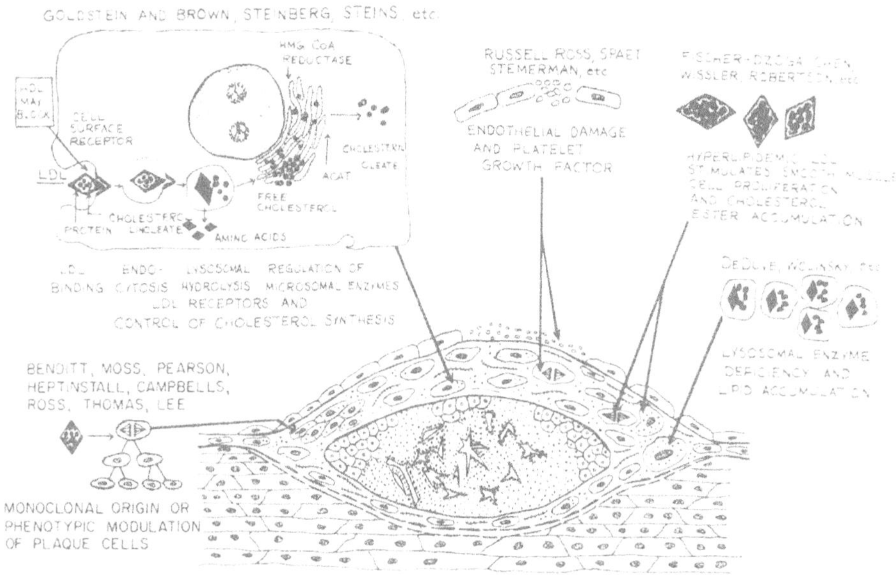

Fig. 3 Some of the major recent developments in understanding a few of the cellular pathobiological reactions that appear to be important in the pathogenesis (and regression) of the atherosclerotic plaque. (Modified from R. W. Wissler, Coronary atherosclerosis and ischemic heart disease, in: "Brain and Heart Infarct.," K. J. Zulch, ed., p. 206, Springer-Verlag, New York, Heidelberg, Berlin, 1977.)

their responses.[39,43-46] Some of the most consistent of these are that about 90% of rhesus coronary artery lesions are eccentric and intimal, while the majority of the cynomolgus lesions (75%), developing in the same length of time, are concentric and transmural. Correlated with this striking difference in lesion configuration at the microscopic level is a remarkable difference in circulating immune complexes. We researched for these because of the resemblance of the arterial involvement to lesions we and others had studied in the serum sickness rabbit model in the forties[47,48] and which Minick and co-workers had combined with atherogenic rations in the sixties and seventies to produce an atheroarteritis.[49,50]

Several other probable consequences of these pathogenetic differences are now being studied in both human and nonhuman primates. These include the incidence of thrombosis associated with each type of lesion which, in the human at least, seems to be much higher in the arteries showing transmural and concentric lesions. On theoretical grounds the eccentric lesions with ulceration should be especially vulnerable to spasm because of the abundant intact arterial medial musculature available to contract.[51]

A major effect of the concentric, transmural lesions is to interfere with regression. Even though copious quantities of lipid may be removed from the lesions when the hypercholesterolemia is corrected, the scarring and contraction of the damaged media may lead to an actual further decrease in lumen size.[43,52,53] We hope that an era is approaching when sophisticated high resolution imaging of human atherosclerotic plaques during life will make it possible to visualize the type of lesions which may be present in coronary or other arteries.

One additional contribution of work with experimental models has been to call attention to the rather remarkable variations in lesion components which can result from feeding various food fats.[54-55] Not only does this present an opportunity to develop lesions with contrasting components of cellular, lipid and fibrous matrix for regression studies, but it also offers an opportunity to learn much more about the pathobiology of lipoproteins and the effects of their fatty acids at the cellular and molecular level.

SUMMARY

Atherosclerosis is a dynamic process in which a number of stimuli to arterial lipid deposition, cell proliferation and cell death, and the synthesis of fiber and matrix proteins by modulated smooth muscle cells are the major factors which can vary to control to process. The circulating levels and interaction of lipoproteins, the integrity of the endothelium, the heart rate and the height of the blood pressure and many incompletely understood arterial wall factors all appear to affect these components. Although there are many unanswered questions, it is clear that immense progress has been made in the past 25 years in developing a reasonable understanding of the cellular pathobiology of the atherosclerotic process. The momentun of this progress is such as to project a very promising future in which the molecular pathology of atherogenesis will be understood well enough to permit prevention, retardation and more effective regression of the dangerous advanced plaque.

ACKNOWLEDGMENTS

The author is grateful to Gertrud Friedman, Joan King and Gwen Matthews who have helped to prepare this manuscript. He also acknowledges the contributions to the results from this laboratory reported or referred to in this paper which have been supported in part by grants from the National Institutes of Health (HL-115062, HL-07237) and which have been made possible by the hard work and enlightened help of Drs. Godfrey Getz, Katti Fischer-Dzoga, Draga Vesselinovitch, Robert Chen, Sandra Bates, Thomas Schaffner, Harry Davis, as well as many students and technologists.

REFERENCES

1. R. W. Wissler, Development of the atherosclerotic plaque, in: Myocardium: Failure and Infarction, E. Braunwald, ed., p. 155, H. P. Publishing Co., New York (1974).
2. R. W. Wissler, The emerging cellular pathobiology of atherosclerosis, Artery 5:409 (1979).
3. R. Ross, Atherosclerosis: A problem of the biology of arterial wall cells and their interactions with blood components, Arteriosclerosis 1:293 (1981).
4. D. Steinberg, Lipoproteins and atherosclerosis: A look back and a look ahead, Arteriosclerosis 3:283 (1983).
5. R. W. Wissler and D. Vesselinovitch, The pathobiology of the artherosclerotic plaque in the mid-1980s, in: "Regression of atherosclerotic lesions: Experimental studies and observations in humans," R. Malinow and V. Blaton, eds., Plenum Press, New York (1984).
6. R. Ross and J. A. Glomset, The pathogenesis of atherosclerosis, New Eng. J. Med. 295:369, 420 (1976).
7. R. W. Wissler, Conference on the Health Effects of Blood Lipids: Optimal Distributions for Populations, Workshop Report: Laboratory-Experimental Section, Prev. Med. 8:175 (1979).
8. V. C. Y. Kao, R. W. Wissler, and K. Fischer-Dzoga, The influence of hyperlipemic serum on the growth of medial smooth muscle cells of rhesus monkey aorta in vitro, Circulation 38 (Suppl. VI):12 (1968).
9. K. Fischer-Dzoga and R. W. Wissler, Stimulation of proliferation in stationary primary cultures of monkey aortic smooth muscle cells, II. Effect of varying concentrations of hyperlipemic serum and low-density lipoproteins of varying dietary fat origins, Atherosclerosis 24:515 (1976).
10. R. W. Wissler, Interactions of low-density lipoproteins from hypercholesterolemic serum with arterial wall cells and their extracellular products in atherogenesis and regression, in: "The Biochemistry of Atherosclerosis," A. Scanu, R. W. Wissler, and G. S. Getz, eds., p. 345, Marcel Dekker, Inc., New York (1979).
11. Y. Yoshida, K. Fischer-Dzoga, and R. W. Wissler, Effects of normolipidemic high-density lipoproteins on proliferation of monkey aortic smooth muscle cells induced by hyperlipidemic low-density lipoproteins, Exp. Mol. Pathol., (In Press, 1984).
12. N. E. Miller, Prevention of coronary heart disease: The role of high-density lipoproteins, Postgrad. Med. J. 56:575 (1980).
13. S. R. Bates, Accumulation and loss of cholesterol esters in monkey arterial smooth muscle cells exposed to normal and hyperlipemic serum lipoproteins, Atherosclerosis 32:165 (1979).
14. S. R. Bates, Effect of HDL on the interaction of hyperlipemic LDL with smooth muscle cells, Artery 7:303 (1980).
15. R. W. Wissler, K. Fischer-Dzoga, S. R. Bates, and R. M. Chen, Arterial smooth muscle cells in tissue culture, in: "Structure and Function of the Circulation," Vol. III, C. J.

Schwartz, N. T. Werthessen, and S. Wolf, eds., p. 427, Plenum Press, New York (1981).
16. R. W. Wissler, Atherosclerosis--its pathogenesis in perspective, *in*: "Comparative Pathology of the Heart (Adv. Cardiol.)," Vol. 13, F. Homberger, ed., p. 10, S. Karger, Basel (1974).
17. R. M. Chen, G. S. Getz, K. Fischer-Dzoga, and R. W. Wissler, The role of hyperlipidemic serum on the proliferation and necrosis of aortic medial cells *in vitro*, *Exp. Mol. Pathol*. 26:359 (1977).
18. W. A. Thomas, J. M. Reiner, R. A. Florentin, K. Janakidevi, and K. J. Lee, Arterial smooth muscle cells in atherogenesis: Births, deaths and clonal phenomena, *in*: "Atherosclerosis IV, G. Schettler, Y. Goto, Y. Hata, and G. Klose, eds., p. 16, Springer-Verlag, Berlin (1977).
19. R. W. Wissler, Principles of pathogenesis of atherosclerosis, *in*: "Heart Disease: A Textbook of Cardiovascular Medicine, second edition, E. Braunwald, ed., p. 1185, W. B. Saunders Co., Philadelphia (1984).
20. W. C. Roberts, The status of the coronary arteries in fatal ischemic heart disease, *Cardiovasc. Clin*. 7:1 (1975).
21. D. B. Zilversmit, Atherogenesis: A postprandial phenomenon, *Circulation Res*. 33:633 (1973).
22. R. W. Mahley, Atherogenic hyperlipoproteinemia, The cellular and molecular biology of plasma lipoproteins altered by dietary fat and cholesterol, *Med. Clin. N. Am*. 66:375 (1982).
23. R. W. Mahley, H. Weisgraber, and T. Innerarity, Canine lipoproteins and atherosclerosis: II. Characterization of the plasma lipoproteins associated with atherogenic and non-atherogenic hyperlipidemia, *Circ. Res*. 35:722 (1974).
24. G. M. Fless, R. W. Wissler, and A. M. Scanu, Study of abnormal plasma low-density lipoproteins in rhesus monkeys with diet-induced hyperlipidemia, *Biochemistry* 15:5799 (1976).
25. L. L. Rudel, L. L. Pitts, II, and C. A. Nelson, Characterization of plasma low-density lipoproteins of nonhuman primates fed dietary cholesterol, *J. Lipid Res*. 18:211 (1977).
26. K. V. Krishnaiah, L. F. Walker, J. Borensztajn, G. Schonfeld, and G. S. Getz, Apolipoprotein B variant derived from the rat intestine, *Proc. Nat. Acad. Sci*. 17:3806 (1980).
27. G. M. Fless, T. Kirchhausen, K. Fischer-Dzoga, R. W. Wissler, and A. M. Scanu, Relationship between the properties of the apo B containing low-density lipoproteins (LDL) of normolipidemic rhesus monkeys and their mitogenic action on arterial smooth muscle cells grown *in vitro*, *in*: "Atherosclerosis V," A. M. Gotto, Jr., L. C. Smith, and B. Allen, eds., p. 607, Springer-Verlag, New York (1980).
28. G. M. Fless, T. Kirchhausen, K. Fischer-Dzoga, R. W. Wissler, and A. M. Scanu, Serum low-density lipoproteins with mitogenic effect on cultured aortic smooth muscle cells, *Atherosclerosis* 41:171 (1982).
29. G. Assmann, Lipid Metabolism and Atherosclerosis, Schauttauer Verlag, Stuttgart (1982).

30. E. P. Benditt, Implications of the monoclonal character of human atherosclerotic plaques, Am. J. Pathol. 86:693 (1977).
31. J. Chamley-Campbell, G. R. Campbell, and R. Ross, The smooth muscle cell in culture, Physiol. Rev. 59:1 (1979).
32. C. Gajdusek, P. DiCorleto, R. Ross, and S. M. Schwartz, An endothelial cell-derived growth factor, J. Cell. Biol. 85:467 (1980).
33. S. J. Leibovich and R. Ross, A macrophage-dependent factor that stimulates the proliferation of fibroblasts in vitro, Am. J. Pathol. 84:501 (1976).
34. E. P. Benditt and J. M. Benditt, Evidence for a monoclonal origin of human atherosclerotic plaques, Proc. Nat. Acad. Sci. 70: 1753 (1973).
35. G. R. Campbell and J. H. Chamley-Campbell, The cellular pathobiology of atherosclerosis, Pathology 13:423 (1981).
36. J. L. Goldstein and M. S. Brown, The low-density lipoprotein pathway and its relation to atherosclerosis, Ann. Rev. Biochem. 46:897 (1977).
37. C. DeDuve, The participation of lysosomes in the transformation of smooth muscle cells to foamy cells in the aorta of cholesterol-fed rabbits, Acta Cardiol. Suppl. 20:9 (1974).
38. J. L. Goldstein, Y. K. Ho, S. K. Basu, and M. S. Brown, A binding site on macrophages that mediates the uptake and degradation of acetylated low-density lipoprotein producing massive cholesterol deposition, Proc. Nat. Acad. Sci. 76:333 (1979).
39. R. W. Wissler and D. Vesselinovitch, Atherosclerosis--relationship to coronary blood flow, Am. J. Cardiol. 52:2A (1983).
40. R. W. Wissler and D. Vesselinovitch, Experimental models of human atherosclerosis, Ann. N. Y. Acad. Sci. 149:907 (1968).
41. T. Schaffner, V. M. Elner, M. Bauer, and R. W. Wissler, Acid lipase: A histochemical and biochemical study using triton X100-naphthyl palmitate micelles, J. Histochem. Cytochem. 26:969 (1978).
42. T. Schaffner, K. Taylor, E. J. Bartucci, K. Fischer-Dzoga, J. H. Beeson, S. Glagov, and R. W. Wissler, Arterial foam cells exhibit distinctive immunomorphologic and histochemical features of macrophages, Am. J. Pathol. 100:57 (1980).
43. D. Vesselinovitch and R. W. Wissler, Correlation of types of induced lesions with regression of coronary atherosclerosis in two species of macaques, in: "Lipoproteins and Coronary Atherosclerosis," G. Noseda, C. Fragiacomo, R. Fumagalli, and R. Paoletti, eds., p. 401, Elsevier, Amsterdam (1982).
44. D. Vesselinovitch and R. W. Wissler, Quantitation of certain qualitative differences in the atherosclerotic process, in: "Atherosclerosis VI," G. Schettler, A. M. Gotto, G. Middelhoff, A. S. Habenicht, and K. R. Jurutka, eds., p. 174, Springer-Verlag, Berlin (1983).
45. H. R. Davis, D. Vesselinovitch, and R. W. Wissler, Reticuloendothelial system response to hyperlipidemia in rhesus and cynomolgus monkeys, J. Leuk. Biol. (In Press, 1984).

46. R. W. Wissler and D. Vesselinovitch, New concepts of factors involved in the natural history and regression of atherosclerosis, Periodica Angiologica 5:178 (1983).
47. A. R. Rich and J. E. Gregory, The experimental demonstration that periarteritis nodosa is a manifestation of hypersensitivity, Bull. Johns Hopkins Hosp. 72:65 (1943).
48. H. C. Hopps and R. W. Wissler, The experimental production of generalized arteritis and periarteritis (periarteritis nodosa), J. Lab. Clin. Med. 31:939 (1946).
49. C. R. Minick, G. E. Murphy, and W. C. Cambell, Experimental induction of atherosclerosis by the synergy of allergic injury to arteries and lipid-rich diet, I. Effect of repeated injection of horse serum in rabbits fed dietary cholesterol supplement, J. Exp. Med. 124:635 (1966).
50. C. R. Minick and G. E. Murphy, Experimental induction of atherosclerosis by the synergy of allergic injury to arteries and lipid-rich diet, II. Effect of repeatedly injected foreign protein in rabbits fed a lipid-rich, cholesterol-poor diet, Am. J. Pathol. 73:265 (1975).
51. L. M. Buja, L. D. Hillis, C. S. Petty, and J. T. Willerson, The role of coronary arterial spasm in ischemic heart disease, Arch. Pathol. Lab. Med. 105:221 (1981).
52. M. L. Armstrong and M. G. Megan, Responses of two macaque species to atherogenic diet and its withdrawal, in: "Atherosclerosis III," G. Schettler and A. Weizel, eds., p. 336, Springer-Verlags, Berlin (1974).
53. W. Hollander, B. Kirkpatrick, B. Paddock, J. Colombo, M. Nagraj, and S. Prusty, Studies on the progression and regression of coronary and peripheral atherosclerosis in the cynomolgus monkey, Exp. Mol. Pathol. 30:55 (1979).
54. D. Vesselinovitch, G. S. Getz, R. H. Hughes, and R. W. Wissler, Atherosclerosis 20:303 (1974).
55. D. Vesselinovitch, R. W. Wissler, T. J. Schaffner, and J. Borensztajn, The effects of various diets on atherogenesis in rhesus monkeys, Atherosclerosis 35:189 (1980).
56. D. Kritchevsky, S. A. Tepper, D. Vesselinovitch, and R. W. Wissler, Cholesterol vehicle in experimental atherosclerosis, Part 13, Randomized peanut oil, Atherosclerosis 17:225 (1973).

SECRETORY FUNCTIONS OF THE MONONUCLEAR PHAGOCYTE

W. A. Scott,†* N. A. Pawlowski†, E. B. Cramer,†† and Z. A. Cohn†

†The Rockefeller University, New York, and ††Department of Anatomy and Cell Biology
Downstate Medical Center, Brooklyn, New York

The functional properties of mononuclear phagocytes include their well-known capacities for phagocytosis and pinocytosis. Work in recent years has provided greater understanding of the effector functions of these cells; in particular, their secretory nature. The versality of the macrophage has been a surprise; over 50 secretory products including mediators, cytocidal factors, and growth-promoting agents have been identified[1] and triggers for some activities described.

I will restrict my remarks to the secretory activities of the mononuclear phagocyte and more specifically to the synthesis of arachidonic acid (20:4) metabolites. Potent inflammatory mediators are derived from the cyclooxygenase and lipoxygenase pathways of 20:4 metabolism (Fig.1). The cyclooxygenase products [prostaglandins (PG), prostacyclin, and thromboxane] have been shown to influence platelet aggregation, smooth muscle tone, and basic aspects of the inflammatory process. The lipoxygenase pathway products include leukotrienes (LT) which possess unique proinflammatory actions. LTB mediates white cell chemotaxis and adhesion to endothelium. LTC mediates increased vascular permeability and smooth muscle contraction. LTC together with its degradation products LTD and LTE, comprise the slow reacting substances of anaphylaxis.

*new address: W. A. Scott, c/o E. R. Squibb, The Institute for Medical Research, P. O. Box 4000, Princeton, New Jersey 08540

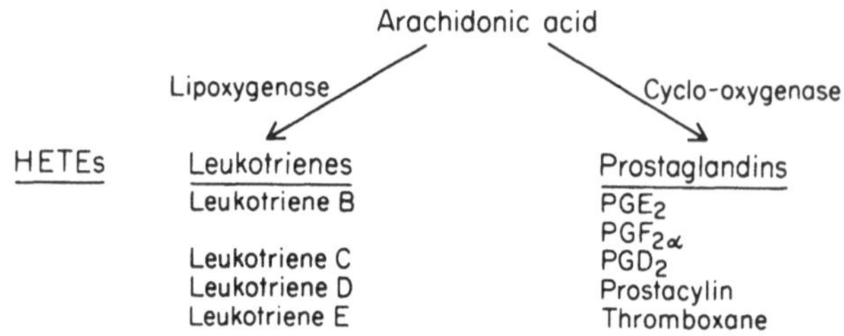

Fig. 1 Cyclooxygenase and lipoxygenase pathways of 20:4 metabolism.

HUMAN CIRCULATING BLOOD MONOCYTES

In man, the circulating blood monocyte can be isolated in quantity by relatively simple techniques, and thus is a pool of readily accessible mononuclear phagocytes. Other laboratories have demonstrated that these cells produce prostaglandins. Our interest in this area stemmed from observations in this laboratory indicating that mouse periotoneal macrophages are rich sources of LTC when challenged with inflammatory stimuli such as IgG,[3] IgE[4] immune complexes or zymosan.[3]

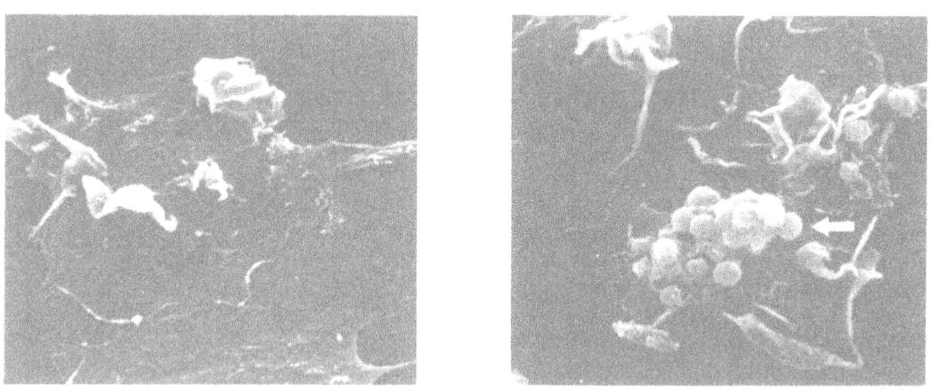

Fig. 2 Scanning electron micrographs of glutaraldehyde-fixed human monocytes. Left: Adherent monocyte culture prepared by conventional density gradient techniques (P-M). Right: Adherent monocytes prepared from monouclear cells washed in serum-EDTA (S-M).

Considering that the macrophage is a potent source of leukotrienes, it was of interest to determine whether this is also true of the macrophage precursor, the circulating blood monocyte. A number of years ago, Stossel et al.[5] found that monocyte phospholipids are rich in 20:4 which indicated that these cells contain considerable substrate for the production of 20:4 metabolites.

In initial experiments, monocytes isolated from Ficoll-Paque gradients contained 3-5 platelets rosetted to their surfaces[6] and Fig.2, as determined by microscopic examination. The rosetted platelets appeared to be activated as evidenced by their swollen appearance and the irregular shape of their surfaces (Fig. 2). This contamination presented a serious problem to the study of monocyte 20:4 metabolism since platelets are potent sources of 20:4 oxygenated products [primarily thromboxane and 12-hydroxy-5,8,10,14-eicosatetraenoic acid (12-HETE). By subjecting mononuclear cell preparatioins to two sequential incubations in neat human serum containing 5 mM EDTA at 37°C, surface contamination was reduced to 1 to 2 platelets per 200 monocytes (Fig. 2). This simple technique provided a rapid and convenient means to eliminate rosetted platelets from monoclear cell preparations.

In order to determine the full spectrum of 20:4 metabolites synthesized by monocytes, cultures were labeled with [^{3}H]20:4 in serum-containing medium, washed, and exposed to a stimulus to initiate 20:4 metabolism in serum-free medium. The radiolabeled products were separated by reverse-phase HPLC and their elution times compared with those of radiolabeled standards. Comparisons of radiolabeled 20:4 metabolites recovered from serum-treated monocytes (S-M), platelet-contaminated monocytes (P-M) and adherent cultures of platelets exposed to A23187 were carried out. Calcium inophore A23187 was the stimulus of choice since this agent promotes 20:4 metabolism in a variety of cell types. The proportions of cyclooxygenase and lipoxygenase products for each of the above cultures differed. In platelet and P-M preparations, 12-HETE accounted for 30 and 21% of the total metabolites (Fig. 3A and 3B). This proportion was reduced to 6-7% of the total in S-M, suggesting that 12-HETE was a platelet-derived product and that platelets contribute to the products in P-M stimulated with A23187. On detachment of P-M from the surface of plastic tissue culture vessels and replating, the percentage of 12-HETE was reduced to 3% of the 20:4 metabolites (Fig. 3C) in the resulting monolayers (D-M). This additional reduction may have resulted from the removal of platelets trapped under adherent P-M. It is not clear at present whether the continued low production of 12-HETE is an indicator of trace platelet contamination or the presence of a 12-lipoxygenase in monocytes.

In these same cultures treated with A23187, 5-hydroxy-6,8,11,14-eicosatetraenoic acid (5-HETE) increased from 0% in adherent platelets to 16 and 37% of the total 20:4 products in P-M and S-M. These data suggested that 5-HETE was monocyte-derived and that the ratio of 5- to 12-HETE is a convenient marker of platelet contamination. While the proportion of cyclooxygenase products decreased as monocyte purity increased, their continued production suggested that these metabolites were also synthesized by monocytes.

Platelet- and monocyte-specific stimuli were helpful in sorting out the products generated by each cell type. Thrombin promoted the release of only thromboxane and 12-HETE by both platelets and P-M. This array of products indicated that this is a platelet-specific

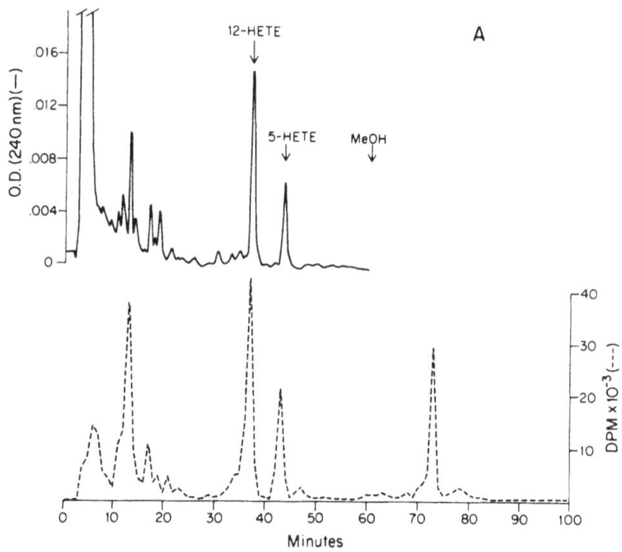

Fig. 3 HPLC profiles of the 20:4 metabolites released by (A) P-M, (B) platelets, and (C) D-M after 20 min incubation with 1 g/ml of A23187. Cultures were labeled for 4 h with $[^3H]$20:4 in medium containing 10% human serum. At the end of the labeling period, the cultures were washed, overlaid with medium without serum and the stimulus applied in ethanol. The media were extracted and subjected to reverse-phase HPLC on a column of Ultrasphere ODS eluted at 1 ml/min with 60 ml of methanol/water/acetic acid (75:25:0.01, vol/vol/vol) followed by 40 ml of methanol/acetic acid (100:0.01, vol/vol). ^{3}H-labeled prostaglandin and thromboxane standards eluted at 4-11 min. Elution times of 15-HETE (31-33 min) 12-HETE (36-38 min), and 5-HETE (42-45 min) were determined using standards. Other 20:4 metabolites included di-HETEs at 12-16 min, HHT at 17-18 min, and unreacted 20:4 at 71-80 min. Reproduced with permission from[6].

Individual cyclooxygenase products were identified by pooling the contents of fractions 4-11 and rechromatography on a Waters fatty acid analysis column as described previously.[4]

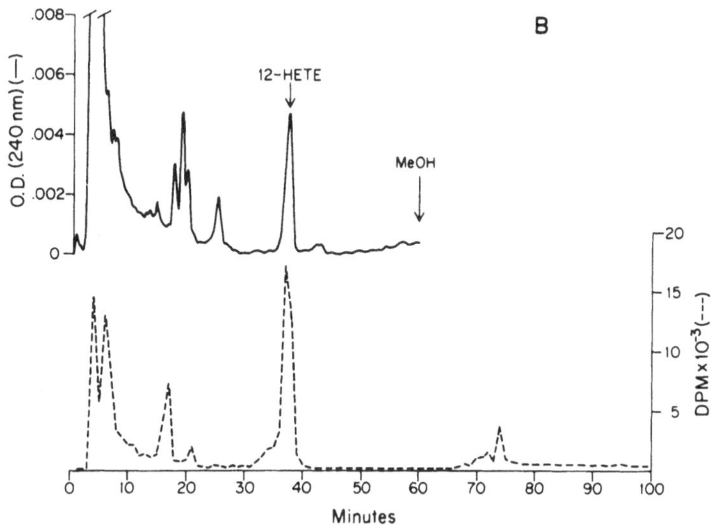

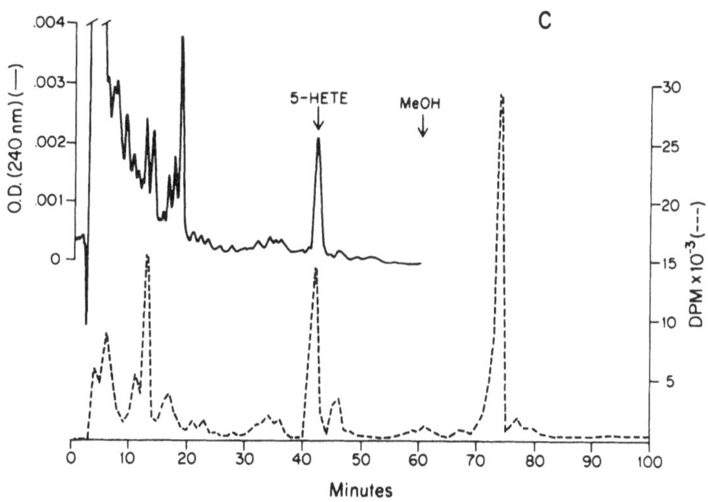

Fig. 3 (continued)

TABLE 1

20:4 METABOLITES SYNTHESIZED BY S-M EXPOSED TO A23187 OR OpZ

20:4 metabolites	Percent of total 20:4 metabolites	
	A23187	OpZ
Cyclooxygenase		
thromboxane	7.1	23.4
6-keto PFG1	1.1	2.0
PFG2	1.5	2.6
PGE2	1.9	2.9
HHT	5.4	16.0
Lipoxygenase		
mono-HETEs	41.3	12.0
di-HETEs	28.9	18.0

Radiolabeled cultures were established as described under Fig. 3. Cultures were exposed to either A23187 (20 min) or OpZ (60 min). The media were extracted and subjected to HPLC. Results are presented as the percent of total 20:4 metabolites recovered.

stimulus. This specificity was further assured by the lack of response (no release) of S-M and D-M to thrombin. In contrast, monocytes, but not platelets, responded to opsonized zymosan (OpZ) or Sephadex beads with IgG immune complexes coated on their surfaces. The percentage of cell-associated radiolabel released with particulate stimuli was comparable (15-18%) to that found on exposure to A23187. However with particulate stimuli, a greater proportion (50%) of the released 20:4 was metabolized via the cyclooxygenase pathway than with an A23187 stimulus (25%). The single major product formed was thromboxane (Table 1). In addition smaller amounts of leukotrienes C and B were detected; however quantitation of these products is incomplete.

These are the first data concerning the spectrum of products formed by human monocytes. It is evident that human monocytes release both cyclooxygenase and lipoxygenase products of 20:4. Previous studies have focused on the production of PGE by monocytes and regu-

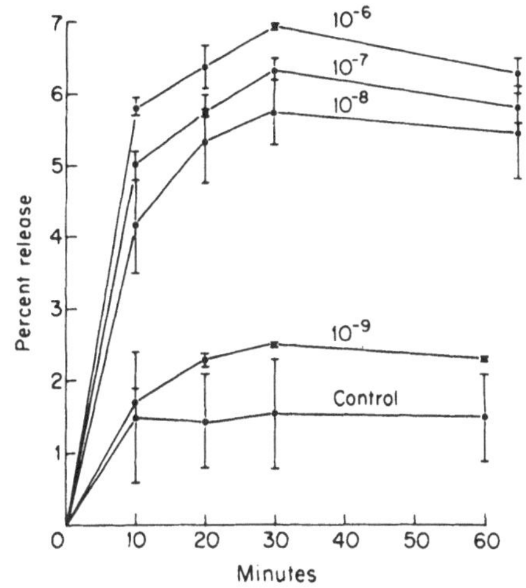

Fig. 4 Time course of 20:4 release by endothelial cells as a function of LTC concentration (M). Cultures were labeled with $[^3H]20{:}4$ for 16 h in medium 199 containing 10% human serum. After washing, the cultures were overlaid with medium 199 without serum and LTC was added. Controls were incubated in medium 199 without additions. Reproduced with permission from[12].

lation of the immune response by the release of this mediator.[7,8] While these cells release low levels of PGE, thromboxane remained the major product regardless of the stimulus (Table 1). From radioimmunoassay measurements thromboxane synthesis by monocytes (0.83 pmol/μg cell protein) stimulated with OpZ compared favorably with that by platelets (0.84 pmol/μg cell protein) treated with thrombin.[6] Neutrophils also release thromboxane[9] although these cells have considerably less synthetic potential (0.003 pmol/μg cell protein). During an inflammatory reaction, all three cell types produce this potent mediator of vasoconstriction and platelet aggregation.

EFFECT OF LEUKOTRIENES ON VASCULAR ENDOTHELIUM

Studies with mouse indicated that macrophages are potent sources of prostacyclin and PGE[10] in addition to LTC. This finding led to our interest in the effects of these agents on the vasculature. Prostacyclin is an important vasodilator, and PGE also can have this effect. In the hamster cheek pouch assay, LTC and LTD produce a transient constriction of arterioles followed by leakage from postcapillary venules.[11] Together these lipid mediators can produce a generous edematous reaction. A number of structurally unrelated vasoactive agents including PGE are reported to promote prostacyclin synthesis by vascular endothelium. We were interested in whether the leukotrienes may have a similar mode of action.

Using cultured human endothelial cells from the vein of umbilical cord, we have monitored the effects of LTC on 20:4 metabolism by these cells.[12] Cultures labeled with [^{3}H]20:4 released radiolabel in a dose-dependent manner in response to a LTC challenge (Fig. 4). Half-maximal stimulation occurred at approximately 5 X 10^{-8} M LTC. At all concentrations (10^{-9} to 10^{-6} M) of the LTC stimulus, release by endothelial cells was linear for approximately 30 min and leveled off thereafter. LTD, but not LTE and LTB, was effective in promoting release within this concentration range.

Comparisons of thrombin- and LTC-mediated 20:4 release indicated that LTC was somewhat less effective than thrombin as a stimulus of endothelial cell 20:4 metabolism. In this in vitro setting, thrombin (1 U/ml) promoted 1.2-2.9 times more 20:4 release than a maximal LTC stimulus.

Reverse-phase HPLC analyses indicated that prostacyclin was the major 20:4 product synthesized by LTC treated endothelial cells. Therefore the leukotrienes can be induced in the list of a number of vasoactive agents such as histamine,[12] and bradykinin[13] which stimulate endothelium cell prostacyclin synthesis. The leukotrienes, histamine, and bradykinin are also known to promote plasma exudation. However, prostacyclin does not have this effect. It has been proposed that a second mediator or mechanism mediates vessel wall permeability and that a combination of this factor and prostacyclin determines the quantity of plasma exudate. While the leukotrienes, histamine, and bradykinin may promote dilation through a common mechanism, it is unknown whether a common mechanism controls vascular permeability.

FUTURE STUDIES

Mononuclear phagocytes are potent sources of 20:4 metabolites and other products which influence vascular tone, permeability, and growth. Others in this conference will discuss macrophage-derived products that may play prominent roles in vascular disease. Rather than being a simple phagocytic cell, the mononuclear phagocyte is an important effector of the vasculature. In this role, these cells may have functions in immediate forms of hypersensitivity, expression of allergic states as well as in delayed types of hypersensitivity. We require specific reagents to control the secretion of individual products in order to delineate their activities.

Possible interactions of the monocyte with other cellular elements of blood such as the platelet may be important in vessel injury. Progress in elucidating factors which control such interactions will offer insights into the physiologic significance of cell-cell communication and the influence of such interactions on the function of individual cell types. Hopefully progress in these areas will provide directed approaches to the control of vascular disease and inflammatory reactions in man.

ACKNOWLEDGMENT

Supported by the National Institutes of Health grants HL-27186, AI-16480, and AI-07012, and a grant-in-aid from the Squibb Institute for Medical Research.

REFERENCES

1. C. F. Nathan, H. W. Murray, and Z. A. Cohn, N. Eng. J. Med. 303: 622-626 (1980).
2. C. A. Rouzer, W. A. Scott, A. L. Hamill, and Z. A. Cohn, J. Exp. Med. 152:1236-1247 (1980).
3. C. A. Rouzer, W. A. Scott, A. L. Hamill, F.-T. Liu, D. H. Katz, and Z. A. Cohn, J. Exp. Med. 156:1077-1086 (1982).
4. C. A. Rouzer, W. A. Scott, Z. A. Cohn, P. Blackburn, and J. M. Manning, Proc. Natl. Acad. Sci., U.S.A., 77:4928-4932 (1980).
5. T. P. Stossel, R. J. Mason, and A. L. Smith, J. Clin. Invest. 54:638-645 (1974).
6. N. A. Pawlowski, G. Kaplan, A. L. Hamill, Z. A. Cohn, and W. A. Scott, J. Exp. Med., In Press (1983).
7. J. S. Goodwin, A. D. Bankhurst, and R. P. Messner, J. Exp. Med. 146:1719-1734 (1977).
8. J. I. Kurland and R. Bockman, J. Exp. Med. 147:952-957 (1978).
9. I. M. Goldstein, C. L. Malmstren, H. Kindahl, H. B. Kaplan, O. Ridmark, B. Samuelsson, and G. Weissman, J. Exp. Med. 148: 787-792 (1978).
10. W. A. Scott, J. M. Zrike, A. L. Hamill, J. Kempe, and Z. A. Cohn, J. Exp. Med. 152:324-335 (1980).
11. S.-E. Dahlen, J. Bjork, P. Hedquist, K.-E. Arfors, S. Hammarstromm, J.-A. Lindgren, and B. Sammuelsson, Proc. Natl. Acad. Sci., U.S.A., 78:3887-3891 (1981).
12. E. B. Cramer, L. Polog, N. A. Pawlowski, Z. A. Cohn, and W. A. Scott, Proc. Natl. Acad. Sci., U.S.A., 80:4109-4113 (1983).
13. S. L. Hong and D. Deykin, J. Biol. Chem. 257:7151-7154 (1982).

RISK FACTORS FOR THE DEVELOPMENT OF PREMATURE CARDIOVASCULAR DISEASE

H. Bryan Brewer, Jr., Dennis L. Sprecher, Richard E. Gregg, and Jeffrey M. Hoeg

Department of Health & Human Services
NIH, National Heart, Lung, and Blood Institute
Bethesda, Maryland 20205

INTRODUCTION

Coronary artery disease is the major cause of death and disability in the United States and in other industrial countries. During the last twenty years smoking, high plasma cholesterol, and hypertension have been identified as major risk factors for the development of premature cardiovascular disease.[1,2] Major insights into the mechanisms involved in the development of vascular disease associated with hypercholesterolemia have occurred due to detailed analyses of plasma lipids, the characterization of plasma lipoproteins, and the identification of changes in the plasma lipoproteins which predispose to vascular disease. Recently research has also focused on the role of receptors and apolipoproteins, the protein moeity of plasma lipoproteins, in lipid and lipoprotein metabolism in normal subjects and patients with dyslipoproteinemia and atherosclerosis. Specific defects in apolipoproteins and receptors are now known to result in the development of dyslipoproteinemias characterized by atherosclerosis. The present review will summarize our current knowledge on the plasma lipoproteins, apolipoproteins, and the risk factors associated with the development of premature atherosclerosis.

APOLIPOPROTEINS

Thirteen major human apolipoproteins† have been isolated and characterized (Table 1).[3-6] The major apolipoproteins associated with

---

†Abbreviations: Apolipoproteins, apo; high density lipoproteins, HDL; low density lipoproteins, LDL; intermediate density lipoproteins, IDL.

TABLE 1

Apolipoprotein	Major Density Class	Approximate Molecular Weight	Major Site of Synthesis in Man
A-I	HDL	28,000	Liver-Intestine
A-II	HDL	18,000	Liver-Intestine
A-IV	Chylomicrons	45,000	Intestine
B-100	VLDL-IDL-LDL	250,000	Liver
B-48	Chylomicrons-VLDL-IDL	160,000	Intestine
C-I	Chylomicrons-VLDL-HDL	6,500	Liver
C-II	Chylomicrons-VLDL-HDL	10,000	Liver
$C\text{-}III_{0\text{-}2}$†	Chylomicrons-VLDL-HDL	10,000	Liver
D	HDL	20,000	?
$E_{2\text{-}4}$*	Chylymicrons-VLDL-HDL	40,000	Liver
F	HDL	30,000	?
G	VLDL	75,000	?
H	Chylomicrons	45,000	?

†Subscript indicates number of sialiac acid residues on the apolipoprotein.
*Subscript denotes the isoforms separable by isoelectrofocusing.

high density lipoproteins are apoA-I and apoA-II, while apoB is the major protein constituent of LDL. Two forms of apoB, designated apoB-48 and apoB-100, are synthesized by the intestine and liver, respectively, in man. The major physiological functions of plasma apolipoproteins include (1) structural constituent of the plasma lipoprotein particle, (2) cofactor for enzymes involved in lipid and lipoprotein metabolism, (3) ligand for interaction with specific cellular receptor sites, thereby directing lipoprotein metabolism and (4) lipid exchange protein, fascilitating the exchange of lipids between lipoprotein particles. The well established functions of the plasma lipoproteins are included in Table 2.

GENERAL OVERVIEW OF LIPOPROTEIN METABOLISM

Triglyceride-rich Lipoprotein ApoB Cascades

A conceptual overview of the metabolism of the plasma lipoproteins is shown in Fig. 1.[5-7] The metabolic relationship of the major plasma lipoproteins containing apoB synthesized by the intestine and liver may be considered to consist of two major "cascades." The first apoB cascade involves chylomicrons secreted by the intestine, containing apoB-48 which functions to transport dietary lipids from the intestine to the liver. The triglyceride-rich lipoproteins acquire other apolipoproteins, particularly apoE and apoC-II from

TABLE 2

PHYSIOLOGICAL FUNCTIONS OF HUMAN PLASMA APOLIPOPROTEINS

Physiological Function	Apolipoprotein
I. Cofactor for Enzyme	
1. lipoprotein lipase	apoC-II
2. lecithin cholesterol acyltransferase (LCAT)	apoA-I
II. Ligand on Lipoprotein Particle for Interaction with Receptor Site on Cells	
1. chylomicron remnant	apoE
2. LDL	apoB-100
3. HDL	apoA-I & apoE
III. Structural Protein on Lipoprotein Particle	
1. intestinal chylomicron	apoB-48
2. hepatogenous VLDL	apoB-100
3. HDL	apoA-I
IV. Lipid Exchange Protein	
1. cholesteryl ester	?apoD

HDL. The triglycerides in chylomicrons undergo hydrolysis to free fatty acids and monoglycerides by lipoprotein lipase. ApoC-II functions as a cofactor for lipoprotein lipase.[8,9] With triglyceride hydrolysis, the chylomicrons are sequentially reduced to "remnants," first having a density of VLDL and finally IDL. Chylomicron remnants are removed from the plasma by binding to liver receptors having an affinity for apoE.

The second apoB cascade involves hydrolysis of triglyceride-rich VLDL containing apoB-100 secreted by the liver. The triglycerides on VLDL also undergo hydrolysis by lipoprotein lipase and are serially converted to lipoproteins with densities of IDL, and finally LDL. During the conversion to IDL, some of the lipoproteins bind to a hepatic receptor and are taken up by the liver. A second enzyme, hepatic lipase, has been proposed to be important in the conversion of IDL to LDL, and may function both as a triglyceryl hydrolase and a phospholipase.[10] During the conversion of IDL to LDL, apoC-II and apoE dissociate from the lipoprotein particles, resulting in apoB-100 being the principal LDL apolipoprotein. The apoB-100 on LDL interacts with receptors (LDL or B,E receptor) on peripheral cells (e.g., fibroblasts and smooth muscle cells)[11] and the liver.[12] The LDL-receptor interaction initiates a receptor mediated endocytosis and catabolism of LDL.[11]

HDL Lipoproteins

HDL arise in plasma by direct synthesis from the liver and intestine, and by transfer of lipids and apolipoproteins to HDL during the catabolism of triglyceride-rich apoB lipoproteins.[6] HDL has been proposed to function as a "reservoir" for apolipoproteins (e.g., apoC-II and apoE) during lipoprotein metabolism, and in the transport of cholesterol from peripheral cells back to the liver by a process termed "reverse cholesterol transport"[13] (Fig. 1). In this process HDL has been proposed to interact with a receptor on peripheral cells and remove free cholesterol from the cell. ApoE or in some species apoA-I may be synthesized by some peripheral cell and possibly facilitate the egress of cholesterol from the cell.[14,15] This cholesterol is then rapidly esterified by the enzyme lecithin cholesterol acyl-transferase (LCAT), and the cholesteryl esters are transferred to the core of the HDL particle, or exchanged to other lipoprotein particles (e.g., VLDL or chylomicrons). A large fraction of the HDL cholesteryl esters may be transported to the liver for ultimate removal from the body.

RISK FACTORS FOR THE DEVELOPMENT OF ATHEROSCLEROSIS

Lipoproteins

LDL. Epidemiological studies have established that the higher the plasma concentrations of total cholesterol and LDL cholesterol, the greater the risk of the development of premature cardiovascular disease.[1,2,16] Two monogenic diseases, familial hypercholesterolemia and combined hyperlipidemia, are characterized by elevated levels of plasma LDL. The molecular defect in familial hypercholesterolemia has been extensively evaluated and shown to be due to a defect in the LDL (apoB,E) receptor, both in the peripheral cell[11,17] and the liver.[12] As a result of the defect in the receptor, LDL catabolism is reduced, and there is also an increased production of LDL.[18] The molecular defect(s) in combined hyperlipidemia is as yet unknown. An increased production of lipoproteins within the apoB-100 cascade has been reported,[19] and hyperapobetalipoproteinemia has also been observed.[20] The mechanism by which LDL induces atherosclerosis is not known; however, recent studies in which modified LDL was rapidly taken up by macrophages may indicate that modification of LDL is an important prerequisite to the atherosclerotic process.[21,22] Regardless of the pathophysiological mechanism involved in the elevation of

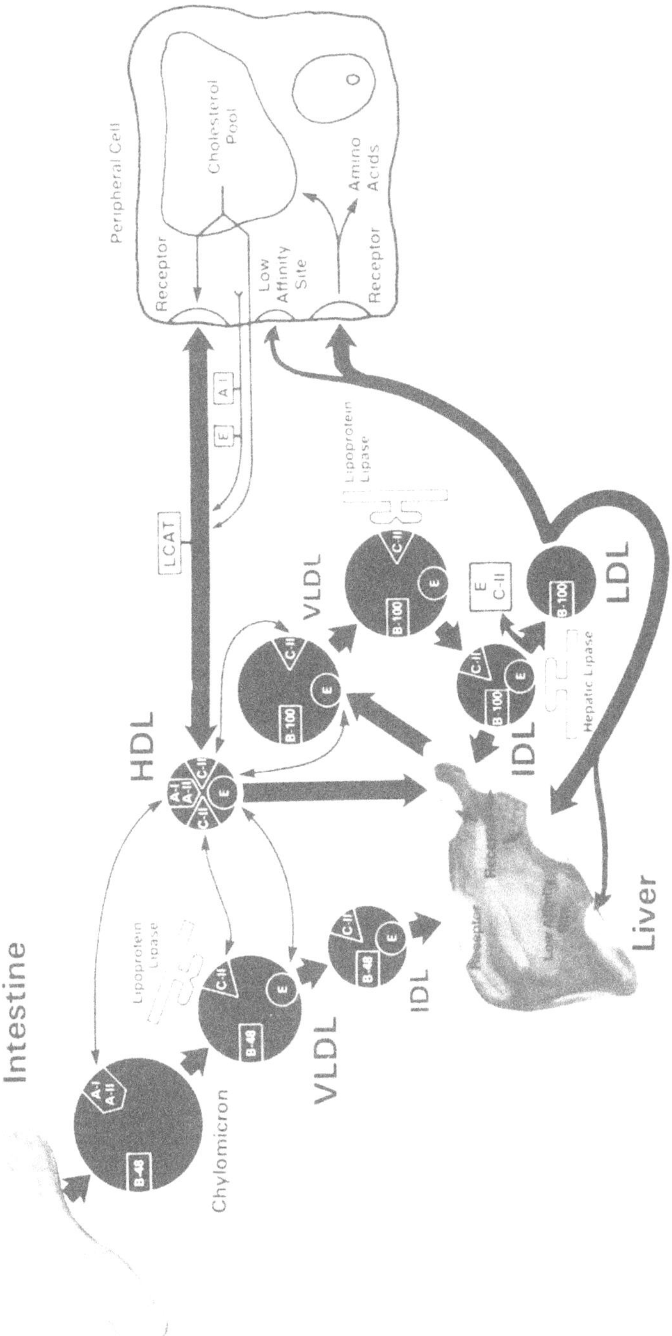

Fig. 1 Schematic model of lipoprotein metabolism (*see* text for details).

plasma levels of LDL, increased atherosclerosis remains a characteristic clinical feature of these diseases.

β-VLDL. Remnants of triglyceride-rich lipoproteins accumulate in patients with type III hyperlipoproteinemia.[7,23] These remnants, separated by ultracentrifugation at density < 1.006 g/ml, migrate into the β position on lipoprotein electrophoresis (β-VLDL), and have been designated floating β lipoproteins. An additional important diagnostic feature of this dyslipoproteinemia is a VLDL cholesterol to plasma triglyceride ratio > 0.3 (normal < 0.3), and an elevated level of plasma apoE.[7,23] These remnants also contain both apoB-100 and apoB-48, indicating that the lipoproteins which accumulate in type III hyperlipoproteinemia are derived from lipoproteins synthesized by both the liver and intestine.[24]

As outlined above apoE has been shown to fascilitate the uptake of triglyceride-rich lipoproteins by an apoE receptor system in the liver. Population studies and structural analyses of apoE have shown that apoE is present at a single genetic locus with three common alleles which have been designated E^2, E^3, and E^4.[25,26] The three E apolipoproteins encoded by these alleles are separable by isoelectrofocusing and are designated $apoE_2$, $apoE_3$, and $apoE_4$. The predominate E phenotype in the normolipidemic population is $apoE_3$. An increased frequency of apoE deficiency (E° allele) or $apoE_2$ phenotype (E^2 allele) has been observed in patients with type III hyperlipoproteinemia.[7,23,27] In early adult life, subjects with the $apoE_2$ pheontype are normolipidemic or hypolipidemic. Individuals with the $apoE_2$ phenotype but without hyperlipidemia are classified as normolipidemic E^2 homozygotes or patients with dysbetalipoproteinemia. In later life, some patients become hyperlipidemic and develop a type III lipoprotein profile. Genetic and kindred studies have suggested that the $apoE_2$ phenotype is a permissive factor and an additional condition (e.g., obesity or separated dyslipoproteinemia) is required for normolipidemic subjects to become hyperlipidemic.[25]

The dyslipoproteinemia associated with type III hyperlipoproteinemia predisposes to the development of premature cardiovascular disease, and the atherosclerotic lesions which develop are indistinguishable from those which are present in patients with elevated levels of LDL.[7]

Lp(a). The third plasma lipoprotein which has been associated with the development of vascular disease is Lp(a).[28,29] Lp(a) is a lipoprotein with a hydrated density of approximately 1.063 g/ml, a pre-β position on electrophoresis, and an apolipoprotein composition of apoB-100 as well as the specific Lp(a) protein.[29] Lp(a) appears to be synthesized and catabolized, independent of other plasma lipoproteins. The mechanisms involved in the development of atherosclerosis due to increased levels of Lp(a) are not completely understood, and a detailed analysis of the atherosclerotic lesions in these patients has not been reported.

TABLE 3

FACTORS AFFECTING THE PLASMA LEVELS OF HDL CHOLESTEROL

Increased Levels	Decreased Levels
Female sex	Male sex
Exercise	Hypertriglyceridemia
Lean body mass	Obesity
Alcohol	Diabetes
Nicotinic acid administration	Types I and V hyperlipoproteinemia
Estrogen administration	Androgen administration
Heparin injection	Familial HDL deficiency (a) Tangier disease
Familial hyperalphalipoproteinemia	(b) ApoA-I + ApoC-III deficiency

HDL. An inverse relation between HDL-cholesterol levels and premature vascular disease has been established by several epidemiological studies.[6,30-32] The HDL_2 subclass was more highly correlated with the severity of atherosclerosis than total HDL.[32] The causal relationship between low HDL and the development of atherosclerosis is unknown. As reviewed above, HDL may function as a circulating lipoprotein receptor of cholesterol from peripheral cells, and it may be hypothesized that high HDL-cholesterol levels reflect an increase in the reverse cholesterol transport from peripheral cells back to the liver (Fig. 1). ApoE containing HDL may also compete with the LDL (apoB,E) receptor, thereby reducing LDL uptake by peripheral cells.[33]

The clinical situations associated with elevated and reduced levels of HDL cholesterol are summarized in Table 3. Of particular interest are the recent studies on Tangier disease which is characterized by markedly reduced levels of HDL, apoA-I, and apoA-II. The molecular defect in Tangier disease is a structural defect in mature apoA-I, resulting in increased catabolism of both proapoA-I and mature apoA-I.[34-36] The proteolytic processing of proapoA-I to apoA-I in plasma and the specific peptidase responsible for this conversion is normal in Tangier disease.[36]

A newly described dyslipoproteinemia characterized by a severe reduction in HDL and premature cardiovascular disease has been shown to be due to a deficiency of apoA-I + apoC-III. Two separate kindreds with this dyslipoproteinemia have been reported; one characterized by an insertion in the apoA-I gene[37] and the other with no apparent insertion or deletion in the apoA-I gene.[38] In both kindreds, apoA-I + apoC-III are deficient, suggesting a linkage of expression of the apoA-I and apoC-III genes.

Apolipoproteins

Recent studies have indicated that plasma apolipoproteins may serve as effective markers for patients with dyslipoproteinemias and atherosclerosis. Studies have established that elevated levels of apoB of LDL,[20,39], and reduced levels of apoA-I of HDL,[39-41] are associated with increased vascular disease. An elevated apoB to LDL cholesterol ratio also has been associated with an increased incidence of angiographically documented coronary artery disease.[20] The plasma concentration of either apoE or its individual isoforms has not been associated with premature vascular disease.[42,43] Recently apoC-II and the ratio of apoC-II to apoA-I have been observed to be effective predictors of patients with angiographically proven coronary artery disease.[44] In this study apoA-I was a better predictor than total plasma, LDL, or HDL cholesterol levels in discriminating individuals with established cardiovascular disease from control subjects.

SUMMARY

The elucidation of the major risk factors for the development of premature atherosclerosis including plasma cholesterol, hypertension, and smoking has permitted the institution of specific therapy to reduce the risk of vascular disease. The further elucidation of LDL and HDL as positive and negative risk factors, respectively, has provided additional insights into the role of lipoproteins in cholesterol transport and atherosclerosis. Analysis of plasma apolipoproteins suggests that they may be even more effective than lipoproteins as predictors of premature vascular disease.

The results of the Lipid Research Clinics Coronary Primary Prevention Trial clearly established the effectiveness of decreasing coronary risk by the reduction of LDL cholesterol in hyperlipidemic subjects.[45,46] Aggressive diet and drug treatment of patients with elevated plasma levels of LDL would be anticipated to have a major impact on the development and/or progression of premature vascular disease.

The implications of reduced levels of HDL on clinical practice is less certain. At present there is no evidence that interventions that change HDL levels will influence the development of vascular disease. In addition, the role of triglycerides and triglyceride-rich lipoproteins as potential risk factors for the development of premature atherosclerosis has not been firmly established. Additional epidemiological studies as well as basic research will undoubtedly provide the answers to these important unresolved questions.

REFERENCES

1. J. Stamler, Circulation 58:3-19 (1978).
2. W. B. Kannel, W. P. Castelli, T. Gordon, and P. M. McNamara, Ann. Intern. Med. 74:1-12 (1971).
3. R. L. Jackson, J. O. Morrisett, and A. M. Gotto, Jr., Physiol. Rev. 56:259-316 (1976).
4. A. M. Scanu and T. Teng, in: "The Biochemistry of Atherosclerosis," A. M. Scanu, ed., Marcel Dekka, Inc., New York, pp. 107-122 (1979).
5. H. B. Brewer, Jr., Klinische Wochenschrift 59:1023-1035 (1981).
6. H. B. Brewer, Jr., E. J. Schaefer, J. C. Osborne, and L. A. Zech, in: "Report of the High Density Lipoprotein Methodology Workshop," K. Lippel, ed., U. S. Department of Health, Education and Welfare, NIH Publication No. 79-1661, pp. 29-41 (1979).
7. H. B. Brewer, Jr., L. A. Zech, R. E. Gregg, D. Schwartz, and E. J. Schaefer, Ann. Int. Med. 98:623-640 (1983).
8. J. C. LaRosa, R. I. Levy, P. Herbert, S. E. Lux, and D. S. Fredrickson, Biochem. Biophys. Res. Commun. 41:57-62 (1970).
9. R. J. Havel, V. G. Shore, B. Shore, and D. M. Bier, Cir. Res. 27:595-600 (1970).
10. W. C. Breckenridge, J. A. Little, P. Alaupovic, C. S. Wang, A. Kuksis, G. Kakis, F. Lindgren, and G. Gardiner, Athero. 45: 161-179 (1982).
11. J. L. Goldstein and M. S. Brown, Ann. Rev. Biochem. 46:897-930 (1977).
12. J. M. Hoeg, S. J. Demosky, E. J. Schaefer, T. E. Starzl, and H. B. Brewer, Jr., J. Clin. Invest. 73:429-436 (1984).
13. J. A. Glomset, J. Lipid Res. 9:155-167 (1968).
14. S. K. Basu, M. S. Brown, Y. K. Ho, R. J. Havel, and J. L. Goldstein, Proc. Natl. Acad. Sci., U.S.A., 78:7545-7549 (1981).
15. M. L. Blue, P. Ostapchuk, J. S. Gordon, and D. L. Williams, J. Biol. Chem. 257:11151-11159 (1982).
16. G. G. Rhoads, C. L. Gulbrandsen, and A. Kagan, N. Engl. J. Med. 294:293-298 (1976).
17. J. L. Goldstein and M. S. Brown, Metabolism 26:1257-1275 (1977).
18. A. K. Soutar, W. B. Myant, and G. R. Thompson, Arteriosclerosis 28:247-256 (1977).
19. U. Beil, S. M. Grundy, J. R. Crouse, and L. A. Zech, Athero. 2:44-57 (1982).
20. A. D. Sniderman, S. Shapiro, D. Marpole, B. Skinner, B. Teng, and P. O. Kwitervich, Jr., Proc. Natl. Acad. Sci., U.S.A., 77:604 (1980).
21. S. K. Basu, M. S. Brown, Y. K. Ho, and J. L. Goldstein, J. Biol. Chem. 254:7141-7146 (1979).
22. A. M. Fogelman, I. Schechter, and J. Seager, Proc. Natl. Acad. Sci., U.S.A., 77:2214-2218 (1980).
23. R. J. Havel, in: "Lipid Disorders," R. J. Havel, ed., The Medical Clinics of North America 106:441-454 (1982).
24. M. Ming, R. E. Gregg, E. J. Schaefer, J. M. Hoeg, and H. B. Brewer, Jr., J. Lipid Res. 24:803-809 (1983).

25. G. Utermann, K. H. Vogelberg, and A. Steinmets, Clin. Genet. 15:37-62 (1979).
26. V. I. Zannis and J. L. Breslow, Biochem. 20:1033-1041 (1981).
27. G. Ghiselli, E. J. Schaefer, P. Gascon, and H. B. Brewer, Jr., Science 214:1239-1241 (1981).
28. K. Berg, G. Dahlen, and M. H. Frick, Clin. Genet. 6:230-235 (1974).
29. J. D. Morrisett, D. Wenkert, A. M. Gotto, Jr., G. H. Dahlen, S. H. Gianturco, C. Herdeman, and J. W. Gaubatz, in: "Proceedings of the Workshop on Apolipoprotein Quantification," U. S. Dept. of Health and Human Services, NIH Publication No. 83-1266, pp. 158-178 (1983).
30. T. Gordon, W. P. Castelli, M. C. Hjortland, W. B. Kannel, and T. R. Dunbar, Am. J. Med. 62:707-714 (1977).
31. T. A. Pearson, B. H. Bulkly, S. C. Aachuff, P. O. Kwitervich, and L. Gordis, Am. J. Epidem. 109:285-295 (1979).
32. B. Lewis, Am. J. Card. 52:5B-8B (1983).
33. T. L. Innerarity and R. W. Mahley, Biochem. 17:1440-1447 (1978).
34. L. L. Kay, R. Ronan, E. J. Schaefer, and H. B. Brewer, Jr., Proc. Natl. Acad. Sci., U. S. A., 79:2485-2489 (1982).
35. E. J. Schaefer, L. L. Kay, L. A. Zech, and H. B. Brewer, Jr., J. Clin. Invest. 70:934-945 (1982).
36. P. Bojanovski, R. E. Gregg, M. Meng, R. Ronan, L. A. Zech, and H. B. Brewer, Jr., Clin. Res., In Press.
37. S. K. Karathanosis, J. McPherson, V. I. Zannis, and J. L. Breslow, Nature 304:371-373 (1983).
38. E. J. Schaefer, W. H. Heaton, M. G. Wetzel, and H. B. Brewer, Jr., Atherosclerosis 2:16-26 (1982).
39. P. Avagaro, B. M. G. Bittolo, G. Cazzalato, G. Quinci, and F. Belussi, Artery 4:385-394 (1978).
40. J. J. Albers, M. C. Cheung, and W. K. Hazzard, Metabolism 27:479-485 (1978).
41. J. J. Maciejko, D. R. Holmes, B. A. Kotfke, A. R. Zinsmeister, D. M. Dinh, and S. J. T. Mao, N. Engl. J. Med. 309:385-389 (1983).
42. M. H. Tan, L. Weldon, J. J. Albers, M. C. Cheung, R. J. Havel, and J. Vigne, J. Clin. and Invest. Med. 3:225-230 (1980).
43. H. J. Menzel, R. G. Kladetzky, and G. Assmann, Arteriosclerosis 3:310-315 (1983).
44. D. L. Sprecher, E. J. Schaefer, R. E. Gregg. P. Wilson, and H. B. Brewer, Jr., Clin. Res. 219A (1983).
45. The Lipid Research Clinics Coronary Primary Prevention Trial Results, I. Reduction in Incidence of Coronary Heart Disease, J.A.M.A. 251:351-364 (1984).
46. The Lipid Research Clinics Coronary Primary Prevention Trial Results, II. The Relationship of Reduction in Incidence of Coronary Heart Disease to Cholesterol Lowering, J.A.M.A. 251:365-374 (1984).

FATE OF CHOLESTERYL LINOLEYL ETHER INJECTED INTO RATS AS CHYLOMICRONS, ACETYLATED LDL AND HDL

Yechezkiel Stein and Olga Stein

Lipid Research Laboratory, Department of Medicine B
Hadassah University Hospital, and Department of
Experimental Medicine and Cancer Research
Hewbrew University-Hadassah Medical School
Jerusalem, Israel

INTRODUCTION

During the past few years we have used cholesteryl linoleyl ether, a nonhydrolyzable analogue of cholesteryl ester, to study cellular uptake of lipoprotein cholesteryl ester in culture[1-3] and in the intact animal.[4-7] In experiments with low density lipoproteins which had been modified by acetylation, and thus targeted for uptake by non-parenchymal cells, the hepatic retention of a labeled ether analogue of triacylglycerol was encountered even several weeks after injection.[8,9] When chylomicrons labeled with [^{14}C]cholesteryl linoleyl ether and retinyl [^{3}H]hexadecyl ether were injected (Fig. 1), loss of both labeled compounds from the liver was encountered already 1 week after injection.[10] The question was whether labeled cholesteryl ether disappears more quickly when injected as part of lipoprotein taken preferentially by hepatocytes and persists much longer in the liver when injected as a part of acetylated LDL, which is taken up preferentially by nonparenchymal cells.[11,12] Groups of rats were injected simultaneously with chylomicrons and acetylated low density lipoprotein labeled with [^{14}C]- or [^{3}H]cholesteryl linoleyl ether and the hepatic retention was monitored up to 70 days after injection. The results obtained provide evidence that cholesteryl linoleyl ether is retained in the liver for many weeks if it is injected as part of acetylated LDL (Fig. 2), and thus taken up mainly by nonparenchymal cells.[11,12] A relatively slow but progressive elimination of the labeled cholesteryl linoleyl ether occurred when it had been injected bound to chylomicrons (Fig. 2), which were taken up and metabolized mainly by hepatocytes.[13,14] The labeled cholesteryl linoleyl ether which was taken up by the hepatocytes was excreted into the bile

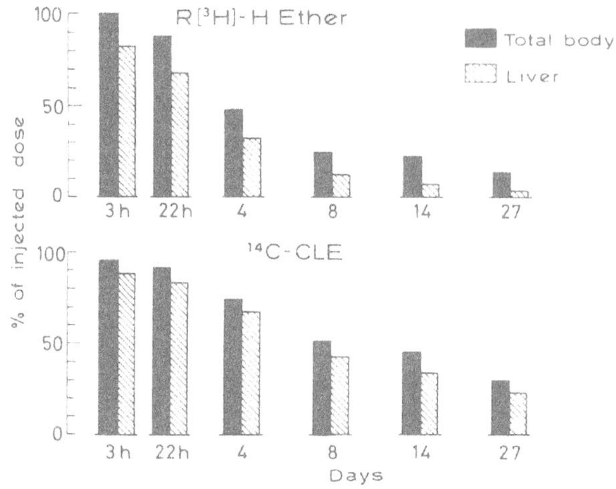

Fig. 1 Loss of R [^{3}H]-H ether and [^{14}C]CLE from liver and body following injection of labeled chylomicrons into rats. The isotopes were injected as retinyl [^{3}H]hexadecyl ether [R^{3}H-H ether] and [^{14}C]cholesteryl linoleyl ether [^{14}C-CLE]. Total body = sum of radioactivity recovered in organs and plasma. Adapted from Goodman et al.[10]

(Fig. 3). The excretion of the compound occurred apparently without prior hydrolysis of the ether bond.

High density lipoprotein (HDL) is the major lipoprotein fraction in rat plasma. In the rat, the half-life in the circulation of radioiodinated HDL protein was found, in three different studies,[15-18] to be about 10 h. However, there is less agreement as to the sites of HDL protein or cholesteryl ester catabolism. Since in the rat there is little or no cholesteryl ester transfer protein,[19] it is possible to follow the fate of injected cholesteryl ether-labeled HDL. We compared in the same set of experiments, the clearance from the circulation and tissue uptake of HDL protein labeled with ^{125}I and of HDL labeled with cholesteryl linoleyl ether. The methodology described previously for the labeling of chylomicrons[6] and very low density lipoprotein[5] was modified to label HDL with cholesteryl linoleyl ether. The modification consisted mainly in the choice of the donor of the labeled compound, and the direction of transfer, i.e., from a neutral lipid-rich particle back to HDL.

To label HDL with [^{3}H]cholesteryl linoleyl ether, we used the d > 1.21 g/ml fraction of rabbit serum which is known to be a rich source of cholesteryl ester transfer protein. The labeled compound was incorporated into Intralipid and then transferred to rat HDL (Fig. 4). In experiments in which a high ratio of Intralipid triacylglycerol to HDL protein was used (10 mg triacylglycerol/1 mg protein),

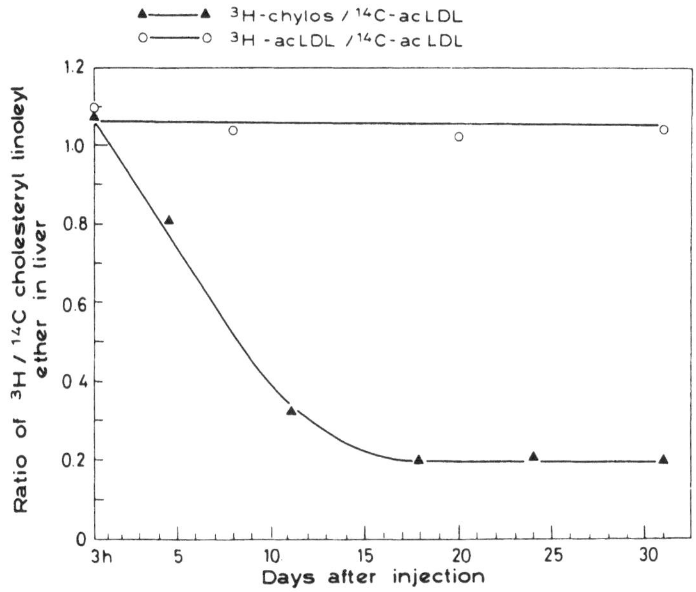

Fig. 2 Ratio of $^3H/^{14}C$ cholesteryl linoleyl ether in the liver after simultaneous injection of: Δ, [^3H]cholesteryl linoleyl ether-labeled chylomicrons plus [^{14}C]cholesteryl linoleyl ether-labeled acetylated LDL (exp. 1); or O, acetylated LDL labeled with [^3H]- and [^{14}C]cholesteryl linoleyl ether (exp. 3). The ratio of the two labels in the tissue was normalized to the ratio of the two labels in the injected material which was taken as 1.0. Adapted from Stein et al.[25]

there was considerable transfer of triacylglycerol to HDL. We used, therefore, a very low ratio of triacylglycerol (TG) to protein (0.012 mg TG/mg protein), in order to minimize the transfer of triacylglycerol to HDL.

Under conditions used, the efficiency of labeling was about 25% and all comigrated with the re-isolated HDL protein on agarose gel electrophoresis (Fig. 5). Rat HDL labeled with [^3H]cholesteryl linoleyl ether or with ^{125}I was injected into groups of rats and the disappearance of each label from the circulation was determined after 4 h. As seen in Table 1, both the ^{125}I- and ^3H-labeled HDL were cleared from the circulation to a similar extent, and only 45 and 40%, respectively, of the injected dose remained in the plasma compartment. Even though the loss from the circulation of the two labels did not differ appreciably, a marked difference was seen in the amount of ^{125}I and ^3H recovered in the liver 4 h after injection. The recovery of only 11% of injected [^{125}I]HDL could indicate that either the protein was not taken up by the liver or that it had been taken up and

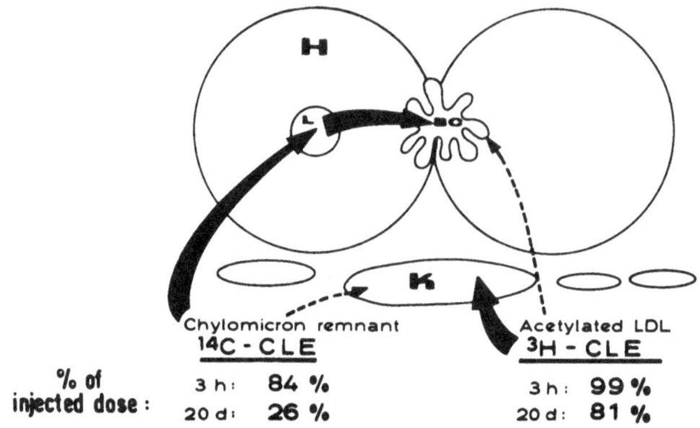

Fig. 3 Divergent metabolic fate in the liver of cholesteryl linoleyl ether injected with chylomicrons or acetylated LDL. H = hepatocytes; L = lysosome; BC = bile canaliculus; K = nonparenchymal cell. Adapted from Stein et al.[25]

was degraded. To eliminate that fraction of the lipoprotein that could have been denatured by the labeling technique, we used the screening procedure.[15] The screening procedure was important also because of the possible transfer of various apolipoproteins between HDL, the d > 1.21 g/ml fraction of serum and Intralipid during the

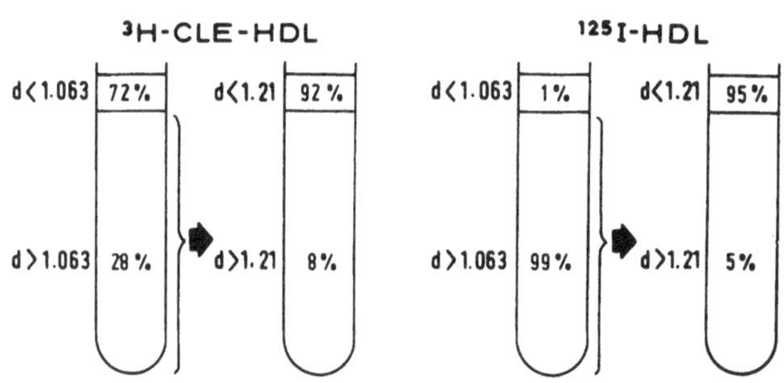

Fig. 4 Labeling of HDL with [^{3}H]cholesteryl linoleyl ether. Conditions: Rat HDL (10 mg protein) was incubated for 18 h at 37°C with 125 μg triacylglycerol Intralipid containing $1.7 \cdot 10^{7}$ dpm [^{3}H]cholesteryl ether and d > 1.21 fraction of rabbit serum. [^{125}I]HDL was incubated under similar conditions (see Materials and Methods). The incubation mixture was brought to density 1.063 g/ml, centrifuged for 24 h and the infranatant was then centrifuged at d = 1.21 g/ml for 48 h. The data for the d = 1.063 g/ml fraction represent distribution of label added to the reaction mixture; the data for the d = 1.21 g/ml fraction give the distribution of label between the top and infranant. Adapted from Stein et al.[23]

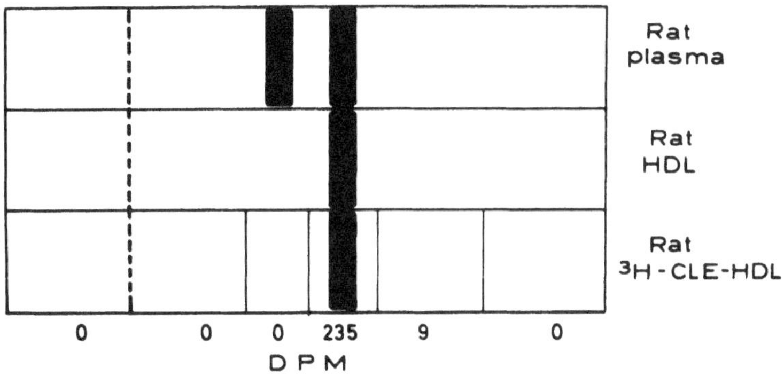

Fig. 5 Agarose gel electrophoresis of rat HDL labeled with [^{3}H]cholesteryl linoleyl ether (CLE). Adapted from Stein et al.[23]

labeling procedure.[20,21] We assumed that any changes in the apolipoprotein composition which might have occurred in the HDL during labeling would have been corrected during the 4 h of screening. The experimental design used permitted a comparison of the removal from the circulation and subsequent fate of the cholesteryl ester and protein moieties of HDL. After injection of the non-screened material, a somewhat more rapid clearance of [^{3}H]cholesteryl linoleyl ether-HDL

TABLE 1

RADIOACTIVITY IN LIVER AND PLASMA AFTER INJECTION OF LABELED HDL INTO RATS

Conditions: Male rats, 250 g body wt. were injected intravenously with 1 mg of labeled HDL protein. 4 h after injection, blood was drawn from the aorta and the serum was used for re-injection. Values are means ± S.E. Numbers in parentheses represent number of rats. ^{125}I values are trichloroacetic acid-precipitable label. Trichloroacetic acid-soluble ^{125}I in tissues was less than 2% of total radioactivity. Adapted from Stein et al.[23]

HDL	Distribution of label after 4 h (% injected dose)	
^{125}I-HDL[5]	44.6 ± 2.3	11.7 ± 0.3
[^{3}H]Cholesteryl linoleyl ether HDL[6]	41.2 ± 1.1	26.3 ± 1.1

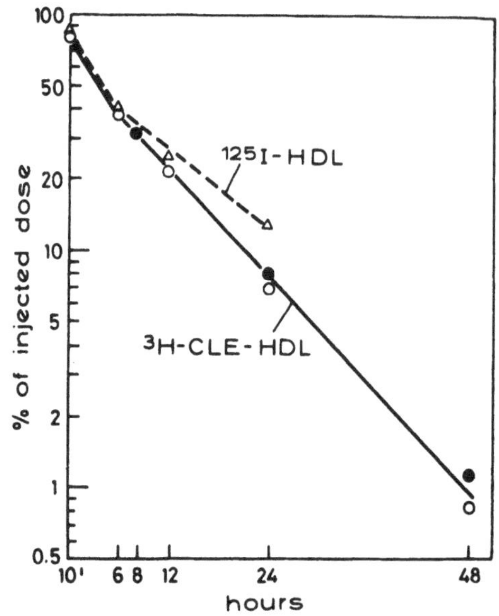

Fig. 6 Removal from plasma of screened [^{125}I]HDL (Δ), and [^{3}H]cholesteryl linoleyl ether-HDL (O,o) after intravenous injection into rats. Each value is a mean of results from three rats: O, Expt.1; o, Expt.2. Adapted from Stein et al.[23]

than of [^{125}I]HDL was seen and this difference was also encountered after injection of the screened HDL. The [^{125}I]HDL was cleared with a $t^{1}/2$ of about 10.5 h, while the $t^{1}/2$ of the [^{3}H]cholesteryl linoleyl ether-HDL was shorter, about 8 h (Fig. 6).

A major fraction of the injected screened [^{3}H]cholesteryl linoleyl ether-HDL was found in the liver (Table 2) and the recovery of the labeled ether at different time intervals after injection in the spleen and adrenals is shown in Table 2. Even though the much lower recovery of ^{125}I-labeled protein than of [^{3}H]cholesteryl linoleyl ether in the liver might indicate that HDL protein was taken up to a lesser extent than was HDL cholesteryl ester, hydrolysis and deiodination of the protein could have contributed also towards the finding of only 9% of labeled [^{125}I]HDL protein in the liver.

The use of the nonhydrolyzable analog of cholesteryl ester permitted not only a better quantification of the uptake of HDL cholesteryl ester by the liver but also localization of the site of uptake to hepatocytes. The loss of the label from the liver 14 and 28 days after injection of [^{3}H]cholesteryl linoleyl ether-HDL (Fig. 7) indicates that over 80% of the label recovered in the liver 48 h after injection had been taken up by hepatocytes. This is in agreement with our

TABLE 2

DISTRIBUTION OF RADIOACTIVITY AFTER INJECTION OF SCREENED HOMOLOGOUS HDL INTO RATS

Conditions: 150 g male rats were injected with 1 ml of rat serum containing screened HDL. Values are means ± S.E. of three rats (trichloroacetic acid-precipitable label; the tricholoroacetic acid-soluble ^{125}I was less than 2% of total radioactivity). From Stein et al.[23]

HDL	Hours after injection	Radioactivity recovered (% injected dose)		
		Liver	Spleen	Adrenal
[^3H]Cholesteyl linoleyl ether-HDL	6	28.3 ± 0.7	1.1 ± 0.14	0.8 ± 0.09
	12	36.4 ± 1.4	1.2 ± 0.3	1.1 ± 0.03
	24	38.6 ± 0.7	1.8 ± 0.09	1.0 ± 0.02
[^{125}I]HDL	6	8.9 ± 0.9	0.5 ± 0.03	0.1 ± 0
	12	8.3 ± 0.7	0.5 ± 0.04	0.1 ± 0.01
	24	6.6 ± 0.3	0.4 ± 0.03	0.06 ± 0.01

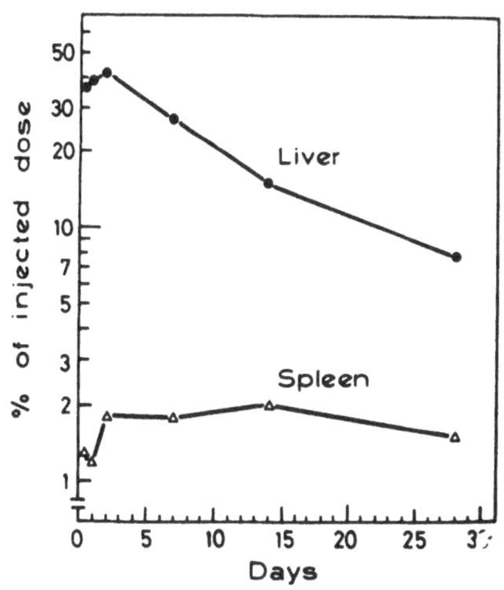

Fig. 7 Loss of [^3H]cholesteryl linoleyl ether-HDL from liver (O) and spleen (Δ). 150-g male rats were injected with 1 ml of rat serum containing screened HDL. Values are means of results from three rats. Adapted from Stein et al.[23]

TABLE 3

EFFECT OF ETHINYL ESTRADIOL ON HEPATIC UPTAKE OF LDL AND HDL LABELED WITH ^{3}H-CHOLESTEROL LINOLEYL ETHER

Conditions: 150 g rats were injected with ^{3}H-cholesteryl linoleyl ether labeled human LDL or with 1 ml rat serum containing [^{3}H]cholesteryl linoleyl ether labeled rat HDL. Ethinyl estradiol, 5 mg/kg, was injected SC for 5 days. The values for LDL were obtained 24 h and for HDL 48 h after injection. Values are means $\pm$ S.E. of 3-5 rats. Adapted from Stein et al.[23,24]

Lipoprotein	Treatment	Liver	Adrenal
		% of injected dose	
LDL	Control	27.2 ± 1.9	0.21 ± 0.03
	Estradiol	81.9 ± 5.5	1.54 ± 0.2
HDL	Control	45.4 ± 2.5	1.00 ± 0.1
	Estradiol	54.8 ± 1.8	5.4 ± 0.9

previous radioautographic studies on [^{125}I]HDL protein uptake by the liver[16] and the results of Glass et al.[22] for apolipoprotein A-I-labeled HDL.

Next we have investigated whether pretreatment of intact rats with a pharmacologic dose of ethinyl estradiol will affect the hepatic uptake of [^{3}H]cholesteryl linoleyl ether HDL. The data in Table 3 compare the effect of estradiol on hepatic uptake of LDL and HDL. While the former was increased about 3-fold, HDL uptake rose only by 20%. In contrast, treatment with ethinyl estradiol increased adrenal uptake of both lipoproteins to a similar extent.

The more rapid clearance of [^{3}H]cholesteryl linoleyl ether than of [^{125}I]HDL from the circulation could be due to removal of some of the cholesteryl ester of HDL independently from the protein moiety. This process could probably take place in the liver, as up to 45% of the injected [^{3}H]cholesteryl linoleyl ether was recovered in that organ.

We have described a method for labeling of lipoproteins with cholesteryl linoleyl ether, a nonhydrolyzable analog of cholesteryl ester. This probe permitted the study of the fate of lipoprotein cholesteryl ester in the intact rat.

ACKNOWLEDGMENTS

This investigation was supported in part by a grant, R01-HL28454, from the NIH.

REFERENCES

1. Y. Stein, G. Halperin, and O. Stein, FEBS Letts. 111:104-106 (1980).
2. T. Chajek-Shaul, G. Friedman, G. Halperin, O. Stein, and Y. Stein, Biochim. Biophys. Acta 666:147-155 (1981).
3. G. Friedman, T. Chajek-Shaul, O. Stein, T. Olivecrona, and Y. Stein, Biochim. Biophys. Acta 666:156-164 (1981).
4. O. Stein, G. Halperin, and Y. Stein, Biochim. Biophys. Acta 620:247-260 (1980).
5. Y. Stein, G. Halperin, and O. Stein, Biochim. Biophys. Acta 663:569-574 (1981).
6. T. Chajek-Shaul, G. Friedman, G. Halperin, O. Stein, and Y. Stein, Biochim. Biophys. Acta 666:216-222 (1981).
7. O. Stein, G. Halperin, and Y. Stein, Biochim. Biophys. Acta 665:477-490 (1981).
8. Y. Kleinman, G. Halperin, O. Stein, and Y. Stein, Atherosclerosis 43:1-6 (1982).
9. Y. Kleinman, O. Stein, and Y. Stein, Isr. J. Med. Sci. 18:819-822 (1982).
10. DeW. S. Goodman, O. Stein, G. Halperin, and Y. Stein, Biochim. Biophys. Acta 750:223-230 (1983).
11. J. L. Goldstein, Y. K. Ho, S. K. Basu, and M. S. Brown, Proc. Natl. Acad. Sci., U.S.A., 76:333-337.
12. R. W. Mahley, K. H. Weisgraber, T. L. Innerarity, and H. G. Windmueller, Proc. Natl. Acad. Sci., U.S.A., 76:1746-1750 (1979).
13. O. Stein and Y. Stein, Lab. Invest. 17:436-446 (1967).
14. O. Stein, Y. Stein, D. S. Goodman, and N. H. Fidge, J. Cell. Biol. 43:410-431 (1969).
15. P. S. Roheim, D. Rachmilewitz, O. Stein, and Y. Stein, Biochim. Biophys. Acta 248:315-329 (1971).
16. D. Rachmilewitz, O. Stein, P.S. Roheim, and Y. Stein, Biochim. Biosphy. Acta 270:414-425 (1972).
17. S. Eisenberg, H. G. Windmueller, and R. I. Levy, J. Lipid Res. 14:446-458 (1973).
18. P. Sigurdsson, S. P. Noel, and R. J. Havel, J. Lipid Res. 20:316-324 (1979).
19. P. J. Barter and J. I. Lally, Metabolism 28:230-236 (1979).
20. J. A. Glomset, C. D. Mitchell, W. C. King, K. A. Applegate, T. Forte, K. R. Norum, and E. Gjone, Ann. N.Y. Acad. Sci. 349:224 (1980).
21. R. B. Weinberg and A. M. Scanu, Atherosclerosis 44:141-152 (1982).

22. C. Glass, R. C. Pittman, and D. Steinberg, Arteriosclerosis 2:440a (1982).
23. Y. Stein, Y. Dabach, G. Hollander, G. Halperin, and O. Stein, Biochim. Biophys. Acta 752:98-105 (1983).
24. Y. Stein, O. Stein, and G. Halperin, Proc. NATO Advanced Study Inst. on Formation and Regression of Atherosclerotic Plaque, Plenum 51:139-155 (1982).
25. Y. Stein, Y. Kleinman, G. Halperin, and O. Stein, Biochim. Biophys. Acta 750:300-305 (1983).

HYPERTRIGLYCERIDEMIA: LIPOPROTEIN RECEPTORS AND ATHEROSCLEROSIS

S. H. Gianturco, A. M. Gotto, Jr., and W. A. Bradley

Baylor College of Medicine and The Methodist Hospital
Department of Medicine
6565 Fannin Street, Houston, Texas 77030

Some forms of atherosclerosis appear to be related to abnormalities in the metabolism of lipoproteins containing apoB and/or apoE. The uptake of these lipoproteins by specific lipoprotein receptors may be involved in atherogenesis. In Houston, we have been particularly interested in the abnormal receptor-mediated cellular uptake of very low density lipoproteins (VLDL) from subjects with hypertriglyceridemia that appears to account for certain VLDL catabolic abnormalties and may be involved in atherogenesis in these subjects.

There are at least 4 different receptors for lipoproteins containing apoB and/or apoE which result in uptake and degradation of the lipoprotein: the LDL-receptor, the acetyl LDL-receptor, the hepatic chylomicron remnant (apoE) receptor and the β-VLDL receptor. Characteristics of these receptors have been described in several excellent recent reviews.[1-3] In this discussion, we will focus on two of these receptors which bind abnormal VLDL--both hypertriglyceridemic (HTG)- and β-VLDL--and might therefore be related to abnormalties that occur in hypertriglyceridemia: First, the classic LDL receptor which Brown and Goldstein defined in cultured human fibroblasts and whose primary role is the catabolism of LDL and, second, the β-VLDL receptor, which Goldstein, Ho, and Brown in collaboration with Innerarity and Mahley first described in murine peritoneal macrophages and whose primary role may be the catabolism of abnormal VLDL.

Several years ago we demonstrated that VLDL from HTG subjects were functionally abnormal: HTG-VLDL, in sharp contrast to normal VLDL, were able to regulate cholesterol synthesis in cultured human fibroblasts because the HTG-VLDL were taken up by the classic LDL receptor pathway.[4] The observation that HTG-VLDL were functionally abnormal was confirmed and extended in Nestel's laboratory, where it was found that human leukocytes degraded HTG-VLDL far more avidly than normal VLDL.[5]

We have extended our studies in cultured cells and found that HTG-VLDL but not normal VLDL not only have the abnormal ability to interact with the classic LDL receptor present on cultured fibroblasts.[4,6,7] but also with β-VLDL receptor of macrophages.[8] We have demonstrated that the abnormal receptor-mediated uptake of HTG-VLDL exerts potentially atherogenic effects in two cell types implicated in atherosclerosis: First, we found that low levels of HTG-VLDL S_f 100-400 (HTG-$VLDL_1$) but not normal $VLDL_1$ were toxic to cultured endothelial cells.[9] Second, we demonstrated that HTG-$VLDL_1$ but not normal $VLDL_1$ produced massive triglyceride engorgement in unstimulated murine peritoneal macrophages, converting these cells into foam cells *in vitro*.[8] Thus, HTG-VLDL might be involved in the pathogenesis of atherosclerosis by initiating foam cell formation and promoting endothelial damage.

In addition, our observations *in vitro* have provided cellular mechanisms to explain several phenomena noted in hypertriglyceridemia. First of all, Reardon, Fidge, and Nestel have shown from *in vivo* turnover studies that in hypertriglyceridemic subjects, as much as two-thirds of the apoB of VLDL disappears directly from the plasma without first being converted to LDL, as it is in normal subjects.[10] Second, some forms of hypertriglyceridemia are associated with premature atherosclerosis.[11] Third, in some forms of hypertriglyceridemia, foam cells accumulate throughout the body.[11] We hypothesize that the abnormal uptake and degradation of HTG-VLDL by the two distinct receptor-mediated pathways can account for the abnormal catabolism of VLDL in hypertriglyceridemia and may be involved in foam cell formation and atherogenesis.

The rest of this paper will focus on studies which, together with our colleagues in Houston, we have carried out to define the binding determinants present in HTG-VLDL but absent in normal VLDL for the two geneticallly distinct receptors that recognize abnormal VLDL: the LDL receptor of fibroblasts and the β-VLDL receptor of macrophages. Major characteristics of these two receptors are summarized in Table 1 and have been reviewed recently.[1-3]

LDL RECEPTOR

General Characteristics

Role. The primary role of the LDL receptor is the catabolism of LDL; Brown and Goldstein demonstrated that approximately two-thirds of plasma LDL is catabolized by this route by comparing LDL turnover rates in normal versus receptor-negative subjects. *In vivo* studies in animals comparing the turnover of LDL with that of modified LDL that are not recognized by the LDL receptor have demonstrated that as

TABLE 1

CHARACTERISTICS OF THE GENETICALLY DISTINCT LDL RECEPTOR AND THE β-VLDL RECEPTOR

Characteristics	RECEPTOR	
	LDL	β -VLDL
Role	LDL catabolism	(abnormal VLDL catabolism)
Relation to atherosclerosis	Defect in FH (severe atherosclerosis)	Foam cell formation (on arterial foam cells and precursors - monocytes/macrophages)
In vitro model	Human skin fibroblasts (normal and mutant)	Murine peritoneal macrophages (no LDL receptors)
Ligands	ApoB and ApoE	ApoB (B-48 or processed ApoB) plus ApoE

much as 50% to 70% of plasma LDL is catabolized by the LDL-receptor mediated pathway. Shephard and Packard, using the reversibly modified cyclohexanedione adduct of LDL estimated that at least one-third of LDL was catabolized by this route in humans. The LDL receptor is present on most cells of the body in order to deliver cholesterol to the cells for membrane or hormone synthesis. Its presence in the liver provides an escape route by which cholesterol can leave the body.

Relation to Atherosclerosis. The critical importance of this pathway in regulating plasma LDL levels is apparent when this receptor pathway is defective or absent, as in familial hypercholesterolemia. Because of the defect in the LDL receptor in this genetic disorder, plasma LDL levels are grossly elevated due to the block in the normal catabolic route and the subjects suffer from massive premature atherosclerosis. Thus, the LDL receptor pathway normally serves a protective role against atherosclerosis by disposing of plasma LDL.

Model System. Brown and Goldstein's discoveries of the LDL receptor and the genetic mutations in subjects with familial hypercholesterolemia have provided the basis for lipoprotein-receptor studies. The ideal model system for studying interactions of lipoproteins with the LDL receptor derives from this work--the cultured human skin fibroblast from normal subjects. Fibroblasts derived from familial hypercholesterolemic homozygotes provide useful experimental controls since these fibroblasts are receptor defective or negative.

Ligands. There are two apoproteins which bind to the LDL receptor. As Goldstein and Brown originally found, the ligand of primary physiological importance is apoB, the apoprotein of LDL. In collaboration with Bersot, Mahley and Innerarity they demonstrated that an abnormal HDL-containing apoE as the only apoprotein also binds avidly to the LDL receptor.[3] Mahley and associates have studied extensively the binding of apoE-containing HDL and apoE/dimiristoyl phosphotidyl choline (DMPC) vesicles to the LDL receptor and these have been recently reviewed.[3]

Lipoproteins that bind to the LDL receptor, in addition to LDL and HDL_c, are IDL (d 1.006-1.03) and small VLDL (S_f 20-60, $VLDL_3$) from both normal and hypertriglyceridemic subjects;[4,6,7] HTG-VLDL S_f 60-400,[6,7] chylomicron remnants,[12] β-VLDL,[3] and Lp(α).[13] Normal VLDL S_f 60-400[6,7] and chylomicrons[12] do not bind to the LDL receptor even though they contain both apoE and apoB.

ApoE MEDIATES BINDING OF HTG-$VLDL_1$ TO THE LDL RECEPTOR

When both apoB and apoE are present in a lipoprotein, as in HTG-

VLDL, which apoprotein mediates the binding of the abnormal VLDL to the LDL receptor?

Using thrombin as a probe, we have demonstrated that the binding of large HTG-VLDL S_f 100-400 (HTG-$VLDL_1$) to the LDL receptor is mediated by apoE.[14] We recently reported that isolated purified VLDL contain serine protease(s) which can cleave apoE thereby causing a loss of LDL receptor binding determinants from the HTG-VLDL.[15] The VLDL-associated protease(s) cleaved a portion of the HTG-VLDL apoE into 2 major fragments; the primary thrombin clip was an arg-ala bond which corresponds to residues 191-192 of the apoE sequence as published by Rall, Weisgraber and Mahley.[16] One of the plasma serine proteases which could produce such a cleavage is thrombin and, in

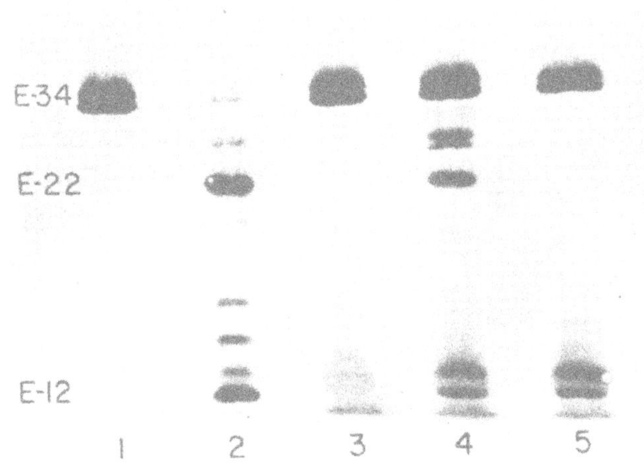

Fig. 1 Immunological identification of apoE fragments in thrombin-inactivated HTG-$VLDL_1$. HTG-$VLDL_1$ were incubated $\pm$ human α-thrombin (50 units/mg) for 2 h at 37°C and tested for reductase suppression $\pm$ recentrifugation. The samples were extracted and electrophoresed on sodium dodecyl sulfate-polyacrylamide gel electrophoresis (12%) before transfer to nitrocellulose paper for immunological detection of apoE and apoE fragments using polycolonal antibodies raised against human apoE. Lane 1, purified total apoE; Lane 2, isolated apoE incubated with thrombin (50 units/mg, 2 h at 37°C); Lane 3, HTG-$VLDL_1$ (starting material); Lane 4, HTG-$VLDL_1$ incubated with thrombin (50 units/mg, 2 h at 37°C; TI HTG-$VLDL_1$); Lane 5, TI HTG-$VLDL_1$ reisolated by flotation through a salt gradient.

fact, purified human α-thrombin produces precisely this same clip when incubated with isolated intact apoE.[15] This raised the question, can thrombin itself cleave apoE of HTG-VLDL and abolish its LDL receptor binding determinants?

Competition experiments[14] show that thrombin treatment of HTG-$VLDL_1$ does indeed abolish its LDL receptor binding determinants. Prior to thrombin treatment, HTG-$VLDL_1$ are effective in competing with the uptake and the degradation of iodinated LDL as LDL itself in normal human fibroblasts. However, after thrombin-treatment the HTG-VLDL are no longer effective competitors of LDL uptake and degradation, indicating loss of the LDL receptor binding determinants. In contrast to the case with HTG-$VLDL_1$, thrombin treatment of LDL had no effect on its ability to bind to the LDL receptor, indicating that the ability of thrombin to abolish receptor binding of HTG-VLDL is due to its effect on apoE rather than to an effect on apoB.[14]

The immunochemical electrophoretic blot shown in Figure 1 demonstrates the effects of thrombin on isolated apoE and on the apoE of HTG-$VLDL_1$. The patterns of intact isolated apoE prior to thrombin treatment (first lane) and after incubation (second lane) demonstrate cleavage into the two major fragments, indicated by arrows. Because of the sensitivity of the technique it is apparent that additional fragments are produced, but from mass analysis 85% of the apoE is converted into the E-22 fragment, the N-terminal two-thirds of the

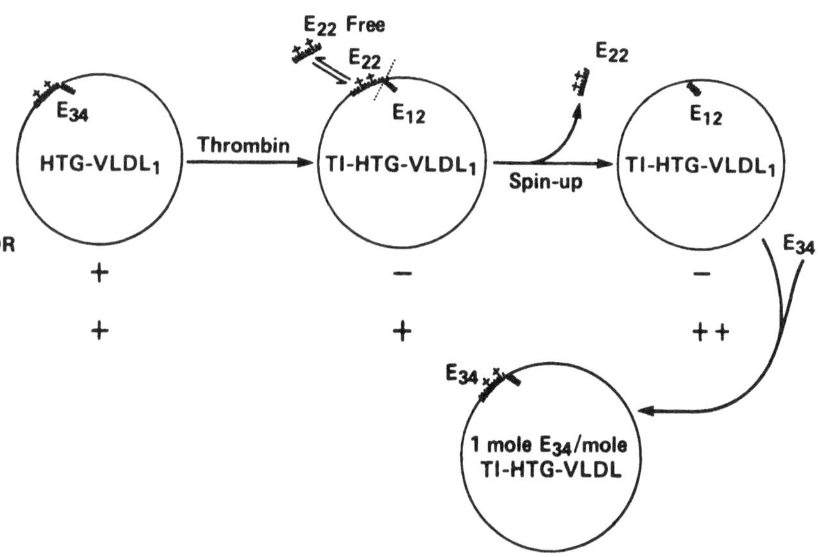

Fig. 2 Schematic summary of the effects of thrombin and apoE reincorporation on the interaction of HTG-$VLDL_1$ with the LDL receptor and the β-VLDL receptor.

molecule, and the E-12 fragment, the carboxy terminal one-third. The third lane is HTG-$VLDL_1$ prior to thrombin treatment. Upon thrombin treatment (lane 4) some, but--it is important to note--not all, of the apoE is converted primarily into the E-22 and the E-12 fragments. It is at this stage that the LDL receptor binding determinants are lost, even though the E-22 fragments are not removed and these fragments contain the mutation sites which are known to affect the binding of the apoE-isoforms to the LDL receptor. The last lane shows that when the thrombin-treated HTG-$VLDL_1$ are reisolated by flotation, all of the large fragments are lost from the lipoproteins, but the smaller, C-terminal fragments remain associated. Thus the large fragment, which contains regions involved in receptor binding, binds very poorly to the VLDL surface; the C-terminal E-12 fragment is the primary lipid-binding region of the apoE molecule. Radioimmunoassays (RIA) indicate a change in expression of apoE epitopes after thrombin treatment of HTG-$VLDL_1$ prior to reisolation (enhanced immunoreactivity). RIA also indicated that approximately 1 mol of apoE was removed per mol of particle when the thrombin-treated HTG-$VLDL_1$ were reisolated, with 2 to 3 mols of apoE remaining on the thrombin-treated, reisolated HTG-$VLDL_1$.[14]

If the cleavage of apoE by thrombin was indeed responsible for the loss of binding determinants, then the reincorporation of apoE into the thrombin-inactivated HTG-$VLDL_1$ should restore receptor recognition, and this is what we found.[14] We used HMG-CoA reductase suppression in normal fibroblasts as a sensitive intracellular endpoint indicating receptor-mediated uptake of the lipoprotein.[14] Thrombin-treated HTG-$VLDL_1$ failed to suppress HMG-CoA reductase activity, indicating that these VLDL no longer bound to the LDL receptor. After reincorporation of intact apoE, the VLDL were essentially as effective as LDL in suppressing reductase activity, indicating that apoE did indeed restore receptor recognition. Reincorporation of approximately 1 mol apoE/mol HTG-$VLDL_1$ was sufficient to restore efficient receptor-mediated uptake. By contrast, the E-12 fragment, as expected, failed to restore uptake and E-22 fragment--either alone or in combination with the E-12 fragment--was only 50% as effective in restoring receptor-mediated uptake as intact apoE. We conclude that--for efficient receptor binding--the intact apoE is required to maintain the appropriate conformation for binding.

Figure 2 summarizes these studies schematically. Native HTG-$VLDL_1$ bind avidly to the LDL receptor via apoE. Thrombin cleaves 1 mol apoE/mol HTG-VLDL into, primarily, the E-22 and the E-12 fragments. This abolishes binding of the particle to the LDL receptor. We have drawn the E-22 fragment as being in equilibrium between the lipoprotein surface and free in solution for two reasons: First, we know from the immunochemical blots that the E-22 fragment is readily removed by flotation and, second, that RIA indicates an increase in apoE immunoreactivity at this point, indicating that more apoE epitopes have been exposed by thrombin treatment, as could occur if the

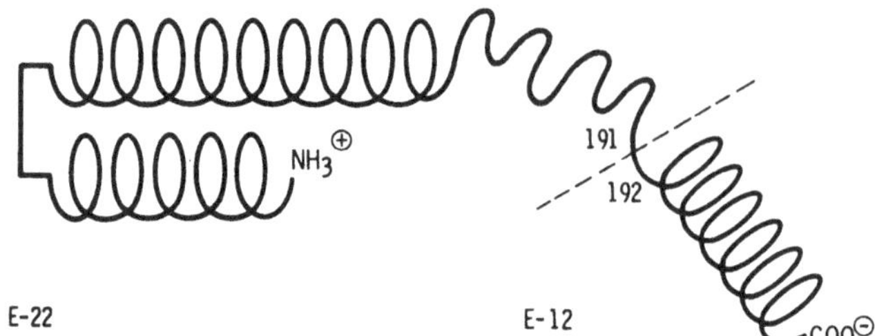

Fig. 3 Schematic model of apoE.

apoE-22 fragment were free in solution rather than associated with the lipoprotein. No E-22 fragments remain associated with the lipoprotein after a 90-minute flotation through a salt gradient, indicating that these fragments bind lipid very poorly. Finally, receptor binding is restored when intact apoE--approximately 1 mol per mol particle--is reincorporated into the thrombin-inactivated HTG-$VLDL_1$, providing compelling evidence that the cleavage of apoE by thrombin was indeed responsible for the loss of receptor binding determinants upon thrombin treatment.

The highly schematic model of apoE in Figure 3 illustrates the two major functional domains of apoE in HTG-$VLDL_1$ which we have identified using thrombin as a probe. To summarize, the primary thrombin clip in apoE is the arg/ala bond at residues 191-192. The E-22 fragment (the N-terminal 22K two-thirds) binds poorly to the VLDL surface but contains a domain that is required for LDL receptor binding. This is consistent with the studies from the Gladstone Foundation which demonstrated that amino acid substitutions in this region affected binding of apoE/DMPC vesicles to the receptor.[3] Our studies indicate, however, that in native VLDL the E-22 fragment by itself is relatively inefficient in binding to the receptor and that intact apoE of an appropriate conformation is required to mediate binding to the receptor.[14]

The E-12 fragment, the C-terminal one-third of the molecule, contains the major lipid binding regions of apoE. This domain anchors apoE to the VLDL particle and is required to maintain the receptor-binding domain of apoE in the appropriate conformation for efficient receptor binding.

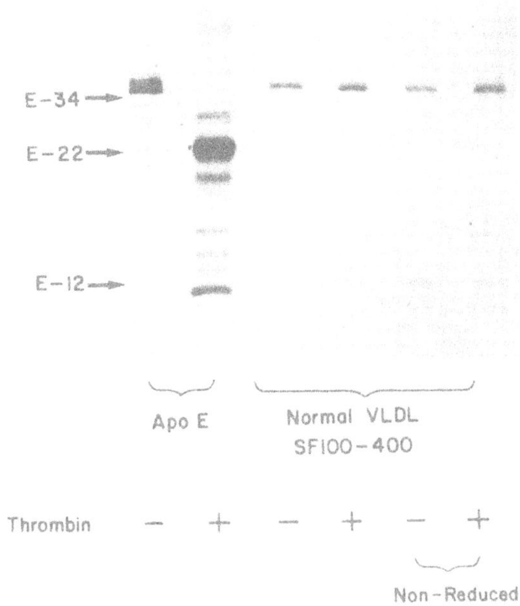

Fig. 4 Immunological techniques indicate that the apoE of normal VLDL is inaccessible to thrombin.

Normal $VLDL_1$ were incubated ± human thrombin, electrophoresed, and blotted as in the legend to Fig. 1. Lane 1, purified apoE; Lane 2, apoE incubated with thrombin; Lanes 3 and 5, normal $VLDL_1$; Lanes 4 and 6, normal $VLDL_1$ incubated with thrombin as in Fig. 1. Samples in Lanes 1-4 were reduced; samples in Lanes 5 and 6 were not.

THE ApoE OF NORMAL $VLDL_1$ IS INACCESSIBLE TO THE LDL RECEPTOR AND TO THROMBIN

These studies again raise the question: Why do not large VLDL from normolipemic subjects bind specifically to the LDL receptor, since normal VLDL contain apoE? Our recent studies using thrombin as a probe have provided an answer to this question. The apoE of normal VLDL is inaccessible to thrombin--it appears to be in a different conformation from that of the apoE of HTG-VLDL that mediates binding to the LDL receptor and is cleaved by thrombin. As shown by immunochemical electrophoretic blots, one of which is shown in Figure 4, the apoE of normal $VLDL_1$ is not cleaved by thrombin under conditions which cleave all of isolated apoE and which inactivate HTG-$VLDL_1$ as

TABLE 2

TWO CONFORMATIONS OF ApoE IN VLDL S_f 60-400

	Normal VLDL	HTG-VLDL
1. Accessible To thrombin To the LDL receptor	–	+
2. Inaccessible To thrombin To the LDL receptor	+	+

The accessible conformation (≥ 1 mol/mol VLDL) is required for LDL receptor binding and can be created in vitro.

shown in Fig. 1. As summarized in Table 2, we have identified two different conformations (populations) of apoE in HTG-$VLDL_1$. One population which is present in HTG-$VLDL_1$ but absent in normal $VLDL_1$ is accessible both to the LDL receptor and to thrombin. The other population of apoE is resistant to thrombin cleavage and is also inaccessible to the LDL receptor. This inaccessible population of apoE is present in both normal $VLDL_1$ and in hypertriglyceridemic $VLDL_1$. For binding to the LDL receptor, large VLDL must contain the accessible conformation, and this can be created by the incorporation of approximately 1 mol apoE/mol of VLDL, either into large normal VLDL S_f 60-400[7] or thrombin-inactivated HTG-$VLDL_1$.[14] The specificity of this phenomenon is demonstrated by the failure of apoA-I to cause normal VLDL[7] or thrombin-inactivated HTG-$VLDL_2$ to bind to the LDL receptor when incorporated into the lipoprotein. This indicates that changes in the conformation of apoB potentially induced by the incorporation of an apoprotein into the particle was not responsible for acquisition of receptor recognition. We conclude that the recognition of large VLDL requires apoE of the accessible conformation. Our radioimmunoassays indicate that there are 1-2 mol apoE/mol normal $VLDL_1$, all inaccessible to thrombin, and at least 2-4 mol apoE/mol HTG-$VLDL_1$, 1-2 of which are accessible to thrombin. Thus RIA indicates that HTG-$VLDL_1$ contain an average of 1-2 mol apoE more than do normal $VLDL_1$ (in terms of percentage of total $VLDL_1$ protein, this is an increase of only 2 to 4% and was not detected by other analytic means); this "extra" apoE in HTG-$VLDL_1$ is in a different conformation from that of normal $VLDL_1$ or the residual apoE of thrombin-treated HTG-$VLDL_1$. In hypertriglyceridemia, there is a shift in the plasma distribution of apoE so that most apoE is in VLDL, not HDL.[17] We suggest that the apoE of HTG-$VLDL_1$ which is accessible to thrombin and to the LDL receptor is acquired in the plasma by transfer during the abnormally long residence time of the VLDL.

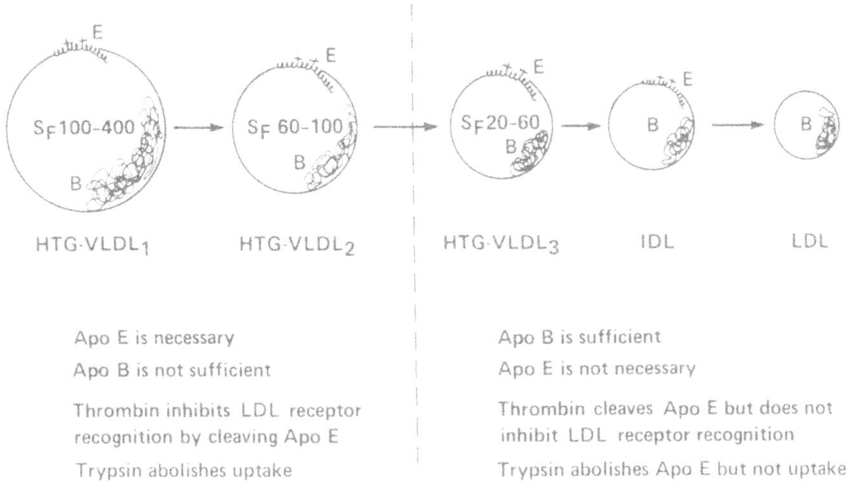

Fig. 5 Schematic summary of protease inactivation of HTG-$VLDL_1$ and HTG-$VLDL_2$ but not HTG-$VLDL_3$, IDL or LDL.

BINDING DETERMINANTS SWITCH FROM ApoE TO ApoB IN THE METABOLIC CASCADE OF HTG-$VLDL_1$ TO LDL

In contrast to large HTG-$VLDL_1$, the binding of LDL is mediated by apoB. This raises the question, where in the metabolic cascade from large HTG-$VLDL_1$ to LDL do the receptor binding determinants switch from apoE to apoB? To answer this question we took advantage of the abilities of thrombin and trypsin to inactivate apoE but not apoB as a receptor-binding site.[14] Many laboratories have shown that the apoB-mediated binding of LDL is not significantly reduced by proteolysis by trypsin or plasmin, and we have demonstrated that LDL binding is also resistant to thrombin treatment as well as to trypsination. By contrast, we have shown that the apoE-mediated binding of large HTG-$VLDL_1$ is abolished by both thrombin and trypsin.[14] We have therefore used thrombin and trypsin as probes to identify the switch point in the metabolic cascade. Figure 5 summarizes our results--that both thrombin and trypsin reduce or abolish uptake of HTG-$VLDL_1$ and HTG-$VLDL_2$ (S_f 60-100), but have little to no effect on the uptake of small VLDL (S_f 20-60, $VLDL_3$), IDL, or LDL.[18] As shown in Figure 6, trypsin abolishes the ability of HTG-$VLDL_1$ and HTG-$VLDL_2$ but not HTG-$VLDL_3$, IDL, or LDL to cause receptor-mediated reductase suppression, even though trypsin abolishes all of the apoE of all lipoproteins as shown by immunochemical blots. This indicates that the uptake of the latter three lipoproteins is mediated by apoB and the binding of the larger VLDL (S_f >60) is mediated by apoE.

Table 3 summarizes the interactions of apoB/E containing lipopro-

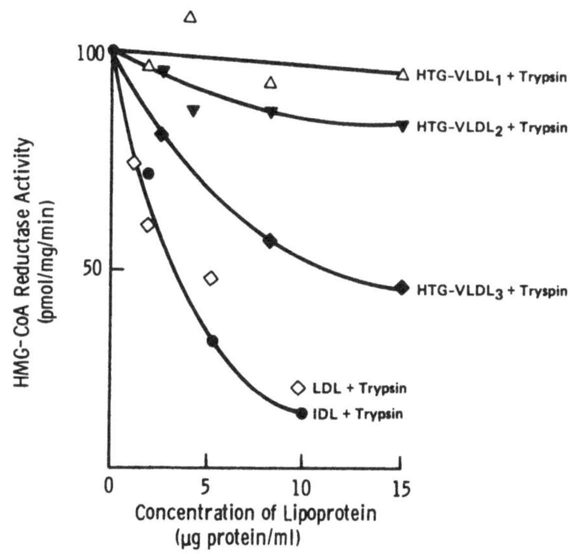

Fig. 6 Effects of Trypsin Digestion on Abilities of HTG-VLDL, IDL and LDL to Suppress Reductase Activity in Normal Fibroblasts.

Cells were grown to approximately 75% confluency in complete medium containing 10% fetal calf serum, washed, and placed on 2 ml of medium containing 5% human lipoprotein deficient serum for 24 h. Indicated amounts of lipoproteins were added to duplicate dishes for 16 h before the cells were washed and harvested. Lipoproteins were incubated with trypsin (GIBCO - Catalog No. 610-5300, 0.1 ml/mg protein, 2 h at 37°C) and reisolated by flotation before testing for reductase suppression in fibroblasts preincubated in lipoprotein-deficient medium. Each data point is the average of duplicate determinations of reductase activity in cells from duplicate dishes. Variation between duplicates was less than 5%. HTG-$VLDL_1$ (▲); HTG-$VLDL_2$, (▼); HTG-$VLDL_3$, (◆); IDL, (◇); and LDL (●).

teins with the LDL receptor. Our studies show that of the large apoB/apoE-containing lipoproteins that bind to the LDL receptor, that binding is mediated by apoE, whereas in the small apoB/E containing lipoproteins, binding is mediated by apoB. Of the large, triglyceride-rich lipoproteins (S_f >60), neither chylomicrons nor normal VLDL bind to the LDL receptor, even though they contain both apoB and apoE. The conformation of these apoproteins is apparently inappropriate for binding to the receptor. Indeed, immunological studies by Schonfeld and colleagues demonstrate that certain antisera to apoB detect major differences in apoB epitope expression in large HTG-VLDL versus small

TABLE 3

INTERACTION OF LIPOPROTEINS WITH THE LDL RECEPTOR AND THE β-VLDL RECEPTOR

Lipoprotein	Thrombin Treatment	Receptor Binding	
		LDL	β-VLDL
Chylomicrons	- +	-	+ ++
HTG-VLDL$_1$	- +	+ -	+ ++
β-VLDL	- +	+ -	+ ++
Normal VLDL	- +	-	- +
IDL	- +	+ +	- -
LDL	- +	+ +	- -
ApoE-HDL	-	+	-

Lipoproteins that bind the β-VLDL receptor have both ApoE and ApoB (B-48 or processed ApoB).

For binding to the LDL receptor, large particles must have thrombin-accessible ApoE (ApoB is insufficient). Small particles may bind via ApoE (HDLc) or via ApoB (IDL, LDL).

VLDL, IDL, and LDL[19] (and this Symposium). In contrast to normal VLDL, both abnormal VLDLs--triglyceride-rich VLDL of S_f >60 from hypertriglyceridemic humans or the cholesteryl ester-rich β-VLDL from Type 3 humans or cholesterol-fed animals--bind to the LDL receptor via apoE. These abnormal VLDL contain a population of apoE of the appropriate conformation for binding; this population is accessible both to thrombin and to the LDL receptor and does not exist in normal VLDL. Of the smaller apoB/E-containing lipoproteins, binding is mediated by apoB. Both normal and HTG-VLDL of S_f 20-60 and intermediate density lipoproteins bind to the LDL receptor primarily via apoB even though apoE is present.

Thus normally, apoB is the physiologically important ligand for the LDL receptor and triglyceride-rich lipoproteins are not catabolized by this route. Blum has shown that in hypertriglyceridemia, however, there is a redistribution of apoE from HDL into VLDL,[17] and we suggest that it is this transferred apoE that produces HTG-VLDL$_1$ and HTG-VLDL$_2$ which have the abnormal ability to interact with the LDL receptor. Uptake of HTG-VLDL by this pathway can account for the direct disappearance of VLDL from plasma in hypertriglyceridemia and, since uptake is toxic to cultured endothelial cells, this could be atherogenic if it also occurs *in vivo*.

β-VLDL RECEPTOR

General Characteristics

Some of the characteristics of the β-VLDL receptor are presented in Table 1 and have been reviewed recently.[2,3] This receptor was first identified in murine peritoneal macrophages and is found in macrophages from other species, including human monocyte-derived macrophages in which it was shown to be genetically distinct from the LDL receptor.[20] The receptor is named after the cholesteryl ester-rich, β-migrating VLDL, isolated from animals fed massive amounts of cholesterol, which was first demonstrated to bind to this distinct receptor on macrophages. After binding to the receptor, the β-VLDL are internalized, hydrolyzed in the lysosomes, and the liberated cholesterol is reesterified with oleate and stored as lipid droplets in the cytoplasm, producing a foam cell morphology (VLDL from normal animals failed to do this). We have demonstrated that HTG-VLDL$_1$ also bind to this receptor, and unlike normal VLDL, produce massive triglyceride engorgement and foam cell morphology in the cells after uptake, lysosomal degradation and reesterification.[8] This sequence is analogous to that which occurs after binding of the cholesteryl ester-rich β-VLDL, except that the cells reesterify and store triglyceride rather than cholesteryl ester, since triglyceride and not cholesteryl ester is the predominant lipid in HTG-VLDL$_1$. Van Lenten and Associates have demonstrated that chylomicrons bind to the receptor whereas normal VLDL do not.[20]

Role. We suggest that the primary role of the β-VLDL receptor *in vivo* may be catabolism of abnormal VLDL, both HTG-VLDL and β-VLDL. Disposal of abnormal VLDL by such a mechanism would serve to protect other cells, such as endothelial cells, from the potentially deleterious effects of uptake and hydrolysis of the abnormal VLDL by the LDL pathway. In pathological states, such as dietary cholesterol insults or in hypertriglyceridemia, the macrophages cannot dispose of the accumulated lipid rapidly enough, and foam cell formation then ensues. Indeed, the β-VLDL receptor has been demonstrated in arterial foam cells by Pitas and colleagues as well as in human monocyte/macrophages, which are probably the precursors to many of the foam cells in early atherosclerotic lesions.

Model System. The ideal model system for studying the lipoprotein binding determinants for this receptor is the unstimulated murine peritoneal macrophage, since these cells--unlike human monocyte/macrophages or long-term cell lines--possess few to no LDL receptors.[2] When cells possess both receptors--both of which bind abnormal VLDL--interpretation of binding and uptake studies is ambiguous and not easily interpreted.

Ligand. Our studies, along with studies from other laboratories, suggest that the apoprotein domains which serve as the ligand for the β-VLDL receptor are more complex than the ligands for the LDL recep-

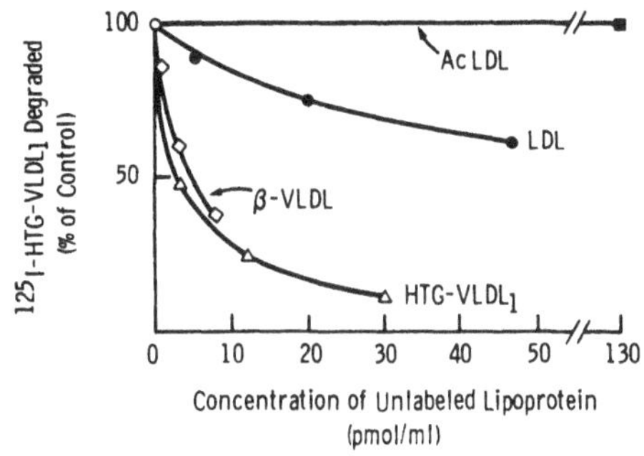

Fig. 7 Specificity of the β-VLDL receptor in murine peritoneal macrophages.

Freshly isolated adherent murine peritoneal macrophages were incubated with 125 I-hypertriglyceridemic $VLDL_1$ (J. P., type 5; 4.6 μg protein/ml, equivalent to 4 pmol $VLDL_1$/ml) and the indicated concentrations of unlabeled lipoproteins for 16 h at 37°C before the media were processed to determine acid-soluble, non-iodide radioactivity: (△) homologous hypertriglyceridemic $VLDL_1$; (◇) cholesteryl ester-rich (β) VLDL from cholesterol-fed rabbits; (●) normal LDL, d 1.02-1.063 acetyl LDL (■). Each point represents the mean from three dishes and is expressed as percent of control, the amount degraded in the absence of competing unlabeled lipoproteins. For the LDL competition curve, this control value was 1757 ng/mg cell protein and standard deviations were less than 12%; for the CER-VLDL curve the control value was 647 ng/dish and standard deviations were less than 5%. Hypertriglyceridemic VLDL was run in each experiment and gave essentially identical competition curves (50% inhibition at 3 pmol HTG-$VLDL_1$/ml).

tor. Some but not all apoB/apoE-containing lipoproteins induce lipid accumulation in macrophages via the β-VLDL receptor pathway: chylomicrons (normal, post-prandial as well as those from fasting Type 5 subjects); HTG-$VLDL_1$ but not normal $VLDL_1$; HTG-$VLDL_2$ is moderately active but normal $VLDL_2$ is inactive; neither HTG nor normal $VLDL_3$ are taken up, and neither IDL nor LDL bind. We have found that Lp (α) also are not taken up by macrophages by any receptor mediated pathway. Likewise, HDL_c containing only apoE do not bind to this receptor. The apoprotein composition of β-VLDL provides a clue to the receptor ligand: the apoproteins of β-VLDL are almost entirely apoB and apoE, with little to no apoC present. Thus we suggest that both an apoB species along with a domain of apoE is required for binding.

Figure 7 summarizes some of our studies on the specificity of the β-VLDL receptor.[8] Because of the differences in sizes and composi-

TABLE 4

THE LIPID WHICH ACCUMULATES IN MACROPHAGES AFTER RECEPTOR-MEDIATED UPTAKE REFLECTS THE COMPOSITION OF THE LIPOPROTEIN

Lipoprotein (β-VLDL Receptor)	Thrombin Treatment	Lipid Accumulated ^{14}C-Oleate Incorporation	
		Cholesterol Ester	Triglyceride
Chylomicrons	−	−	+
	+	−	++
HTG-VLDL	−	−	+
	+	−	++
Normal VLDL	−	−	−
	+	−	+
β-VLDL	−	+	−
	+	++	−
(Scavenger Receptor) Acetyl LDL	−	+	−
	+	+	−

tions of HTG-$VLDL_1$, β-VLDL and LDL it is necessary to compare these lipoproteins on a particle rather than a protein basis for competition studies to be meaningful. On a particle basis, HTG-$VLDL_1$ and β-VLDL are equally effective in competing for the uptake and degradation of iodinated HTG-$VLDL_1$, indicating that these lipoproteins bind to the same receptor (on a protein basis HTG-$VLDL_1$ appears to be more effective than β-VLDL). By contrast, neither LDL nor acetyl LDL compete effectively with the abnormal VLDL for uptake.

As summarized in Table 4, the lipid which accumulates in marcophages reflects that of lipoprotein internalized by the cells.[2,8] Thus when cholesteryl ester-rich lipoproteins are taken up by macrophage receptors, cholesteryl esters accumulate in the cytoplasm of the cell and the activity of acyl-cholesteryl ester transferase (ACAT) is stimulated, so that exogenous oleate is incorporated into the cellular cholesteryl ester. This oleate incorporation is used as one measure of the increase in cellular cholesteryl ester produced by the receptor-mediated uptake of the lipoprotein.[2] For example, uptake of acetyl-LDL by the scavenger pathway or uptake of β-VLDL by the β-VLDL pathway results in the stimulation of oleate incorporation into cellular cholesteryl esters and accumulation of these esters in the cytoplasm. We have shown that, analogously, when triglyceride-rich chylomicrons and HTG-$VLDL_1$ are taken up by the β-VLDL receptor pathway of macrophages, this produces triglyceride engorgement in the cell and stimulates the incorporation of exogenous oleate into cellular triglyceride.[8] Likewise, Van Lenten, Fogelman, Edwards and their col-

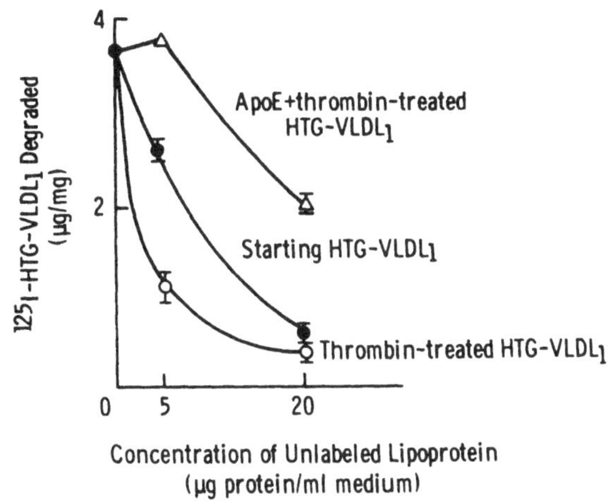

Fig. 8 Competitive uptake and degradation studies show that thrombin enhances binding of HTG-$VLDL_1$ to the β-VLDL receptor, and that reincorporation of apoE reverses this effect.

Immediately after nonadherent cells were removed, the adherent macrophages were incubated with I-125-labeled HTG-$VLDL_1$ (5 μg/ml) alone or with the indicated quantities of unlabeled lipoproteins for 18 h before the cells and media were processed to determine uptake and degradation as described in methods. Each point is the average of values from duplicate dishes (range is shown by error bars). HTG-$VLDL_1$ (●); thrombin-treated, reisolated HTG-$VLDL_1$ (O); thrombin-treated HTG-$VLDL_1$ plus apoE (100 μg apoE/500 μg apoVLDL). (△).

leagues demonstrated that chylomicrons are avidly taken up by the β-VLDL receptor of human monocyte/macrophages[20] with no cholesteryl ester accumulation resulting.

We demonstrated that VLDL from normal, fasting subjects do not produce triglyceride reesterification or accumulation in unstimulated murine peritoneal macrophages. Consistent with our findings, Van Lenten and co-workers found that normal fasting VLDL do not compete effectively for the β-VLDL receptor of human monocyte/macrophages. Thus our studies[8] and those of Van Lenten et al.[20] using human triglyceride-rich lipoproteins are consistent with the earlier studies of Brown, Goldstein, Ho, Innerarity and Mahley which showed that normolipemic animal VLDL failed to induce lipid accumulation in macrophages.[2,3] Under different culture conditions, normal VLDL has been shown to produce lipid accumulation in certain macrophages, via secreted lipoprotein lipase or by phagocytosis,[21,22] and these alternate mechanisms may also play a role in the atherogenic process.

ApoE MODULATES INTERACTION OF HTG-$VLDL_1$ WITH THE β-VLDL RECEPTOR

Table 3 summarizes results of experiments which we have recently performed using thrombin as a probe to determine the role of apoE in recognition of HTG-VLDL and β-VLDL by the β-VLDL receptor of macrophages. In sharp contrast to the effects of thrombin on recognition of HTG-$VLDL_1$ by the LDL receptor, we have found that thrombin treatment of apoB/apoE-containing lipoproteins enhances their uptake by the β-VLDL receptor of macrophages.[23] Thus chylomicrons, HTG-VLDL, and β-VLDL cause even greater triglyceride (cholesteryl-ester β-VLDL) reesterification and accumulation after thrombin cleavage of a portion of the apoE of the lipoproteins; reincorporation of apoE reversed these effects.

Competition studies provide further evidence that apoE cleavage causes the enhanced uptake of thrombin-treated HTG-$VLDL_1$ and, moreover, indicate that the observed enhanced uptake of thrombin-treated-$VLDL_1$ is due to enhanced uptake by the SAME receptor, rather than by some alternate mechanism, such as by phagocytosis or by a different receptor. Iodinated HTG-$VLDL_1$ were incubated with macrophages in the presence and absence of unlabeled HTG-$VLDL_1$ (Fig. 8). The middle curve shows that these homologous HTG-$VLDL_1$ effectively competed with the uptake and degradation of the labeled HTG-$VLDL_1$. When these VLDL were treated with thrombin and reisolated, they were even more effective in competing for receptor-mediated uptake and degradation (lower curve, Fig. 8). This indicates that the enhanced triglyceride uptake and reesterification observed after thrombin treatment is due to enhanced uptake via the same receptor. The upper curve shows that when apoE was added to the thrombin-treated HTG-$VLDL_1$, this actually decreased its ability to compete for the receptor, indicating that the thrombin-accessible apoE can modulate and even inhibit binding to the macrophage receptor.

These studies are summarized schematically in Figure 2. Native HTG-$VLDL_1$ bind to both the LDL receptor of fibroblasts and the β-VLDL receptor of macrophages. Thrombin cleaves approximately 1 mol apoE/mol HTG-$VLDL_1$ into the E-22 and the E-12 fragments. This abolishes binding to the LDL receptor but has little to no effect on binding of the particle to the β-VLDL receptor. Removal of the E-22 fragment by centrifugation results in enhanced uptake by the β-VLDL receptor; these particles still do not bind to the LDL receptor. Reincorporation of apoE reverses both of these functional changes, so that the reconstituted particle again binds to both the LDL receptor and the β-VLDL receptor with affinities resembling that of the native HTG-$VLDL_1$.

We conclude from these studies that the thrombin-accessible apoE that mediates the binding of HTG-$VLDL_1$ to the LDL receptor is not required for binding of the particle to the β-VLDL receptor. Rather this thrombin-accessible apoE can modulate the binding of the particle to the β-VLDL receptor, and, in some cases, reincorporation of apoE actually inhibits the β-VLDL receptor, as shown in Figure 8.

Cleavage of the accessible apoE of HTG-$VLDL_1$ by thrombin has two functional effects: it abolishes binding to the LDL receptor and enhances binding to the β-VLDL receptor. Thus thrombin could, in effect, route HTG-$VLDL_1$ to the β-VLDL receptor of macrophages for catabolism, diverting the HTG-VLDL away from cells which possess LDL receptors. This could serve a protective function _in vivo_ by preventing uptake and potential toxicity of the HTG-$VLDL_1$ in cells which process LDL receptors. For example, we have shown that HTG-$VLDL_1$ (but not normal $VLDL_1$) are toxic to cultured endothelial cells.[9] If overloaded, however, as in extreme hypertriglyceridemia, routing of VLDL to the β-VLDL receptor of macrophages could potentiate foam cell formation and possibly contribute to the pathogenesis of atherosclerosis. Indeed, foam cells accumulate throughout the body in Types 1, 3, and 5 hyperlipoproteinemia.[11] The foam cells isolated from diabetics with hypertriglyceridemia and eruptive xanthomas contain triglyceride as the predominant lipid. During therapy and resolution of the hypertriglyceridemia and the lesions, triglyceride disappears first, leaving cholesterol-rich foam cells until these too finally resolve.[24] We suggest that such a sequence could occur in atherogenesis associated with hypertriglyceridemia.

So what does mediate binding of abnormal VLDL to the β-VLDL receptor? The apoE of HTG-$VLDL_1$ that mediates binding to the LDL receptor and is cleaved by thrombin apparently alters domains involved in binding to the β-VLDL receptor. We suggest that a domain of an apoB species not present in normal VLDL or LDL along with a domain of apoE may be involved in recognition by the β-VLDL receptor. Studies from several laboratories suggest that intestinally-derived apoB-48 might be involved in binding to the β-VLDL receptor. β-VLDL from animals fed cholesterol and from Type 3 subjects contain particles that were relatively enriched with an apoB species with B-48 mobility showed enhanced uptake by macrophages.[3] Similarly, Van Lenten and co-workers demonstrated that chylomicrons, which contain B-48, bound to the β-VLDL receptor, and normal fasting VLDL, which do not contain B-48, were ineffective in competing for this receptor.[20] We find that HTG-$VLDL_1$ also contain apoB species in addition to apoB-100, and some of these species have mobilities similar to B-48, B-74, B-26, as well as other species.

THROMBIN PROCESSES ApoB-100 OF ALL ApoB/ApoE-CONTAINING LIPOPROTEINS INTO SMALLER SPECIES

As we have reported, thrombin treatment of LDL has no effect on its ability to bind to the LDL receptor.[14] Likewise, many laboratories have found that trypsinization of LDL does not abolish its

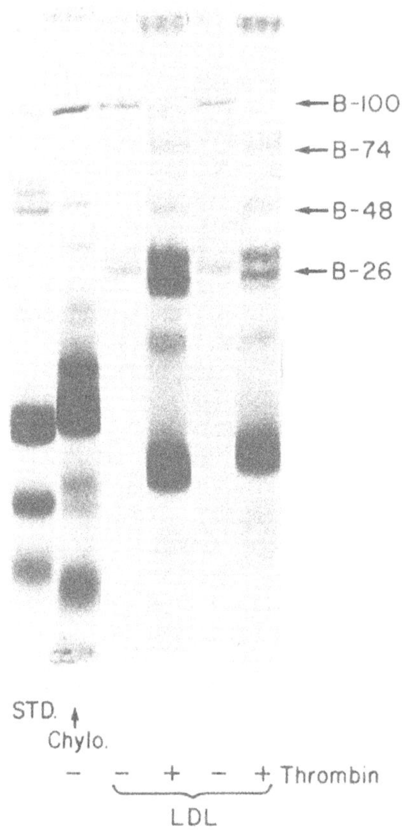

Fig. 9 3% SDS page of thrombin-treated LDL (d = 1.03-1.05): The first gel shows molecular weight markers, the second gel is plasma chylomicrons. The top band is apoB-100 and the second band is apoB-48, the intestinally derived apoB. The third and the fifth gels are two different normal LDL preparations, d 1.03-1.05, washed at each density. These LDL preparations consist primarily of B-100, with some B-74 and B-26 present, which Kane has suggested represent breakdown products of B-100.[26] Gels 4 and 6 are the LDLs after incubation with thrombin. Virtually all of the apoB-100 has been converted into species with electrophoretic mobilities in these 3% gels that are remarkably similar to B-74, B-26, and B-48, with several additional bands apparent. The lowermost band in each of gels 4 and 6 is thrombin itself.

ability to interact with the LDL receptor, although trypsin cleaves apoB.[25]

RIA detected no changes in apoB of HTG-VLDL after thrombin treatment, and pore-gradient gels also failed to detect changes in apoB with thrombin treatment. So it at first appeared that thrombin had no effect on apoB. Electrophoresis in 3% SDS polyacrylamide gels or immunochemical blots of 5% slab gels, however, demonstrate that thrombin can convert apoB-100 of all apoB-containing lipoproteins into new species; the mobilities of three of these are similar to B-48, B-74, and B-26.

Figure 9 illustrates that maximal changes in electrophoretic mobilities in 3% SDS PAGE that can be produced in apoB-100 of LDL upon treatment with purified human α-thrombin. The first gel shows molecular weight markers, the second gel is plasma chylomicrons. The top band is apoB-100 and the second band is apoB-48, the intestinally derived apoB. The third and the fifth gels are two different normal LDL preparations, d 1.03-1.05, washed at each density. These LDL preparations consist primarily of B-100, with some B-74 and B-26 present, which Kane has suggested represent breakdown products of B-100.[26] Gels 4 and 6 are the LDLs after incubation with thrombin. Virtually all of the apoB-100 has been converted into species with electrophoretic mobilities in these 3% gels that are similar to B-74, B-26, and B-48, with several additional bands apparent. The lowermost band in gels 4 and 6 is thrombin itself. The degradation of B-100 is dependent on thrombin concentration and on the time of incubation. Virtually the same patterns are produced when VLDL or IDL are incubated with thrombin.

THROMBIN ENHANCES UPTAKE OF NORMAL VLDL BUT NOT LDL BY THE -VLDL RECEPTOR OF MACROPHAGES

Processing of apoB of normal VLDL by thrombin results in an important functional change: after, but not prior to, thrombin treatment, normal VLDL can cause receptor-mediated triglyceride accumulation in murine peritoneal macrophages.[27] Thrombin processing of each of the VLDL subclasses--S_f 100-400, S_f 60-100, and S_f 20-60--causes each to stimulate the incorporation of oleate into cellular triglyceride. By contrast, thrombin treatment of LDL fails to produce uptake as measured by cholesterol reesterification, even though its apoB-100 was processed by thrombin. This suggests that another VLDL component, in addition to processed apoB, is required for interaction with the β-VLDL receptor.

We suggest that for binding to the β-VLDL receptor, a lipoprotein must contain a specific apoB domain along with another VLDL component. The required apoB domain is absent in normal VLDL but present in HTG-VLDL and chylomicrons and in thrombin processed normal VLDL. Since apoE is virtually the only other apoprotein present in β-VLDL, we suggest that a domain of the inaccessible apoE that is present in all VLDLs is required in conjunction with the correct apoB domain for binding to the β-VLDL receptor.

TABLE 5

DIFFERENCES IN RECEPTOR RECOGNITION DETERMINANTS IN NORMAL-VLDL AND HTG-VLDL

VLDL Sf60-400	Normal		HTG	
Thrombin Treatment	–	+	–	+
Receptor β-VLDL	–	+	+	++
LDL	–		+	–
Apoprotein differences				
ApoE				
1. Accessible to thrombin, LDL receptor	–	–	+	–
2. Inaccessible to thrombin, LDL receptor	+	+	+	+
ApoB				
ApoB-100	+	+	+	+
ApoB-48 like species	–	+	+	+
Processed ApoB	–	+	+	+

Table 3 summarizes the interactions of lipoproteins with the LDL and the β-VLDL receptor before and after thrombin processing. Chylomicrons do not bind to the LDL receptor but do bind to the β-VLDL receptor; this binding is enhanced by thrombin treatment. Both abnormal VLDLs--HTG and β--bind to both receptors; thrombin treatment reduces or abolishes their binding to the LDL receptor but enhances binding to the β-VLDL receptor. Native, large normal VLDL bind to neither receptor; after thrombin cleavage of the apoB, normal VLDL acquire the ability to interact with the β-VLDL receptor but not the LDL receptor. IDL and LDL both bind to the LDL receptor but not to the β-VLDL. Thrombin treatment of these lipoproteins does not change either of these interactions. Table 5 summarizes the structural differences in normal and hypertriglyceridemic VLDL that account for their functional differences. Normal VLDL S_f >60 do not bind to the LDL receptor of fibroblasts because they lack the population of apoE of the appropriate conformation for binding--apoE that is accessible both to thrombin and to the receptor and is present in HTG-VLDL S_f >60). This apoE can be incorporated into the normal VLDL _in vitro_. Normal VLDL do not bind to the β-VLDL receptor of macrophages because they do not contain the appropriate domain of apoB required for this binding. Thrombin treatment of normal VLDL confers upon the VLDL the ability to bind to the β-VLDL receptor; since thrombin processes apoB but not apoE of normal VLDL we conclude that the processed apoB (along with the inaccessible apoE) allows receptor binding. Native HTG-VLDL isolated in the presence of serine protease inhibitors and hirudin, contain the processed apoB species as well as the appropriate apoE.

We have made several observations *in vitro* which suggest that thrombin or other plasma proteases can route VLDL to macrophages for catabolism. First, thrombin cleavage of apoE of HTG-VLDL abolishes its binding to the LDL receptor and enhances binding to the β-VLDL receptor. Second, thrombin cleavage of apoB of normal VLDL causes uptake by the β-VLDL receptor of macrophages. We hypothesize that thrombin or other plasma protease can route apoB/E-containing lipoproteins to macrophages for uptake, and this could enhance foam cell formation in pathological states where the system is overloaded.

SUMMARY

We have shown first, that apoB mediates the binding of small VLDL S_f 20-60 and IDL, as well as LDL, to the LDL receptor. Second, apoE of an appropriate, accessible conformation is required for the binding of large VLDL to the LDL receptor; HTG-VLDL S_f >60 but not normal VLDL S_f >60 have this apoE population. Third, the same population of apoE that mediates binding of HTG-VLDL S_f >60 to the LDL receptor modulates its binding to the β-VLDL receptor, but it is not required for the latter interaction. Fourth, a domain of processed apoB or apoB-48 in association with a domain of the inaccessible apoE is required for binding to and uptake by the β-VLDL receptor. Fifth, our observations suggest that the abnormal catabolism of VLDL that occurs in hypertriglyceridemia may be explained by the abnormal uptake of HTG-VLDL by either the LDL or the β-VLDL receptor pathway. Finally, we suggest that plasma proteases may route apoB/E-containing lipoproteins to macrophages for disposal, and this results in foam cell formation.

ABBREVATIONS

HTG-VLDL, hypertriglyceridemic very low density lipoproteins; $VLDL_1$, S_f 60-100; $VLDL_3$, S_f 20-60; IDL, intermediate density lipoproteins; TI, thrombin inactivated; HMG-CoA, 3-hydroxy-3-methylglutaryl CoA; LDL, low density lipoproteins; apoE, apolipoprotein-E; E-12, Mr 12,000 carboxy terminal fragment of apoE; E-22, Mr 22,000 amino terminal fragment of apoE; EDTA, ethylenediaminetetraacetic acid; SDS, sodium dodecylsulfate.

ACKNOWLEDGMENTS

We are most grateful to Dr. John W. Fenton for his generous gift of purified human α-thrombin and to Dr. Duane L. Peavy for many helpful discussions.

This work was supported in part by a Specialized Center of Research (SCOR) in Arteriosclerosis Grant No. HL-27341 and a grant from the American Heart Association (80-875).

REFERENCES

1. J. L. Goldstein and M. S. Brown, Ann. Rev. Biochem. 46:897-930 (1977).
2. M. S. Brown and J. L. Goldstein, Ann. Rev. Biochem. 52:223-61 (1983).
3. R. W. Mahley and T. L. Innerarity, Biochim. Biophy. Acta 737: 197-222 (1983).
4. S. H. Gianturco, A. M. Gotto, Jr., R. L. Jackson, J. R. Patsch, H. D. Sybers, O. D. Taunton, D. L. Yeshurun, and L. C. Smith, J. Clin. Invest. 61:320-328 (1978).
5. A. Poyser and P. J. Nestel, Artery 6:122-143 (1979).
6. S. H. Gianturco, C. J. Packard, J. Shepherd, L. C. Smith, A. L. Catapano, H. D. Sybers, and A. M. Gotto, Jr., Lipids 15:456-463 (1980).
7. S. H. Gianturco, F. B. Brown, A. M. Gotto, Jr., and W. A. Bradley, J. Lipid Research 23:984-993 (1982).
8. S. H. Gianturco, W. A. Bradley, A. M. Gotto, Jr., J. D. Morrisett, and D. L. Peavy, J. Clin. Invest. 70:168-178 (1982).
9. S. H. Gianturco, S. G. Eskin, L. T. Navarro, C. J. Lahart, L. C. Smith, and A. M. Gotto, Jr., Biochim. Biophys. Acta 618:143-152 (1980).
10. J. F. Reardon, N. H. Fidge, and P. J. Nestel, J. Clin. Invest. 61:850-860 (1978).
11. D. S. Fredrickson, J. L. Goldstein, and M. S. Brown, in: "The Metabolic Basis of Inherited Diseases," J. G. Stanbury, M. F. Wyngaarden, and D. S. Fredrickson, eds., McGraw Hill, New York, 4th edition, pp. 604-655 (1978).
12. C. H. Floren, J. J. Albers, B. J. Kudchodkar, and E. L. Bierman, J. Biol. Chem. 256:425-433 (1981).
13. F. Krempler, G. M. Kostner, A. Roscher, F. Haslauer, K. Bolzano, and F. Sandhofer, J. Clin. Invest. 71:1431-1441 (1983).
14. S. H. Gianturco, A. M. Gotto, Jr., S.-L. C. Hwang, J. B. Karlin, A. H. Y. Lin, S. C. Prasad, and W. A. Bradley, J. Biol. Chem. 258:4526-4533 (1983).
15. W. A. Bradley, E. B. Gilliam, A. M. Gotto, Jr., and S. H. Gianturco, Biochem. Biophys. Res. Comm. 109:1360-1367 (1982).
16. S. C. Rall, Jr., K. H. Weisgraber, and R. W. Mahley, J. Biol. Chem. 257:4171-4178 (1982).
17. C. B. Blum, L. Aron, and R. Sciacca, J. Clin. Invest. 66:1240-1250 (1980).
18. S. H. Gianturco, A. M. Gotto, Jr., J. B. Karlin, S. C. Prasad, and W. A. Bradley, Fed. Proc. 42: Abstract No. 366 (1983).
19. G. Schonfeld, W. Patsch, B. Pfleger, J. L. Witztum, and S. W. Weidman, J. Clin. Invest. 65:1288-1297 (1979).
20. B. J. VanLenten, A. M. Fogelman, M. M. Hokom, L. Benson, M. E. Haberland, and P. A. Edwards, J. Biol. Chem. 258:5151-5157 (1983).

21. P. Lindqvist, A. M. Ostlund-Lindqvist, J. L. Witztum, D. Steinberg, and J. A. Little, J. Biol. Chem. 258:9086-9092 (1983).
22. S. R. Bates, P. L. Murphey, Z. Feng, T. Kanazawa, and G. S. Getz, Arteriosclerosis Vol. 4, In Press (1984).
23. W. A. Bradley, D. L. Peavy, J. D. Morrisett, A. M. Gotto, Jr., and S. H. Gianturco, Fed. Proc. 42: Abstract No. 367 (1983).
24. F. Parker, J. D. Bagdade, G. F. Odland, and E. L. Bierman, J. Clin. Invest. 49:2172-2187 (1970).
25. K.-S. Hahm, M. J. Tikkanen, R. Darger, T. G. Cole, J. M. Davie, and G. Schonfeld, J. Lipid Res. 24:877-885 (1983).
26. J. P. Kane, D. A. Hardman, and H. E. Paulus, Proc. Natl. Acad. Sci., U.S.A., 77:2465-2469 (1980).
27. W. A. Bradley, A. M. Gotto, Jr., D. L. Peavy, and S. H. Gianturco, Circulation 68:III-216 (1983).

HYPERTRIGLYCERIDEMIA AND ATHEROSCLEROSIS
ANALYSIS OF AN ABNORMAL LIPOPROTEIN SYSTEM AND POTENTIAL BENEFICIAL EFFECTS OF TRIGLYCERIDE LOWERING THERAPY

Shlomo Eisenberg

Lipid Research Laboratory, Department of Medicine B
Hadassah University Hospital
Jerusalem, Israel

INTRODUCTION

Hypertriglyceridemia is the most common form of lipid transport disorders. In spite of insufficient markers for accurate diagnosis, hypertriglyceridemic states can be divided by several criteria. For example, high plasma triglyceride levels are often found in humans with a variety of diseases, and in such subjects the hypertriglyceridemic state reflects the status of the underlying disease. Diabetes mellitus, nephrotic syndrome, various forms of renal diseases (including hemodialysis and renal transplantation), and hypothyroidism are a few examples. Primary hypertriglyceridemic state consists of several forms of familial diseases. The commonest types are familial hypertriglyceridemia (FHTG) and familial combined hyperlipoproteinemia (FCHL).[1-3] Rarer forms of hypertriglyceridemia are lipoprotein lipase (or apo C-II deficiency) syndromes[4,5] and familial dysbetalipoproteinemia ("type III hyperlipoproteinemia"), a distinct disease entity that reflects combination of genetic absence of apo E-3 and E-4[6-8] together with a second metabolic disease.[9] Sporadic, polygenic and ill-defined syndromes also contribute a large number of subjects to total hypertriglyceridemic population.

In spite of the marked heterogeneity of the hypertriglyceridemia syndrome several features seem to prevail in many instances. Association of accelerated atherosclerosis and hypertriglyceridemia is one of the more disputable issues in today's medicine. Yet, several established facts must serve as guidelines in this dispute. In most, if not all retrospective and prospective studies, a definite association exists between plasma triglyceride levels, the prevalence of hypertriglyceridemia and the risk to develop arteriosclerosis, especially of the coronary arteries. Hulley and his associates, for example, cite no less than 28 such studies, reported by 1979.[10] Many more similar reports have been published since that time. In some defined conditions, that association is very strong and suggests a cause-effect relationship. These include both secondary (e.g., renal diseases)[11] and primary forms of hypertriglyceridemia (e.g., FCHL[1-3] and type III disease).[6-9] Thus, although in some other hypertriglyceridemic states no evidence of accelerated coronary disease has been detected (e.g., FHTG), it is necessary to define working hypotheses that will provide the metabolic basis between hypertriglyceridemia and atherosclerosis, if it exists. This is especially important from the therapeutic point of view: both diets and drugs are extremely effective in reducing elevated plasma triglyceride levels.

Previous attempts to relate hypertriglyceridemia and atherosclerosis have been largely unsatisfactory. It is almost certain that the triglyceride molecule by itself is non-atherogenic, and if it enters cells, it is rapidly degraded to glycerol and free fatty acids. Hulley and associates have carried out a multivariance analysis of their own data.[10] The analysis showed that the power of plasma triglyceride levels to predict the development of IHD (significant in univariant analysis) decreases considerably when corrected for plasma cholesterol levels, and disappears when the low levels of HDL cholesterol associated with high plasma triglyceride levels[13,14] are taken into consideration. Yet, this analysis may be partially invalid, as in hypertriglyceridemia increasing proportions of plasma cholesterol are present in the triglyceride-rich lipoproteins (predominately VLDL), and as the low plasma HDL cholesterol are probably a direct consequence of the higher triglyceride levels.

In the present text, we wish to present a hypothesis that may provide a metabolic basis for the presence of accelerated atherosclerosis on hypertriglyceridemic states, and thereby provide a rationale for triglyceride lowering therapy. The hypothesis is based on our own observations on the nature of the plasma lipoprotein system in a group of hypertriglyceridemic patients before and after institution of triglyceride-lowering therapy (bezafibrate, 600 mg/day), and on known metabolic pathways. The fundamental assumption of the hypothesis is that the mere presence of high plasma triglyceride levels induces alterations of all plasma lipoprotein classes and that such alterations reflect activities of existing metabolic pathways and result in abnormal metabolism of the lipoproteins. These abnormalities, in turn, are potentially atherogenic.

THE LIPOPROTEIN SYSTEM IN HYPERTRIGLYCERIDEMIA

The composition and structure of lipoproteins isolated from the plasma of human subjects with hypertriglyceridemia (HTG) is considerably different from that found in normotriglyceridemic (N) subjects.

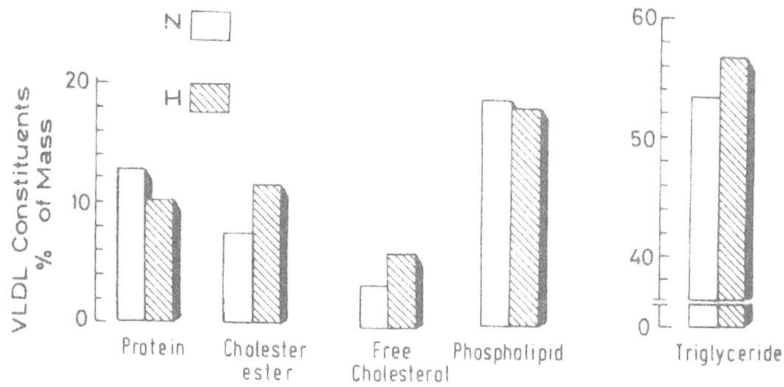

Fig. 1 Chemical composition of VLDL (d < 1.006 g/ml) from human subjects with normotriglyceridemia (N) and hypertriglyceridemia (H).

Very Low Density Lipoproteins

Figure 1 contrasts the composition of HTG-VLDL and N-VLDL. Four abnormalities are apparent: low total protein content, high free cholesterol and cholesteryl ester content, and low triglycerides.[15] Similar observations were recently also reported by other investigators.[16] In our study, all four abnormalities were strongly and significantly related to plasma triglyceride levels, and reversed towards normal when triglyceride lowering therapy was instituted. Could these abnormalities reflect altered VLDL sub-population distribution, such as predominance of large-sized and less dense particle population, or contamination of the VLDL with chylomicrons? We believe not, as with these two instances, it is possible to explain only the low protein content of HTG-VLDL but not the lipid abnormalities. In fact, light VLDL fractions and chylomicrons contain more triglycerides and less cholesterol (free and esterified) than the denser populations.[17] In addition, we were not able to detect large amounts of B-48 (a marker of intestinal lipoproteins) in HTG-VLDL, in agreement with a recently published report.[18] Finally, when N- and HTG-VLDL are fractionated to several density sub-populations, the differences between the two are largely confined to the large-sized and lighter fractions VLDL-I and VLDL-II.[19] Hence, it is the abnormal composition of VLDL-I and VLDL-II, but not their relative contribution to total VLDL that is responsible for the abnormalities of the HTG-VLDL. Because VLDL-I and VLDL-II are preferred acceptors for transferred cholesteryl ester,[20] we suggest that this abnormal composition reflects the prolonged exposure of the VLDL to the core-lipid transfer reaction. This, in turn, reflects the long circulation time of VLDL in hypertriglyceridemia,[21-23] due to absolute, or relative decrease of the lipoprotein lipase activity.[15,24,25]

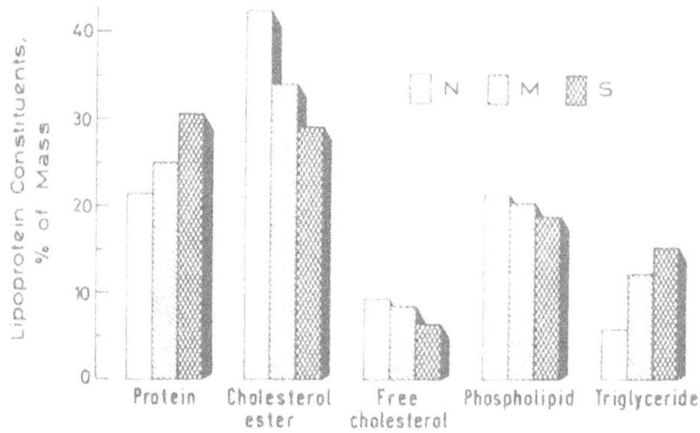

Fig. 2 Chemical composition of LDL (homogeneous zonal fraction) from human subjects with normotriglyceridemia (N), moderate hypertriglyceridemia (M), and severe hypertriglyceridemia (S).

Low Density Lipoproteins

Several abnormalities were found in HTG-LDL (Fig. 2). When separated on a zonal ultracentrifugation system, HTG-LDL (d 1.006-1.063 g/ml) always included an abnormally higher proportion of IDL, and is composed of several LDL fractions.[15] The main LDL fraction, corresponding to N-LDL, was further analyzed. HTG-LDL (main fraction) was denser than N-LDL, relatively enriched with protein and triglycerides and contained significantly less cholesteryl ester and free cholesterol.[15,16,26] As well, HTG-LDL was smaller (by electron microscopy) than N-LDL, and LDL-diameters smaller than 170 A (N = 210-220 A) were observed.[15] Again, all these abnormalities were strongly and significantly related to the degree of triglyceridemia, and tended to revert towards normal when plasma triglycerides were reduced. The change of the LDL core-volume and the cholesteryl ester to protein ratio (based on regression analysis of the data) is shown in inserts to Fig. 3. Comparing LDL at plasma triglyceride levels of 100 mg/dl to 500 mg/dl, both are reduced by about 70%. The observed abnormalities of the composition, structure and size of HTG-LDL are best explained by continued activity of the core-lipid transfer proteins, followed by partial hydrolysis of the transferred triglycerides.[15,26,27] Because we have not found increased activity in hypertriglyceridemic plasma (when using a standardized assay system, unpublished), we suggest that the "overactivity" is due to the presence of a large pool of triglyceride-rich lipoproteins in a system with normal, or even low rates of LDL production.

High Density Lipoproteins

HTG-HDL in many respects is similar to HTG-LDL. HTG-HDL belongs

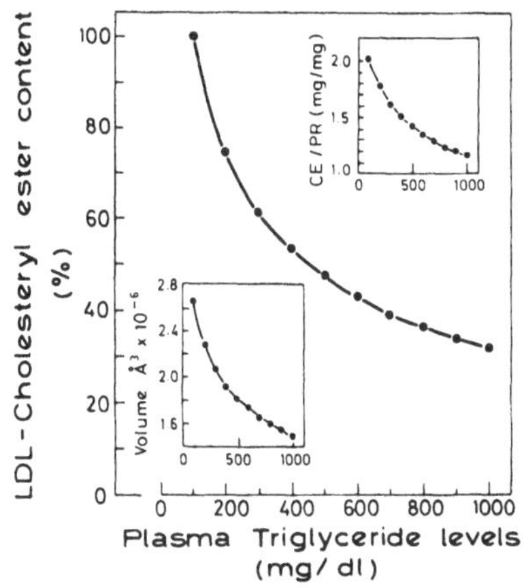

Fig. 3 Relationships between plasma triglyceride levels and LDL cholesteryl ester content. Inserts show the change of LDL core-volume, and cholesteryl ester to protein (CE/PR) ratio with increasing plasma triglyceride levels. Cholesteryl ester content in LDL has been calculated from the volume and composition values. Value of plasma triglyceride level of 100 mg/dl is taken as 100%. The figure and inserts are based on regression equations.

predominantly to the denser HDL_3 sub-population, and the lipoprotein is relatively enriched with proteins and triglycerides, but contains subnormal amounts of cholesteryl esters.[15,26] As for LDL, we found a markedly decreased cholesteryl ester to protein ratio in HTG-LDL, and markedly increased triglyceride to protein ratios. These abnormalties again are compatible with higher than normal core-lipid transfer between HDL and an expanded pool of triglyceride-rich lipoproteins, possibly followed by partial hydrolysis of the transferred triglycerides, and they also tended to revert towards normal with therapy.

CHOLESTERYL ESTER DISTRIBUTIONS IN HYPERTRIGLYCERIDEMIA

Most, if not all, of the compositional abnormalities of HTG-lipoproteins can be attributed to intraplasma metabolic events. Circulating lipoproteins are exposed in the plasma compartment to the activity of several enzymes and lipid transfer proteins. These include extrahepatic lipoprotein lipase (LPL), the heparin-releasable hepatic triglyceride hydrolase (H-TGL), the lecithin:cholesterol acyltransferase (LCAT), and the recently discovered lipid transfer proteins (LTP). The effects of the three enzmes (LPL, H-TGL and LCAT) on the lipoprotein systems were reviewed in detail[28,29] and should not be reiterated. The consequences of the lipid transfer reaction,

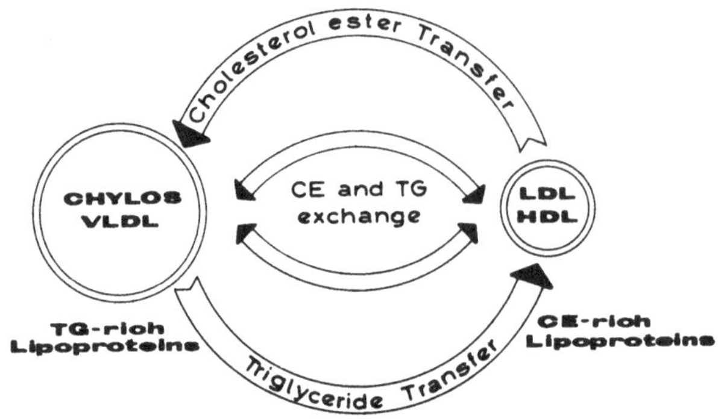

Fig. 4 Schematic representation of the lipid transfer reaction between triglyceride-rich and cholesterol-rich lipoproteins. The figure shows a small component of lipid exchange, and a component of lipid transfer.

however, are not clear. The reaction is catalyzed by a protein that circulates in plasma with a subpopulation of HDL. The protein (M.W. ~61,000 daltons) has been purified by several investigators[30-33] and is distinctly different from any known apolipoprotein. When assayed _in vitro_, the LTP reaction catalyzes exchange and transfer of cholesteryl esters, triglycerides and phospholipids between lipoproteins. After incubation of two lipoproteins with similar core-lipid composition, e.g., LDL and HDL - the main effect of the LTP reaction is exchange. When, however, lipoproteins of _different_ core-lipid composition are incubated, e.g., VLDL and LDL or VLDL and HDL - the LTP reaction causes a very substantial change of the lipid composition of lipoproteins.[27,34] Triglyceride-rich lipoproteins (chylomicrons or VLDL) become enriched with cholesteryl esters and lose triglycerides, while cholesteryl ester molecules in LDL or HDL are replaced by triglycerides. In our experiments, we were able to transfer more than 50% of the cholesteryl ester of LDL or HDL to VLDL.[27,34] When we investigated the capacity of different VLDL populations to serve as acceptors for cholesteryl esters (transferred from HDL), we found (as expected) that the larger particles were preferable to the smaller-sized populations.[20] Thus, more cholesteryl esters were transferred to VLDL-I than to VLDL-II, VLDL-II was superior to VLDL-III, while no transfer to LDL could be detected. This situation is represented graphically in Fig. 4.

"Overactivity" of the LTP reaction is most probably responsible for the abnormal composition of HTG-lipoproteins. In fact, the similarities between _in vivo_ and _in vitro_ observations strongly support the suggestion that the same processes must be involved in the two situations. Thus, we suggest that in hypertriglyceridemia, VLDL clearance is delayed, each particle circulates for a longer period of time, and VLDL (in particular, the large-sized and light particles) become excessively enriched with cholesteryl esters. The high content of apo E in such VLDL particles may reflect abnormal associations of this apoprotein with the cholesteryl ester-enriched VLDL. The source of cholesteryl esters are LDL and HDL. In face of an expanded pool of triglyceride-rich lipoproteins and continuous LTP activity, both LDL and HDL donate cholesteryl ester to VLDL (and chylomicrons) and become enriched with triglycerides. Because transferred triglycerides in LDL and HDL are susceptible to lipase activities,[27,34] both become smaller and denser than the corresponding N-lipoproteins. Hence, increased LTP activity followed by lipase action can adequately explain the abnormalities of HTG-lipoproteins. The observation that all of these abnormalties are reversible with institution of triglyceride lowering therapy (bezafibrate, a drug that increases lipoprotein lipase activity)[15] strongly supports our hypothesis.

METABOLISM OF HYPERTRIGLYCERIDEMIC LIPOPROTEINS

Do the compositional and structural alterations of lipoproteins have metabolic consequences, and if so, are such metabolic consequences likely to play a causal role in atherogenesis? We believe that this is indeed the case.

Metabolism of HTG-VLDL

VLDL-apo B kinetics in humans with hypertriglyceridemia has been reported by several investigators.[21-23] Regardless of the source of patients, experimental procedures and methods of analysis, two abnormalties are consistently observed. The first is slow delipidation rate and the second is decreased fractional conversion of VLDL to LDL. The first abnormality reflects the pathogenesis of hypertriglyceridemic states, absolute, or relative (to increased synthetic rates) decreased rate of VLDL clearance from the plasma.[35,36] We suggest that the second abnormality, i.e., incomplete conversion of VLDL to LDL, is due to the excessive content of cholesteryl esters in HTG-VLDL. To test this hypothesis, we have recently determined the structure and composition of "*in vitro* LDL" produced by nearly complete triglyceride hydrolysis of VLDL subfractions obtained from normo- and hypertriglyceridemic human subjects.[19] Three VLDL preparations were studied: large-sized and light VLDL-I, medium-sized and intermediately dense VLDL-II, and small-sized, dense VLDL-III populations. In VLDL obtained from normotriglyceridemic subjects (plasma triglyceride levels 50-150 mg/dl), LDL-like particles (by density, diameter and lipid and protein composition) were produced from all VLDL populations. In hypertriglyceridemic subjects, in contrast, LDL-like particles were found only after lipolysis of VLDL-III. Neither VLDL-I nor VLDL-II (especially the former) produced LDL-like particles, in spite of almost complete triglyceride hydrolysis (>95%). Post-lipolysis VLDL-I and VLDL-II in such patients were enriched with cho-

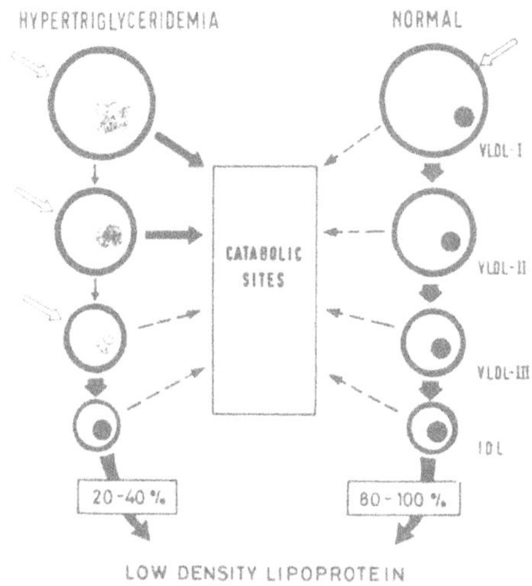

Fig. 5 Schematic representation of VLDL metabolism in normo (NTG) and hyper (HTG)-triglyceridemic humans. In NTG, VLDL enters the plasma compartment mainly with the large-sized, light VLDL-I population. Almost complete (80-100%) conversion of VLDL populations, IDL and LDL is achieved. Only few particles (at the VLDL-III and IDL stage) are cleared from plasma. In HTG, the situation is different. VLDL-I and VLDL-II are cholesteryl ester-rich lipoproteins and cannot complete the conversion pathway. Therefore, "remnants" of these VLDL populations are cleared from plasma and do not form IDL or LDL. That accounts for the low conversion of VLDL to LDL (20-60%). VLDL-III is apparently synthesized independently of VLDL-I or VLDL-II, and is the predominant precursor of IDL and LDL.

lesteryl esters, less dense and much larger than LDL. We suggest that the bulk of hypertriglyceridemic VLDL-I and VLDL-II also behave similarly _in vivo_ and because of the excess cholesteryl ester content cannot form LDL. Such VLDL particles are apparently degraded independently of LDL, as discussed below. Hence, in hypertriglyceridemic humans only VLDL-III is the source of LDL.

This hypothesis, shown schematically in Figure 5 explains not only the reduced VLDL ➡ LDL conversion in hypertriglyceridemia but also the increased LDL levels found when triglyceride levels are reduced by therapy.[15] We suggest that with therapy, VLDL delipidation is accelerated, less cholesteryl ester molecules are transferred to the VLDL (especially VLDL-I and VLDL-II), and more VLDL particles complete the VLDL ➡ LDL conversion pathway.

Metabolism of HTG-LDL and HTG-HDL

The data discussed in the previous section indicates that LDL catabolism must be abnormal in hypertriglyceridemia, and that this abnormality must reflect the loss of cholesteryl esters from the LDL. This is expected even on theoretical grounds alone. It is well established that the regulation of the LDL receptor activity - the major pathway of LDL catabolism - depends on the amount of cholesterol that enters cells with LDL.[37] As HTG-LDL is a cholesterol-poor lipoprotein, the LDL should regulate the receptor activity less effectively than N-LDL and therefore should be degraded from plasma (by the receptor pathway) at an accelerated rate. Recently, we initiated an investigation on the ability of cholesteryl ester-depleted, triglyceride-enriched LDL to down regulate LDL receptor activity and cholesterol synthesis in cultured fibroblasts.[38] For the study, we have used normal LDL modified _in vitro_ by incubation with VLDL and purified core lipid transfer proteins. Moderate depletion of cholesteryl esters was achieved, and the LDL became enriched with triglycerides. Binding internalization and degradation of the modified LDL were similar (though not identical) to those of the control LDL. Yet, the capacity of the modified LDL to down regulate receptor activities and sterol synthesis was substantially less than that found with control LDL. These observations support our hypothesis that LDL catabolism may be accelerated in hypertriglyceridemia in proportion to the depletion of cholesteryl esters from the particle.

Less is known about HDL metabolism in hypertriglyceridemia. This lack of knowledge undoubtedly reflects the uncertainties concerned with regulation of HDL catabolism in general. Although the liver and intestine seem to be the major sites of HDL degradation, it is yet unknown whether these degradative events are determined by specific receptors, and whether such receptors, if they exist, are regulated by the lipid composition of the HDL particle. Yet, similar to LDL, we must assume that the amount of cholesterol cleared from plasma when HDL particles are degraded is substantially less than that cleared with N-HDL.

HYPERTRIGLYCERIDEMIA, CHOLESTERYL ESTER RE-DISTRIBUTIONS AND ATHEROSCLEROSIS

The considerations discussed above all point towards abnormal plasma cholesteryl esters transport in hypertriglyceridemia, due to "overactivity" of the core lipid transfer reaction. Figure 6 illustrates the effects of cholesteryl ester redistribution on plasma cholesterol clearance in normo- and hypertriglyceridemic subjects. Let us begin with LDL and HDL. In normotriglyceridemic subjects, an amount of cholesterol and cholesteryl ester (estimated to be 1.5 to 2.5 g/day) is cleared from the plasma with irreversible degradation of LDL and HDL. In hypertriglyceridemia, however, considerably less

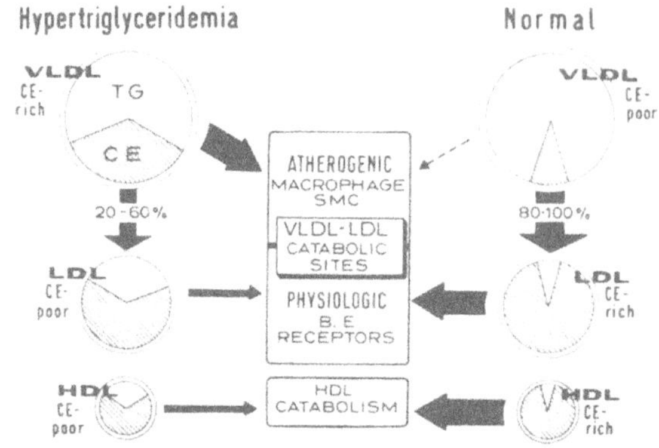

Fig. 6 Effects of cholesterol redistribution on lipoprotein degradation and atherogenesis. The figure compares the lipoprotein system in normotriglyceridemic and hypertriglyceridemic human subjects. In NTG, VLDL to LDL conversion is nearly complete, and cholesterol (free and ester) leaves the plasma predominantly with LDL and HDL catabolism. It is suggested that these routes are non-atherogenic. In HTG in contrast, both LDL and HDL contain subnormal amounts of cholesterol and do not clear from plasma as much cholesterol as NTG lipoproteins. Excess cholesterol (predominantly esterified) is present in VLDL. Such VLDL particles do not complete the VLDL ➡ LDL conversion path and are cleared from plasma by alternate routes (? macrophages; ? smooth muscle cells) that are potentially atherogenic.

cholesterol must be cleared from the plasma with these two lipoproteins. Therefore, in hypertriglyceridemia, an additional pathway for removal of cholesterol from plasma must exist, and the amounts of cholesterol cleared by that pathway must be quite substantial. Our own studies indicate that direct catabolism of cholesterol and cholesteryl ester-rich VLDL or VLDL-remnants, in hypertriglyceridemia provides an "escape" mechanism responsible for the clearance from plasma of cholesterol that normally is catabolized with LDL and HDL. Indeed, both fibroblasts and macrophages were shown to degrade large-sized VLDL particles (VLDL-I and VLDL-II) isolated from hypertriglyceridemic but not normotriglyceridemic humans.[39-41] Degradation of Type III B-VLDL in macrophages[42,43] may represent the extreme situation of inefficient VLDL ➡ LDL conversion, and LDL-independent VLDL catabolism. Figure 3 suggests that the pathway is atherogenic. That suggestion, however, remains to be tested.

ACKNOWLEGMENT

Some of the studies described in the manuscript were supported by a U.S. PHS grant No. HDL 28017.

REFERENCES

1. J. L. Goldstein, H. G. Schrott, W. R. Hazzard, E. L. Bierman, and A. G. Motulsky, J. Clin. Invest. 52:1544-1568 (1973).
2. E. A. Nikkila and A. Aro, Lancet 1:954-958 (1973).
3. J. D. Brunzell, J. J. Albers, A. Chait, S. M. Grundy, E. Groszek, and G. B. McDonald, J. Lipid Res. 24:147-155 (1983).
4. D. S. Fredrickson, R. I. Levy, and F. T. Lindgren, J. Clin. Invest. 47:2446-2457 (1968).
5. W. C. Breckenridge, A. Little, G. Steiner, A. Chow, and M. Poapst, N. Engl. J. Med. 298:1265-1273 (1978).
6. D. S. Fredrickson and R. I. Levy, in: "The Metabolic Basis of Inherited Disease, J. B. Stanbury, J. B. Wyngaarden, and D. S. Fredrickson, eds., pp. 545-614, McGraw-Hill, New York (1972).
7. G. Utermann, K. H. Vogelberg, A. Steinmetz, W. Schoenborn, N. Pruin, M. Jaeschke, M. Hees, and H. Canzler, Clin. Genet. 15:37-62 (1979).
8. H. B. Brewer, Jr., L. A. Zech, R. E. Gregg, D. Schwartz, and E. J. Schaeffer, Ann. Int. Med. 98:623-640 (1983).
9. R. J. Havel, Med. Clin. N. America 66:441-454 (1982).
10. S. B. Hulley, R. H. Rosenman, R. D. Bawol, and R. J. Brand, N. Engl. J. Med. 302:1383-1389 (1980).
11. P. J. Nestel, N. H. Fidge, and M. H. Tan, N. Eng. J. Med. 307: 329-333 (1982).
12. J. D. Brunzell, H. G. Schrott, A. G. Motulsky, and E. L. Bierman, Metabolism 25:313-320 (1976).
13. E. J. Schaeffer, D. W. Anderson, H. B. Brewer, R. I. Levy, R. N. Danner, and W. C. Blackwelder, Lancet ii:391-392 (1978).
14. N. R. Phillips, R. J. Havel, and J. M. Kane, Amer. J. Epidemiol. 116:302-313 (1982).
15. S. Eisenberg, D. Gavish, Y. Oschry, R. Deckelbaum, and T. Olivecrona, Arteriosclerosis 3:500a (1983).
16. N. Vakakis, T. G. Redgrave, D. M. Small, and W. P. Castelli, Biochim. Biophys. Acta 751:280-285 (1983).
17. Z. Kuchinskiene and L. A. Carlson, J. Lipid Res. 23:762-769 (1982).
18. M. S. Meng, R. E. Gregg, E. J. Schaeffer, J. M. Hoeg, and H. B. Brewer, Jr., J. Lipid Res. 24:803-809 (1983).
19. Y. Oschry, S. Eisenberg, R. Deckelbaum, and T. Olivecrona, Arteriosclerosis 2:442a (1982).
20. S. Eisenberg, Biochim. Biophys. Acta, In Press (1984).
21. S. Eisenberg, D. W. Bilheimer, F. T. Lindgren, and R. I. Levy, Biochim. Biophys. Acta 326:361-377 (1973).
22. M. Berman, S. Eisenberg, M. Hall, R. I. Levy, D. W. Belheimer, R. D. Phair, and R. H. Goebel, J. Lipid Res. 19:38-56 (1978).
23. M. F. Reardon, N. H. Fidge, and P. J. Nestel, J. Clin. Invest. 61:850-860 (1978).
24. J. K. Huttunen, C. Ehnholm, M. Kekki, and E. A. Nikkila, Clin. Science & Mol. Med. 50:249-260 (1976).

25. J. Boberg, M. Boberg, R. Gross, J. D. Turner, J. Augustin, and W. V. Brown, Upsala J. Med. Sci. 84:215-227 (1979).
26. R. Deckelbaum, S. Eisenberg, E. Granot, and Y. Oschry, Arteriosclerosis 3:499a (1983).
27. R. Deckelbaum, S. Eisenberg, Y. Oschry, and T. Olivecrona, J. Biol. Chem. 257:6509-6517 (1982).
28. S. Eisenberg and R. I. Levy, Adv. Lipid Res. 13:1-89 (1975).
29. S. Eisenberg, Klin. Wochenschr. 61:119-132 (1983).
30. D. B. Zilversmit, L. B. Hughes, and J. Balmer, Biochim. Biophys. Acta 409:393-398 (1975).
31. J. Ihm, J. A. K. Harmony, J. Ellsworth, and R. L. Jackson, Biochem. Biophys. Res. Commun. 93:1114-1120 (1980).
32. R. E. Morton and D. B. Zilversmit, J. Lipid Res. 23:1058-1067 (1982).
33. J. Ihm, J. L. Ellsworth, B. Chataing, and J. A. K. Harmony, J. Biol. Chem. 257:4818-4827 (1982).
34. R. Deckelbaum, S. Eisenberg, E. Granot, Y. Oschry, and T. Olivecrona, Arteriosclerosis 2:437a (1982).
35. S. M. Grundy, H. Y. I. Mok, L. Zech, D. Steinberg, and M. Berman, J. Clin. Invest. 63:1274-1283 (1979).
36. M. Kekki, Ann. Clin. Res. 12:64-76 (1980).
37. J. L. Goldstein and M. S. Brown, Medical Clinics N. Amer. 66: 335-362 (1982).
38. S. Eisenberg, A. Chait, A. Steinmetz, J. J. Albers, and E. Bierman, Arteriosclerosis 3:490a (1983).
39. S. H. Gianturco, A. M. Gotto, Jr., R. L. Jackson, J. R. Patsch, H. D. Sybers, O. D. Taunton, D. L. Yeshurun, and L. C. Smith, J. Clin. Invest. 61:320-328 (1978).
40. S. H. Gianturco, W. A. Bradley, A. M. Gotto, Jr., J. D. Morrisett, and D. L. Peavy, J. Clin. Invest. 70:168-178 (1982).
41. S. H. Gianturco, A. M. Gotto, Jr., S.-L. C. Hwang, J. B. Karlin, A. H. Y. Lin, S. C. Prasad, and W. A. Bradley, J. Biol. Chem. 258:4526-4533 (1983).
42. M. Fainaru, R. W. Mahley, R. L. Hamilton, and T. L. Innerarity, J. Lipid Res. 23:702-714 (1982).
43. M. S. Brown and J. L. Goldstein, Ann. Rev. Biochem. 52:223-261 (1983).

THE ROLE OF HYDROPHOBICITY IN THE STRUCTURE OF THE HUMAN PLASMA LIPOPROTEINS

Henry J. Pownall and Antonio M. Gotto, Jr.

Baylor College of Medicine, Methodist Hospital
6535 Fannin
Houston, Texas 77030

INTRODUCTION

The plasma lipoproteins can be divided into three major classes based upon their size, structure, density and function. Each of these classes plays an important role in the balance of vascular and intracellular lipid synthesis. In our study of relationship between lipoprotein composition and structure and the dynamics of lipid and protein transport among lipoproteins and cells, we have noted a number of correlations between lipoprotein structure and the transfer of lipoprotein components, within the lipoprotein or to cell membranes. Much of this discussion will focus upon the high-density lipoproteins (HDL), since their structure and properties have been relatively amenable to scientific probes. It is hoped that these studies will be useful in understanding the properties and behavior of the other lipoproteins.

THE THERMODYNAMICS OF LIPOPROTEIN FORMATION

Our understanding of the forces that stabilize the structure of lipoproteins has benefited greatly from studies of reassembled lipoproteins, since these permit systematic identification of the thermodynamic contribution of each apoprotein or lipid to the stability of the macromolecule. The magnitude of the free energy that keeps the apoprotein or lipid bound to the lipoprotein, or that which is required to transfer the molecule from the lipoprotein to the aqueous phase, can be determined by well known equilibrium methods. For some components of HDL, these are readily measured, and for others the values may be calculated. In Table 1 we list some values for the free energy of transfer of some HDL components

TABLE 1

Component	$-\Delta G_a$, kcal/mole	Reference
Apo A-I[a]	9.6	1
Apo A-II[b]	16	2
Apo C-III	10	3
lysopalmitoyl phosphatidylcholine	9.2	4
1,2-dipalmitoyl phosphatidylcholine	15.1	5
cholesterol[c]	13.5	6
cholesteryl oleate.[d]	>24	

[a]Calculated from the solubility of monomeric protein, [P] according to $\Delta G = -RT \ln[P]$

[b]An upper limit calculated by doubling the value of that of reduced and carboxymethylated A-II.

[c]Upper limit; recent evidence suggests that some radioactive impurities might have contributed to this value.

[d] Calculated value that must exceed the sum of the ΔG_a oleic acid and of cholesterol.

from water to a lipid or a lipoprotein environment. Though water soluble, some of some the components self-associate,[7] and it is well known that phospholipids self-assemble into closed structure. Thus, the surface components of HDL might be viewed as being held together by forces similar to those that lead to mixed micelle formation. Less soluble lipophiles, such as cholesteryl esters and triglycerides, associate with lipoproteins as a separate core phase and cannot form HDL-like structures with proteins unless phospholipids are included.

The free energy of association of lipids with micelles or lipoproteins can be estimated on the basis of the thermodynamic model summarized by Tanford.[8] In this model, each part of a molecule contributes to the total free energy of transfer of the molecule from an aqueous to a hydrocarbon phase. For example, each methylene unit contributes roughly -750 cal, whereas the polar moieties contribute a positive free energy increment. The contributions of these may be summed, and a fairly good estimate of the total free energy of association with a lipoprotein can be calculated from

$$\Delta G_a = \Sigma_{i=1}^{N} \delta G_i \qquad (1)$$

where δG_i is the free energy of transfer of the ith functional group from water to hyrodcarbon.

Equation 1 works fairly well for lipids and hydrocarbons, but is unsuitable for apoproteins, due perhaps to the structure of apolipoproteins in water and at the lipoprotein surface. As first hypothesized by Segrest et al.,[9] apolipoproteins form α-helices at the surface of lipoproteins. The helices have polar and nonpolar sides, with the polar face penetrating the lipoprotein and the nonpolar face oriented toward the external aqueous phase. Spectroscopic evidence suggests that the association of an apolipoprotein with a lipoprotein involves the transfer of the hydrophobic residues from the aqueous to a hydrocarbon-like phase. This transfer contributes to the total free energy of association. The transfer of the polar amino acids from the aqueous phase to the lipoprotein surface may also contribute a free energy increment; quantitative measurements of ΔG_a suggest that this contribution is relatively small. The environment of the polar residues does not appear to change with their transfer from water to the lipoprotein; their role may be an expression of their unfavorable free energy of transfer from water to the hydrocarbon phase. This hydrophilicity keeps the polypeptide in contact with water and, in coordination with the hydrophobic residues, orients the apoprotein at the surface.

The transfer of the nonpolar residues to the lipid while simultaneously keeping the polar residues in contact with water forms a helix at the lipoprotein-water interface, making it much easier to rationalize the discrepancy between the measured and calculated ΔG_a (equation 1). If the polar residues keep the apoprotein at the surface, the hydrophobic residues cannot penetrate the most hydrophobic region of the lipid but are retained close to the surface where there is some penetration of water into the lipid. To derive maximal free energy from the hydrophobicity, the nonpolar residues must be transferred to a hydrocarbon phase. Any addition of polar molecules, such as water, to the hydrophobic phase will reduce the ΔG_a. As a consequence, the water-soluble apolipoproteins are loosely bound to the surface of a lipoprotein, as shown in Figure 1 for $HDL_{2,3}$.[10] Their location at the surface is probably important to activation of enzymes and exposure of the determinants for receptor-mediated uptake. Moreover, the low affinity of the apolipoproteins for lipid permits their spontaneous transfer between lipoprotein classes, so that when activation is required for degradation of a newly formed lipoprotein, the longer-lived HDL_3 can serve as an immediate source. This process may facilitate the activation of lecithin:cholesterol acyltransferase (LCAT) by apoA-I or apoC-I and of lipoprotein lipase (LPL) by apoC-II.

A QUANTITIVE MODEL FOR LIPID-APOLIPOPROTEIN ASSOCIATION

Recently, Eisenberg et al.[11] described a vector method, using the helical hydrophobic moment, for classifying proteins on the basis of their primary structure. We modified the method and applied it to the structure of apolipoproteins. Assuming an α-helical conformation, we calculated the mean residue helical amphipathic moment from

$$\langle \mu_A \rangle = \Sigma_{i=1}^{N} \delta G_i / N \tag{2}$$

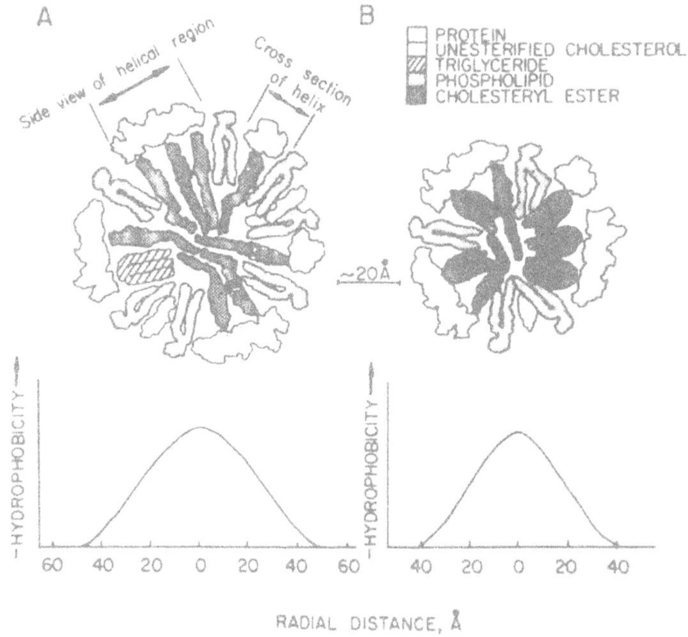

Fig. 1 Schematic representation of the binding of an apolipoprotein to a lipid surface containing a hydrophobic gradient extending from the polar surface to a relatively polar and more hydro-phobic region at the methyl terminus of the phospholipid fatty acyl chain. The α-helical arrangement of the apoprotein as originally proposed by Segrest et al.[9] places the hydrophobic residues, which can penetrate only as far as the first few methylene units of the lipid surface, on one face of the helix.

and the mean residue hydrophobicity from

$$\langle H\rangle = \Sigma_{i=1}^{N} \delta G_i / N \tag{3}$$

where δG_i is the free energy transfer of the ith residue from water to a nonpolar environment and N is the number of amino acid residues. The values for δG_i were selected from Levitt,[12] although other scales give similar results. Our model also permits us to calculate, for all or any amino acid residues, the point along the helical axis at which the $\langle \mu_A \rangle$ is exerted. We obtain the hydrophile-lipophile balance (H/L) from the ratio of the projections of the respective vectors of the polar and nonpolar amino acid residues onto the resultant vector of all residues. One might hypothesize that the perfect surface-associating peptide would be one in which the polar and nonpolar vectors are collinear and located at the midpoint of the helical axis.

From the vector model, we can evaluate the essential features of a lipid- or surface-associating peptide. The alignment of the polar and nonpolar residues can be evaluated by 1) α_d, the angular defect, which is the angle between the polar and nonpolar vectors, 2) Δ[Bond], the number of amide bonds separating the polar and nonpolar vectors, and 3) F, the fractional distance of the helical length at which $\langle\mu_A\rangle$ is exerted. Using these three definitions, the perfect surface-associating peptide is one in which $\alpha_d = 0°$, Δ[Bond] = 0, and F = 0.5. The importance of H/L is difficult to estimate at this time, but we anticipate that this quantity and $\langle\mu_A\rangle$ correlate with the lipophilicity of a peptide. Figure 2 contains an illustration of the model for a lipid-associating region of a native apolipoprotein, apoA-II, 7-31, and for a synthetic lipid-associating peptide designed by Sparrow et al.[13,14]

In Figure 2 the individual vectors, δG_i, are drawn as they would appear if the peptides were in an α-helical conformation. For simplicity the δG_i of the polar residues are drawn as dashed lines in a direction that is 180° out of phase with their actual contribution to $\langle\mu_A\rangle$. The heavy arrow in each panel represents the direction of $\langle\mu_A\rangle$ for all amino acid residues. Hypothetically, when the peptide is bound to a lipoprotein, this vector should be orthogonal to the lipoprotein-water interface. In the native apoprotein, the polar residues on one side of the helical axis reinforce the nonpolar residues that are on the opposite face of the helix, since they have δG_i of the opposite sign. Two places where polar and nonpolar vectors appear to oppose each other in apoA-II (7-31) are at the pairs Leu-10/Lys-28 and Glu-8/ Met-26. However, as this model indicates, these pairs appear at the edges that separate polar and nonpolar sides of the α-helix. Therefore, the side chains of these residues can probably undergo some conformational changes so that they orient toward the side of the lipid-water interface that minimizes their free energy.

In addition to the two-dimensional representations of helical structures proposed by Eisenberg et al.,[11] we have determined the direction and magnitude of the vectors along the axis of the helix and applied this approach to an analysis of the structure of lipid-associating peptides. Figure 3 contains some examples of this part of the model as applied to apoA-II, residues 7-31, and the synthetic lipid-associating peptide,[12] having the sequence

ValSerSerLeuLysGluTyrTrpSerSerLeuLysGluSerPheSer

We can discuss the figure in terms of α_d, Δ[Bond] and F as defined above and given in Table 2. Not unexpectedly, this fragment of apoA-II appears to have good lipid-associating features when evaluated with the helical moment model. For apoA-II, 7-31, the calculated alignment of the polar and nonpolar components is nearly perfect ($\alpha_d = 3°$), such that they reinforce each other very well. The

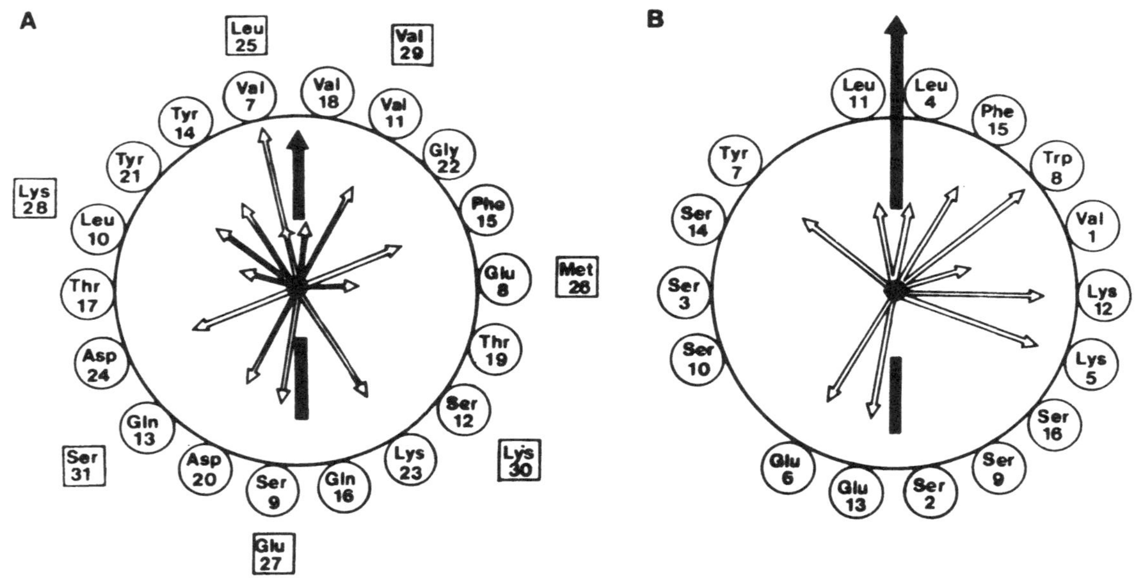

Fig. 2 Two-dimensional representation of the helical amphipathic moment for apoA-II, residues 7-31 (A) and for a synthetic model apolipopeptide (B). The δG_i for the polar residues represented by a dashed arrow are positive; their contribution to $\langle \mu_A \rangle$ reinforces the negative δG_i on the opposite side of the helix. For simplicity, the $\delta G_i \leqslant 0.3$ kcal are not shown but have been included in the calculation of $\langle \mu_A \rangle$.

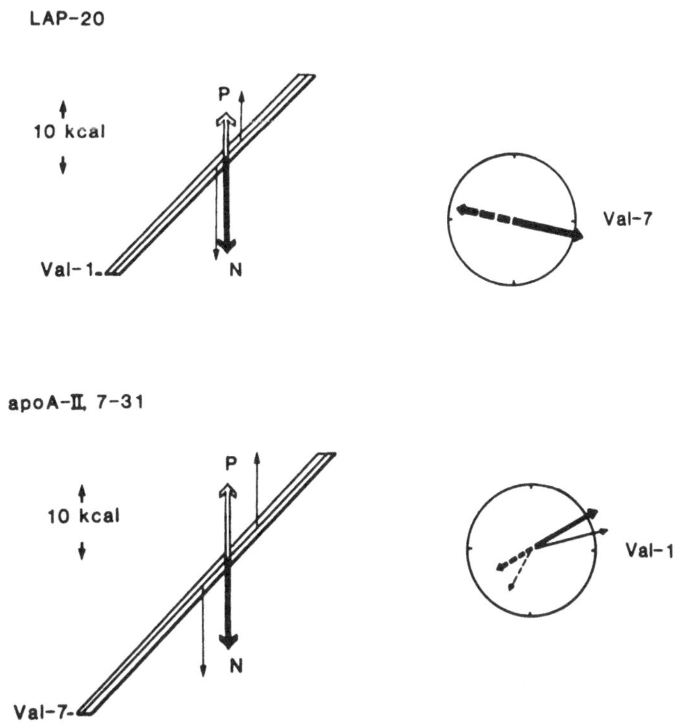

Fig. 3 Schematic representation of the helical amphipathic moment along the axis of the helix. N and P represent the directions of the vectors corresponding to the nonpolar and polar residues, respectively. An end-on view of the helix showing the orientation of $\langle\mu_A\rangle$ is shown at the right. The polar and nonpolar components are represented as fine arrows and $\langle\mu_A\rangle$ is indicated by a bold arrow. The fine arrows are absent for apoA-II, 7-31, since their directions are coincident with that of $\langle\mu_A\rangle$. The left hand panels illustrate the Δ[Bond] and F parameters, whereas the right hand panels show the alignment of the polar and nonpolar components of $\langle\mu_A\rangle$ about the helical axis.

The relative lengths of the dashed and solid portions of the resultant vector shown in bold lines are proportional to their contribution to $\langle\mu_A\rangle$.

distance between the polar and nonpolar components of $\langle\mu_A\rangle$ is Δ[Bond] = 5.4 amide bonds and the location of $\langle\mu_A\rangle$ is near the middle of the helical axis (F = 0.55). The relative lengths of the broken and continuous portions of the bold arrow that represents $\langle\mu_A\rangle$ correspond to the hydrophile-lipophile ratio given by H/L = 0.83. The value of $\langle\mu_A\rangle$ = 0.88 cal/mole is relatively high as pre-

TABLE 2

Peptide	Polar (bond)	Nonpolar (bond)	Resultant (bond)	Angle	Summary
ApoA-II,7-31	10.0 (16.8)		12.1 (11.4)		$<\mu_A>=0.88$ 14H/L=0.83 11Δ[Bond]= 22.1(13.8) 12F=0.55, $\alpha_d=3°$
Sparrow-Gotto LAP-20	7.7(12.5)		13.4(16.2) $\alpha_d=44°$		$<\mu_A>=0.98$ 301H/L =0.43 345Δ[Bond] =2.3 19.6(11.1) 329F=0.58,

dicted by Eisenberg et al.[11] for surface-associating proteins, and the mean residue hydrophobicity, <H> = 0.05 cal/mole, is considerably greater than those of integral membrane proteins of known sequence, for which this parameter is negative. The separation of the polar and nonpolar components is fairly large, although not nearly as great as that of mellitin or other peptides with a polar end that can be exposed to the aqueous phase and a nonpolar end inserted into a membrane with its helical axis perpendicular to the lipid-water interface. A value of F = 0.55 demonstrates that $<\mu_A>$ is close to the middle of the helical axis, suggesting that the amphipathic moment does not favor the preferential association of either end of the helical axis with the lipid surface.

For LAP-20, α_d (=44°) shows misalignment of the polar and nonpolar vectors. However, $<\mu_A>$ is high (0.98 kcal/mole), and <H> corresponds to a peptide that has more hydrophobic than hydrophilic components. The Δ[Bonds] = 2.3 show that alignment along the axis is relatively good and the value of F(=0.58) is fairly close to the middle of the hexical axis. It appears that the synthetic lipid-associating peptide, although originally designed on the basis of a qualitative model, shows some features of native lipid-binding proteins that can be recognized in a more quantitative way by the use of the helical amphipathic moment model. More importantly, the model should be helpful in designing better lipid-associating peptides, which have α_d, F, Δ[Bond], <H>, and $<\mu_A>$ optimized.

LIPID AND APOPROTEIN TRANSFER AMONG PLASMA LIPOPROTEINS AND CELL MEMBRANES

Martin and McDonald[15] provided the first evidence for the spontaneous monomeric transfer of a lipid between the surfaces of an artifical membrane. In this early report they noted that the rate of transfer of dimyristoyl lecithin was faster than that of dipalmitoyl lecithin. Figure 4 contains a schematic representation of the additional multiple equilibria that might be involved in the partitioning of the sparingly soluble components of HDL between water and the lipoprotein surface. These components include cholesterol, fatty acids, mono- and diacyl glyceryl lipids, apolipoproteins (but not the B-protein), triglycerides, and cholesteryl esters, all of which are very insoluble in water.

All of the work to date suggests that the sparingly soluble components of membranes and lipoproteins transfer among cell or lipoprotein surface via the aqueous phase in a process that involves rate-limiting desorption from the surface of the donor into the surrounding aqueous phase. The criteria for this mechanism are that the rate constant is independent of (1) the identity concentration of the acceptor, (2) the donor/acceptor ratio, and (3) the concentration of the transferring species in the donor lipoprotein. Moreover, the rate constants for transfer to water and to acceptor molecules should be indistinguishable.

More recently, some of the structural determinants that regulate the transfer rate have been identified. Pownall et al.[16] compared the transfer behavior of a series of pyrene-labeled lipophiles of different chain lengths. These included fatty acids, their methyl esters, alcohols and alkanes. Within each class, the rate constant

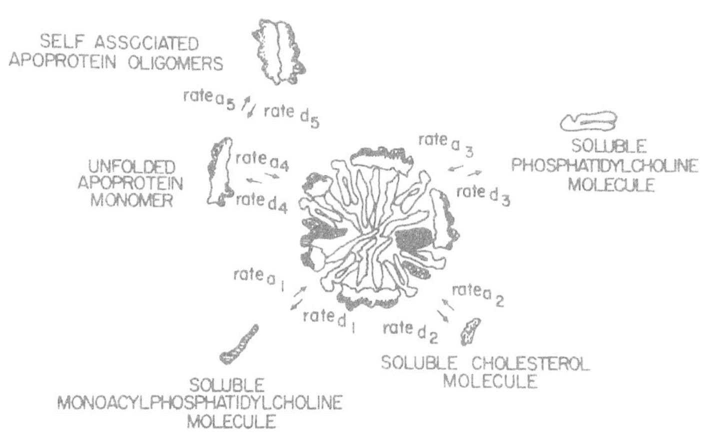

Fig. 4 Schematic representation of the equilibria involved in the distribution of biological lipophiles between a lipid surface and the surrounding aqueous phase. Although represented as a high density lipoprotein in this illustration, the lipid surface might just as easily be a cell membrane or an artificial membrane or lipoprotein.

decreased with increasing chain length. Again, the aforementioned criteria indicated that the mechanism involved monomeric transfer through the aqueous phase. Using absolute rate theory, they determined that each methylene unit contributed 700-800 cal/mole to the free energy of activation for transfer of these lipophiles from one lipid surface to another; a hydrophilic functional group, such as carboxylate, decreased the activation free energy. Thus the rate of desorption of molecules out of a lipoprotein appears to increase with its aqueous solubility. Similarities between kinetic and equilibrium data suggest that the activated state for lipid transfer is similar if not identical to bulk phase water. The rate constants for lipophile transfer out of a number of macromolecular species are given in Table 3.

We can now speculate upon the physiological relevance of these processes to membrane and lipoprotein metabolism. First, transfer rates increase with increasing solubility. The differences in the abundance, solubility and transfer rates of different lipids probably determine whether a specific protein carrier is necessary to maintain lipoprotein and membrane integrity. There is always a high concentration of the fatty acid in serum carried by albumin. The albumin is not required to catalyze fatty acid transfer, since these are transferred on a millisecond time scale (Table 3); in fact, it is probably because of the rapid spontaneous desorption of fatty acids, the products of lipolysis, that a large concentration of a

TABLE 3

Molecule	Transfer Halftime	Solubility[b]	Reference
1-palmitoyl-2-oleoyl phosphatidyl choline	2 da	SS	20
fatty acid/lysopalmitoyl phosphatidyl choline	~40ms	S	21
cholesterol	2.5 hr	SS	20
cholesteryl oleate	>1 year	I	estimated
triglyceride	>1 year	I	estimated
diglyceride		SS	22
Acyl CoA	~500 ms	S	23
Acyl carnitine	~500 ms	S	23

[a]Donors in each case were single bilayer liposomes of 1-palmitoyl-2-oleoyl phosphatidylcholine.

[b]Measured in 100 μM NaCl 10μM Tris pH 7.4.

[c]I, insoluble ($<10^{-12}$M); SS, sparingly soluble ($\sim 10^{-10}$M); S, soluble ($>10^{-6}$M)

fatty acid carrier is needed. The albumin functions largely as a buffer and accepts cytotoxic lipids such as fatty acid and lyso phosphatidylcholine that are released during lipolysis or by the action of lecithin:cholesterol acyltransferase (LCAT). The presence of high concentrations of albumin prevents the aqueous phase solubility of these monoacyl lipids from exceeding their critical micelle concentration, the concentration at which they can disrupt cell membranes. Within the cell, the fatty acid binding protein, which binds to acyl CoA, acyl carnitine and fatty acid, provides the same kind of buffering action[17]. It should be noted though that this buffering capacity is dominant in instances of wide variations in the metabolic state of the system, resulting in rapid increases and decreases in the concentration of these monoacyl lipids.

The very insoluble components such as cholesteryl esters and triglycerides are known to be transported between lipid surfaces *in vivo*, although *in vitro* studies have shown their rates of spontaneous transfer to be immeasurably slow. Since the initial discovery of a cytoplasmic phospholipid transfer factor by Wirtz and Zilversmit,[18,19] numerous other proteins from serum and the cell cytoplasm have been identified. These factors are present *in vivo* in concentrations much lower than those reported for the fatty acid binding protein or albumin. In contrast, their role is not that of a buffer for excess lipids but as a catalyst to either exchange or transfer the insoluble or sparingly soluble lipids. Net transfer might provide essential exogenous lipids to organelles not having a given lipid synthesizing apparatus.

In the plasma compartment, net transfer by a specific carrier protein may provide a route for the appearance of cholesteryl esters in very low density lipoproteins, even though they are synthesized in HDL by LCAT. Finally, an exchange of lipids would provide cell membranes and lipoproteins with a mechanism by which the "quality" of the lipid-water interface is maintained. Scrambling the fatty acid composition of different lipoprotein surfaces removes one determinant that might lead to the preferential association of an enzyme with surfaces having different compositions, and therefore different structures.

Finally, it is probable that spontaneous transfer is important to the transport of some lipid-soluble drugs, vitamins, anesthetics, pesticides and carcinogens. The plasma lipoproteins are not active carriers but rather are some of the many lipid surfaces with which these agents can associate. In contrast, these agents may be cholesteryl esters or an insoluble xenobiotic; neither of which spontaneously transfers. In this case, they can concentrate at some locus within the cell in a process that may have begun with alimentation and ended as an initiating factor in atherogenesis or carcinogensis, respectively. Additional studies of various transfer mechanisms will be needed to validate these hypotheses. It is anticipated that the development of better models for molecular transport will contribute to a better understanding of this process in lipid metabolism.

REFERENCES

1. H. J. Pownall, Q. Pao, M. Rohde, and A. M. Gotto, Jr., Biochem. Biophys. Res. Comm. 85:408-414 (1978).
2. H. J. Pownall, D. L. Hickson, and A. M. Gotto, Jr., J. Biol. Chem. 256:9849-9854 (1981).
3. H. J. Pownall, Q. Pao, D. L. Hickson, J. T. Sparrow, and A. M. Gotto, Jr., Biophys. J. 37:175-176 (1982).
4. M. E. Haberland and J. A. Reynolds, J. Biol. Chem. 250:6636-6639 (1975).
5. R. Smith and C. Tanford, J. Mol. Biol. 67-75 (1972).
6. M. E. Haberland and J. A. Reynolds, Fed. Proc. 32:639 (abs.) (1973).
7. J. C. Osborne and H. B. Brewer, Adv. Protein Chem. 31:253-231 (1977).
8. C. Tanford, "The Hydrophobic Effect," Second Edition, Wiley Interscience, New York (1980).
9. J. P. Segrest, R. L. Jackson, J. P. Morrisett, and A. M. Gotto, Jr., FEBS Lett. 38:247-258 (1974).
10. H. J. Pownall, D. L. Hickson, and A. M. Gotto, Jr., J. Biol. Chem. 256:9849-9854 (1981).
11. D. Eisenberg, R. M. Weiss, and T. C. Terwilliger, Nature 299:371-374 (1982).
12. M. Levitt, J. Mol. Biol. 104:59-107 (1976).
13. J. T. Sparrow and A. M. Gotto, Jr., Ann. N.Y. Acad. Sci. 348:187-208 (1980).
14. J. T. Sparrow, J. D. Morrisett, H. J. Pownall, R. L. Jackson, and A. M. Gotto, Jr., Peptides: Chemistry, Structure and Biology, Proc. 4th Am. Peptide Symp., in: "Ann Arbor Science," R. Walter and J. Meienhofer, eds., pp. 597-602, Ann Arbor, Michigan (1975).
15. F. J. Martin and R. C. McDonald, Biochemistry 15:321-327 (1976).
16. H. J. Pownall, D. L. Hickson, and L. C. Smith, J. Amer. Chem. Soc. 105:2440-2445 (1983).
17. S. Mishkin and R. Turcotte, Biochem. Biophys. Res. Comm. 60:376-381 (1974).
18. D. B. Zilversmit, L. B. Hughes, and J. Palmer, J. Biochim. Biophys. Acta 409:393-398 (1978).
19. K. W. A. Wirtz, H. H. Kamp, and L. L. M. Van Deene, Biochim. Biophys. Acta 274:606-617 (1972).
20. L. R. McLean and M. C. Phillips, Biochemistry 20:2893 (1981).
21. M. C. Doody, H. J. Pownall, Y. J. Kao, and L. C. Smith, Biochemistry 19:108-116 (1980).

22. J. B. Massey, A. M. Gotto, Jr., and H. J. Pownall, Biochemistry, 21:3630-3636 (1982).
23. P. Wolkowicz, H. J. Pownall, and J. McMillan-Wood, unpublished.

METABOLISM OF APOLIPOPROTEINS AND THE METABOLIC HETEROGENEITY OF APO B IN THE RAT

Julian B. Marsh

Department of Physiology and Biochemistry
The Medical College of Pennsylvania
Philadelphia, Pennsylvania 19129

The metabolism of the apolipoproteins covers a very broad subject area. I would like to discuss it, in the main, from the somewhat narrower focus of VLDL catabolism in the rat. I would like to point out that it may be rather artificial to consider apolipoprotein metabolism apart from lipoprotein metabolism, but it is becoming increasingly apparent that apolipoproteins may also have a life of their own. In the beginning, of course, there is DNA and messenger RNA which code for the primary sequence of the apolipoproteins and, after signal peptide cleavage, these traverse the cisternae of the endoplasmic reticulum, ending up in the Golgi where much of the final assembly of VLDL takes place, as seen by electron microscopic studies.[1] The liver is the main organ of lipoprotein synthesis, and probably also of catabolism, and it can synthesize all of the known major apolipoproteins: A-I, A-II, A-IV, B, C-I, C-II, C-III, and E. The small intestinal mucosal cells secrete far less apolipoproteins, but the work of Wu and Windmueller[2] has shown that about half of the plasma A-I, and about two-thirds of apo A-IV, are derived from the intestine, which secretes VLDL and HDL as well as chylomicrons.[3] There have been some recent exciting developments bearing on the question of the synthesis of different apolipoprotein isoforms, such as those of apo A-I[4,5] and on the involvement of tissues other than liver and intestine which I will only mention briefly. Blue, Williams and coworkers[6,7] have found that rooster kidney can synthesize apo B and that human kidney and adrenals can make apo E. Schackelford and Lebherz have shown that chick heart muscle can secrete apo A-I[8]; Basu, Brown and Goldstein[9,10] have found that macrophages from cholesterol-fed mice can synthesize apo E. In this study, they were able to dissociate cholesterol secretion from apo E secretion so that the secretion of an apolipoprotein in association with phospholipid occurred. The point is that not all synthesis and secretion of apolipoproteins is tied to the assembly of a complete lipoprotein particle of the kind found in the circulation, as I have pointed out some time ago.[11] Quarfordt et al.[12] and Havel and co-workers[13,14] have found that chylomicrons and VLDL can bind apo C and apo E when incubated in plasma, and it is probable that all apolipoproteins, with the exception of apo B, can move on and off lipoprotein particles in the circulation. The exposure of lipoproteins to endothelial-bound lipases, and to soluble or complexed plasma LCAT (lecithin-cholesterol acyl transferase) and to lipid transfer proteins, makes it difficult to sort out the complex apolipoprotein associations during lipoprotein catabolism.

Apo B metabolism, in particular, has received a great deal of attention, for several reasons, the most important being that it is virtually the only apoprotein of LDL, presumed to be the atherogenic culprit. In 1978, Godfrey Getz and co-workers,[15] briefly reported that the apo B of intestinal chylomicrons had a faster mobility on SDS gels and this was the first clue, in the rat, that there was a difference between apo B secreted by the liver, and that secreted by the intestine. Hepatic VLDL is converted to LDL in the circulation.[16] In rats and mice, the liver secretes both forms of apo B, whereas in all other mammals so far studied, including man, only the higher molecular weight form of apo B is made by the liver.[17] For the sake of simplicity, we shall call this form B_H in contrast to

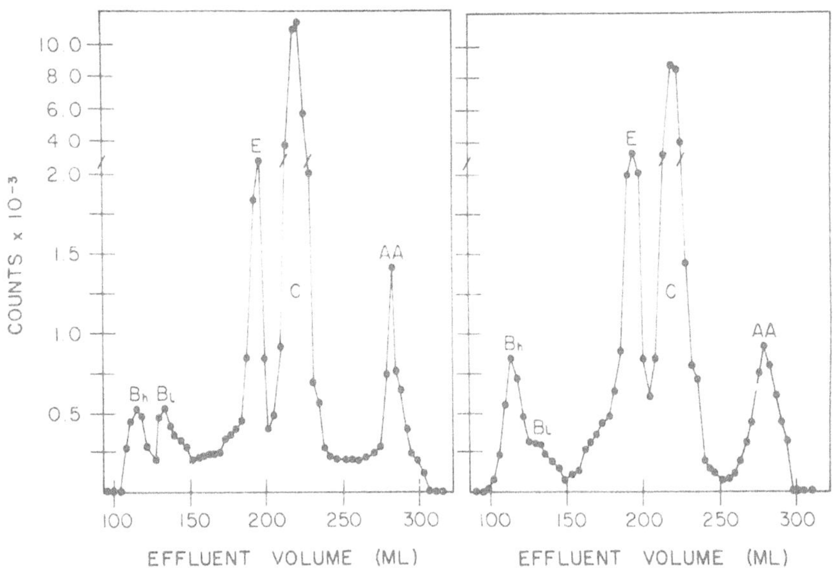

Fig. 1 Representative SDS-column chromatogram of ^{3}H-amino acid labeled VLDL from fasted (left panel) and fed (right panel) liver perfusates.[37]

the intestinal form of lower molecular weight B_L. At present, monoclonal antibodies to B_L, have all been found to react with B_H but not vice-versa[18], so that it is possible that B_L is a cleavage product of B_H. Malloy et al.,[19] have reported one person in which B_L but not B_H was present, raising the possibility of two separate gene products.

As I indicated, in the rat both B_H and B_L are secreted by the liver, as shown by work from this laboratory and by Wu and Windmueller[20] and by Bell-Quint and Forte.[21] They are also both present

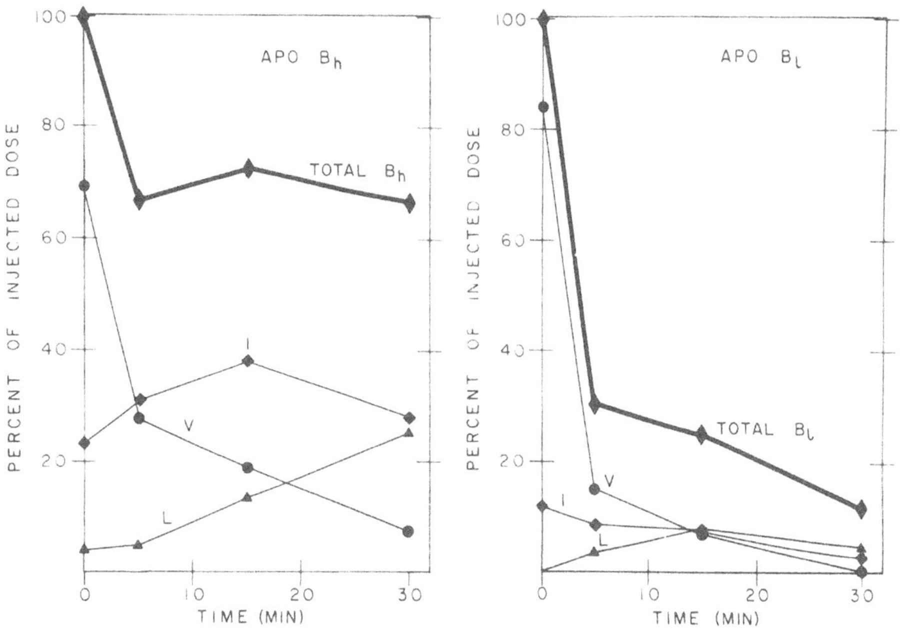

Fig. 2 The percent of injected ^{125}I-apo B_H and ^{125}I-apo B_L radioactivity remaining in plasma (total, -♦-) and remaining in plasma VLDL (V, ●-●-●), IDL (I, ♦-♦-♦) and LDL (L, ▲-▲-▲) 5, 15, and 30 min after injection of hepatic ^{125}I-VLDL. The initial injected dose of ^{125}I-apo B_H and of ^{125}I- apo B_L was determined by SDS-column chromatography of 0-min plasma and radioassay of the appropriate effluent fractions. The concentration of ^{125}I-apo B_H and ^{125}I-apo B_L radioactivity in 1 ml of plasma or of lipoprotein in 1 ml of plasma of timed samples was determined by similar column analyses. The total plasma or lipoprotein radioactivity was calculated by multiplying radioactivity/ml times the plasma volume, assumed to be 4.2% of the body weight. Labeled apo B_H and apo B_L of plasma or lipoprotein divided by the initial injected dose in plasma for each apo B times 100 gave the percent of injected dose remaining.[23]

in the Golgi.[22] The pertinent experiment from our laboratory is shown in Fig. 1 which is an SDS-agarose column chromatogram of the ^3H-amino acid-labeled apoproteins isolated from the VLDL fraction after a single-pass perfusion of the liver. We do not know whether both apo B's are present on the same or different particles. We do know that the proportions of B_H to B_L secreted by rat liver are subject to metabolic regulation, since in 24 hr-fasted rats, in which there was a 30% decrease in total apolipoprotein synthesis, all of the density classes secreted were enriched in apo B_H. Further progress in the area of the biosynthesis of apo B appears to await the molecular biologic approach, which may also lead to knowledge of the primary sequence of apo B which has so far resisted direct sequencing.

When we isolated VLDL from perfused rat liver, labeled it with ^{125}I, and injected it into intact rats, we found that the two forms of apo B disappeared from plasma at different rates.[23] Two-thirds of the apo B_H remained in plasma after 5 min, while only 30% of apo B_L remained. Apo B_L continued to decline during the next 25 min, while apo B_H remained constant. When the individual density fractions of plasma were isolated by ultracentrifugation, as shown in the right-hand panel of Fig. 2, it can be seen that apo B_L rapidly disappeared from VLDL, made a brief appearance in IDL and LDL, and continued to

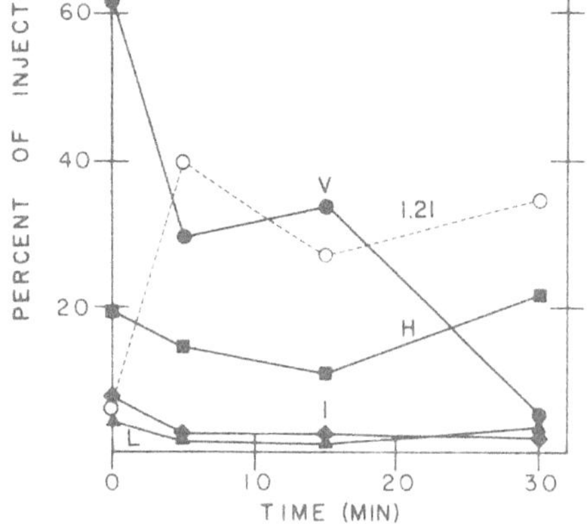

Fig. 3 The percent of injected ^{125}I-apo E remaining in plasma. Conditions are the same as those for Fig. 2.

be lost from all density fractions so that none of it was left in VLDL by 30 min. In contrast, apo B_H, while also rapidly disappearing from VLDL, begins to accumulate in IDL and LDL in 15 min. At 30 min, the amount of labeled B_H in LDL was double that at 15 min. The behavior of the labeled apo E was quite different, as shown in Fig. 3. At 5 min, most of it was lost from the VLDL and appeared in the d > 1.21 fraction and, after 15 min, in the HDL fraction as well. However, most of it remained in plasma at 30 min. To digress for just a moment, I would like to point out the difference in distribution of B_H vs. B_L between VLDL and IDL as shown by the zero time points in Fig. 2. When the original hepatic VLDL was added to carrier plasma and subjected to ultracentrifugation, which was the way the zero time point was obtained, 25% of B_H was in the IDL density range (1.006-1.020), while only 12% of apo B_L was in that fraction. Perhaps there is a slight difference in density between particles containing B_H, and those containing B_L, supporting the view that two types of VLDL particles may be secreted by the liver. To return to the main point, we see then that apo B_H is on its way to LDL, in agreement with the fact that in all mammalian species so far studied, LDL contains almost entirely apo B_H. It should be pointed out that in the rat, most of the VLDL is taken up by the liver and is not converted to LDL,[24] while in humans, most of it does become LDL. This can now be best explained by the fact that approximately two-thirds of the apo B in rat VLDL is apo B_L.[25]

These studies with labeled hepatic VLDL just described were very similar to the results we obtained earlier using plasma VLDL from sucrose-fed rats, as shown in Fig. 4. Again, we see the faster disappearance of apo B_L from plasma. Elovson and co-workers,[22] and Wu and Windmueller[20] using different approaches and techniques, have also concluded that apo B_L has a faster catabolic rate than apo B_H. All three laboratories carried out their experiments at about the same time. Looking again at Fig. 4, it can be seen that the time course of the disappearance of apo E and apo C was quite different from that of apo B_H and apo B_L. By 1 hr, 60% of the injected dose of apo E and 75% of that of apo C remained in the plasma. When we homogenized the liver in SDS and applied samples to our SDS-agarose columns in these experiments, we obtained the results shown in Fig. 5. This shows dramatically the greater hepatic accumulation of apo B_L during the first 15 min, followed by a rapid loss between 15 and 30 min, due to complete catabolism of the bound apo B. Apo E does not behave in this way, indicating that most of it is not internalized and degraded by the liver in the course of VLDL catabolism.

How can we explain the differential catabolism of apo B_L? There is a considerable body of evidence pointing to a critical role of apo E in VLDL and chylomicron catabolism by the liver. Sherrill, Innerarity, and Mahley[26] have shown rapid hepatic clearance of canine lipoproteins containing only apo E. Havel et al.[27] have shown that in Type III dysbetalipoproteinemia, where the E-3 isoform is absent, there is a defective chylomicron remnant clearance, and Cooper

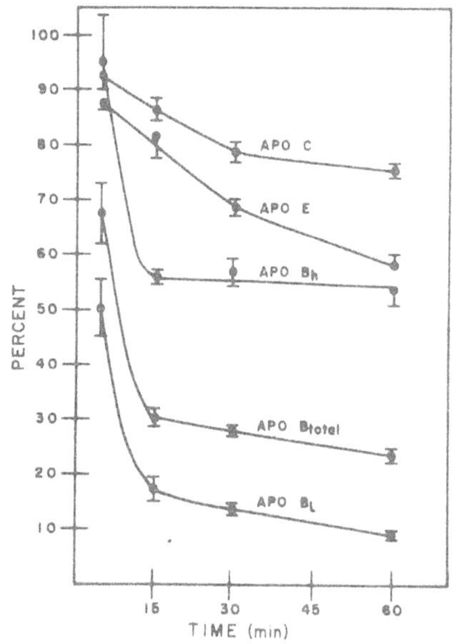

Fig. 4 Time course of the disappearance of individual labeled apoproteins of injected ^{125}I-labeled TRL from rat plasma. Values are expressed as the percent of initial plasma ^{125}I-labeled apoprotein present at the given time point. Each point represents averages of SDS-column analyses of delipidated and non-delipidated plasma of two individual rats amounting to four column analyses per time point. The SE of the four column analyses is indicated by the brackets. Each apoprotein decay curve is designated above the curve as apo C, apo E, apo B_H, apo B_{total}, and apo B_L to identify individual apoproteins disappearance.[38] The values were calculated as described in Table 2.

et al.[28] found that chylomicron remnants bound to liver membranes in relation to their content of apo E. Gianturco et al.[29] found that apo E mediates the uptake of $VLDL_L$ by fibroblasts. The so-called chylomicron remnant receptor, then, may be recognizing an E isoform and may be identical to the E receptor described by Mahley et al.[30] This receptor is not the LDL receptor of Brown and Goldstein since WHHL rabbits, which lack the LDL receptor, have a normal chylomicron clearance rate.[31] We have suggested[23] that there may be an additional B receptor in liver which recognizes B_L after apo E has directed the particle to the liver. A possible alternative explanation which does not invoke a new receptor mechanism is that B_L and B_H-rich particles or remnants bind different amounts of apo E, and therefore different amounts of apo B_H or apo B_L bind to the liver and are subsequently

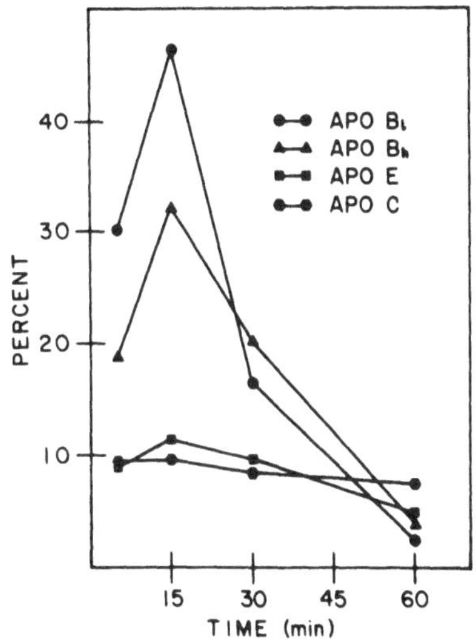

Fig. 5 Time course of the appearance of individual labeled apoproteins of injected ^{125}I-labeled TRL in the liver. Values are calculated as the percent of initial injected plasma ^{125}I-labeled apoproteins present in the liver at the given time point as described in Table 2. Each point represents the average value of two individual rat liver analyses. Individual apoprotein hepatic appearance curves are indicated as apo B_L (●——●), apo B_H (▲——▲), apo E (■——■) and apo C (⬢——⬢).[38]

internalized and degraded. In the case of either hypothesis, it seems clear that the bulk of apo E is not internalized and degraded with the rest of the particle.

VLDL catabolism begins with lipolysis by lipoprotein lipase. We carried out an experiment in which native or lipase-treated VLDL was perfused through rat livers. As can be seen from the right-hand panel of Fig. 6, when VLDL and plasma is presented to rat liver in the absence of lipase activity, a differential uptake of apo B_L does not occur for the first half hour, even though there is considerable hepatic binding during this time. In this half hour, there was a 44% increase in labeled iodopeptides, iodotyrosine, and free iodide in the recirculating perfusate. However, during the second half hour, there was an acceleration of apo B_L disappearance, compared to that of apo B_H and apo E and this was accompanied by an 88% increase in the appearance of labeled small molecules. We attribute this to the action of hepatic lipase during the perfusion. When the labeled VLDL was first incubated with plasma from rats injected with heparin, shown in the left-hand panel of Fig. 6, there was an immediate differential uptake of apo B_L, with a 143% increase in labeled small mol-

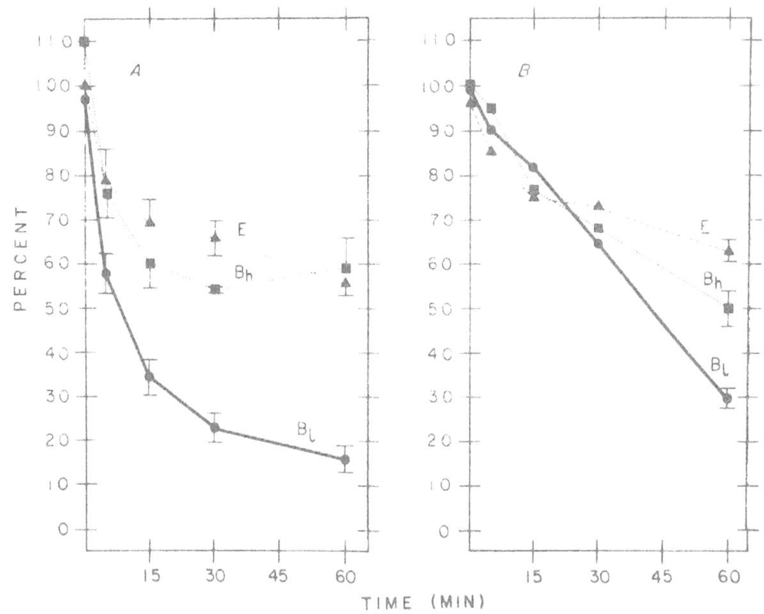

Fig. 6 The removal of labeled apo B_H (——■——), apo B_L (——●——), and apo E (——▲——) in rat liver perfusion of remnant ^{125}I-TRL (A) and control ^{125}I-TRL (B). ^{125}I-TRL was added to postheparin plasma and the mixture was incubated at 37°C for 30 min. The mixture (remnant ^{125}I-TRL) was then quantitatively added to the perfusate to be studied (panel A). Control ^{125}I-TRL experiments (panel B) consisted of identical incubations of ^{125}I-TRL with postheparin plasma except that the postheparin plasma had been heat-inactivated prior to incubation with ^{125}I-TRL as described in Methods. The percent of apoprotein radioactivity concentration remaining in the perfusate after addition of ^{125}I-TRL was calculated as follows: at each time point, 1 ml of perfusate was chromatographed and the radioactivity present in apo B_H, apo B_L, and apo E column regions was calculated. Apoprotein radioactivity/ml perfusate was multiplied by the perfusate volume, giving the total apoprotein radioactivity, and at each time point this value was expressed as percentage of the radioactivity present initially (-10 min). A single error bar indicates one SD. The mean bracketed by double error bars is discrete ($P < 0.05$) from mean values at a given time. Means bracketed by single error bars are not discrete from each other at a given time. The absence of error bars indicates that there were no significant differences in mean values of apo B_H, apo B_L, and apo E at a given time.[38]

ecules in the first half hour and a further increase of 92% in the second half hour. Thus, in an isolated liver perfusion system, we have duplicated our in vivo results and conclude that the first catabolic step must be lipolysis, with both peripheral and hepatic lipases participating, since it has been shown[32] that administration of antihepatic lipase antibodies to rats causes an elevation of plasma VLDL levels in vivo. During lipolysis, apo C leaves VLDL and becomes associated with HDL. Similarly, our experiments show that apo E must do the same. There is much evidence that apo E can readily leave VLDL. Even ultracentrifugal isolation results in loss of apo E, as shown by Mahley and Holcombe.[33] Van't Hooft and Havel found that labeled apo E dissociates from VLDL, when injected into the rat, and its subsequent catabolism parallels that of HDL.[14] It has been shown by Quarfordt et al.[12] and by Havel et al.[13] that hepatic uptake of triglyceride-rich lipoproteins is inhibited by apo C and enhanced by apo E. If apo E is the initial hepatic recognition protein and only the internalization mechanism is specific for apo B_L, direct binding studies with apo B_L may not be revealing. If differential E-binding by B_L and B_H-rich particles occurs, one must first separate such particles in rat VLDL in order to demonstrate this point. There seems little doubt, however, that we are dealing here with the problem of the chylomicron remnant receptor. Our version of VLDL catabolism in the rat is shown in Fig. 7.

It follows from this general scheme that deficiencies of lipoprotein lipase or of hepatic lipase will be associated with elevated VLDL and/or chylomicron levels. Such a situation seems to occur in experimental nephrosis in the rat. Administration of puromycin amino-

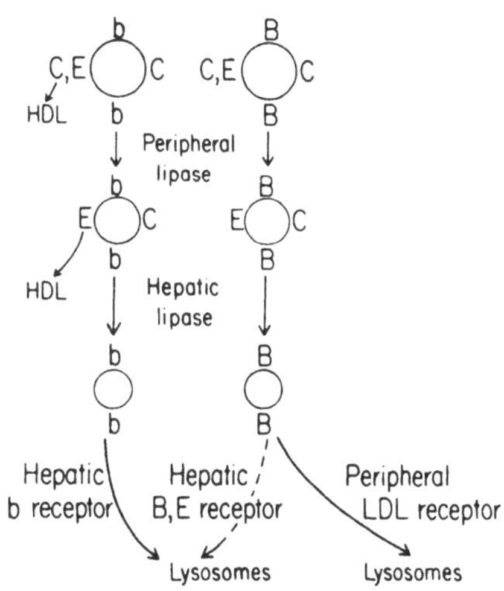

Fig. 7 A scheme of rat VLDL catabolism. The b corresponds to apo B_L (B-48) and the B to apo B_H (B-100). The appearance of two apo B or apo b symbols does not imply the presence of more than one apo B per particle.

TABLE 1

POST-HEPARIN LIPASE ACTIVITY IN PAIR-FED RATS

	Lipoprotein Lipase units/ml	Hepatic Lipase units/ml
Control (4)	80.2 ± 5.15	73.6 ± 0.99
Nephrotic (4)	18.5* ± 2.30	26.8* ± 2.21

*Significantly different from controls (P < .001)

nucleoside to rats produces a severe nephrotic syndrome with an elevation of all classes of plasma lipoproteins. In nephrosis, hepatic overproduction of lipoproteins occurs[40] and this is the primary cause of hyperlipemia. However, we have recently found that nephrosis is accompanied by a deficiency of heparin-releasable peripheral and hepatic lipases, as shown in Table 1. One of the most striking aspects of the hyperlipoproteinemia in nephrosis is the abnormal composition of HDL, which we have found contains almost no apo A-IV or apo E. This can now be clearly related to the decreased lipase activity since we have found that injection of heparin into nephrotic rats stimulates lipolysis and partially restores apo A-IV and apo E to the high density fraction as shown in Table 2. This seems to me to provide a clear-cut _in vivo_ demonstration of the fact that in the rat, apo A-IV and apo E seen in HDL are a consequence of the rapid lipolysis of chylomicrons and VLDL. However, this statement needs amplification because earlier work from this laboratory[34] and by Hamilton et al.[35] indicated that rat liver secretes an HDL which is rich in free cholesterol and in apo E. It is a good substrate for plasma LCAT, and is remodeled as cholesteryl esters are formed. In the past, we assumed that apo E remained with the particle, thus accounting for apo E in HDL but in view of the fact that the nephrotic rat

TABLE 2

EFFECT OF HEPARIN _IN VIVO_ ON APOPROTEIN COMPOSITION OF HDL

	A-IV	E	A-I	C
	Percent of total apolipoprotein			
Normal Rat	16.9	8.1	53.8	11.2
Nephrotic	< 0.3	< 0.3	89.4	9.9
Nephrotic + Heparin	3.8	5.2	82.4	8.6
Nephrotic + Heparin	6.1	4.9	75.6	13.4

also secretes apo E in its nascent HDL, it would appear that the apo E cannot remain associated with HDL but, we suggest, returns to VLDL during remodeling. Therefore, we propose an apo E cycle operating between VLDL and HDL. In LCAT deficiency, large dense molecules containing apo E are found.[36]

I would like to conclude, therefore, that apolipoproteins do have a life of their own, both in synthesis and catabolism, apart from their life in an identifiable lipoprotein particle.

ACKNOWLEDGMENTS

A great deal of the work described in this paper was carried out in collaboration with Dr. Charles E. Sparks. I also wish to acknowledge the participation of Oleh Hnatiuk and Daniel Rader. The more recent studies were carried out by Dr. David W. Garber and Mrs. Betty Gottlieb. I also owe a great deal for helpful advice to Dr. Jane Glick and Dr. A. Catharine Ross, and for enzymes to Dr. Jane Glick. I also wish to thank Drs. George Chacko, Michael Phillips and George Rothblat for helpful discussions. Mrs. Arline Ritz and Mrs. Sarah Massey gave expert technical assistance. Financial support was provided by Program Project Grant HL22633 from the National Institutes of Health.

REFERENCES

1. K. E. Howell and G. E. Palade, Heterogeneity of Lipoprotein Particles in Hepatic Golgi Fractions, J. Cell Biol. 92: 833-845 (1982).
2. A.-L. Wu and H. G. Windmueller, Relative contributions by liver and intestine to individual plasma lipoproteins in the rat, J. Biol. Chem. 254:7316-7322 (1979).
3. G. P. Forester, A. R. Tall, C. L. Bisgaier, and R. M. Glickman, Rat intestine secretes spherical high density lipoproteins, J. Biol. Chem. 258:5938-5943 (1983).
4. G. Ghiselli, H. B. Brewer, Jr., and H. G. Windmueller, Apolipoprotein A-I Isoprotein synthesis by the perfused rat liver, Biochim. Biophys. Res. Commun. 107:144-149 (1982).
5. V. I. Zannis, S. K. Karathanasis, H. T. Kentmann, G. Goldberger, and J. L. Breslow, Intracellular and extracellular processing of human apolipoprotein A-I: Secreted apolipoprotein A-I isoprotein 2 is propeptide, Proc. Natl. Acad. Sci., USA, 80:2574-2578 (1983).
6. M. L. Blue, A. A. Protter, and D. L. Williams, Biosynthesis of apolipoprotein B in rooster kidney, intestine, and liver, J. Biol. Chem. 255:10048-10051 (1980).
7. M. L. Blue, D. L. Williams, S. Zucker, S. A. Khan, and C. B. Blum, Apolipoprotein E synthesis in human kidney, adrenal

gland, and liver, Proc. Natl. Acad. Sci., USA, 80:283-287 (1983).
8. J. E. Shackelford and H. G. Lebherz, Synthesis and secretion of apolipoprotein A-I by chick breast muscle, J. Biol. Chem. 258:7175-7180 (1983).
9. S. K. Basu, J. L. Goldstein, and M. S. Brown, Indepedent pathways for secretion of cholesterol and apolipoprotein E by macrophages, Science 219:871-873 (1983).
10. S. K. Basu, M. S. Brown, Y. K. Ho, R. J. Havel, and J. L. Goldstein, Mouse macrophages synthesize and secrete a protein resembling apolipoprotein E, Proc. Natl. Acad. Sci., USA, 78: 7545-7549 (1981).
11. J. B. Marsh, Biosynthesis of serum lipoproteins, in: "Structural and Functional Aspects of Lipoproteins," A. M. Scanu, ed., Academic Press, New York, pp. 445-462 (1969).
12. F. Shelburne, J. Hanks, W. Meyers, and S. Quarfordt, Effect of apoproteins on hepatic uptake of triglyceride emulsions in the rat, J. Clin. Invest. 65:652-658 (1980).
13. E. Windler, Y. Chao, and R. J. Havel, Determinants of hepatic uptake of triglyceride-rich lipoproteins and their remnants in the rat, J. Biol. Chem. 255:5475-5480 (1980).
14. F. Van't Hooft and R. J. Havel, Metabolism of chromatographically separated rat serum lipoproteins specifically labeled ^{125}I-apolipoprotein E, J. Biol. Chem. 256:3963-3968 (1981).
15. K. V. Krishnaiah, J. Ong, L. F. Walker, J. Borensztajn, and G. S. Getz, Contribution of intestine to plasma apolipoprotein B in the rat, Fed. Proc. 37:257 (Abstract) (1978).
16. D. W. Bilheimer, S. Eisenberg, and R. I. Levy, The metabolism of very low density lipoprotein proteins I. Preliminary in vitro and in vivo observations, Biochim. Biophys. Acta 260: 212-221 (1972).
17. J. P. Kane, Apolipoprotein B: structural and metabolic heterogeneity, Ann. Rev. Physiol. 45:637-650 (1983).
18. Y. L. Marcel, M. Hague, R. Theolis, Jr., and R. W. Milne, Mapping of antigenic determinants of human apolipoprotein B using monoclonal antibodies against low density lipoproteins, J. Biol. Chem. 257:13165-13168 (1982).
19. M. J. Malloy, J. P. Kane, D. A. Hardman, R. L. Hamilton, and K. Dalal, Normotriglyceridemic abetalipoproteinemia. Absence of the B-100 apolipoprotein, J. Clin. Invest. 67:1441-1450 (1981).
20. A.-L. Wu and H. G. Windmueller, Variant forms of plasma apolipoprotein B, J. Biol. Chem. 256:3615-3618 (1981).
21. J. Bell-Quint, T. Forte, and P. Graham, Synthesis of two forms of apolipoprotein B by cultured rat hepatocytes, Biochem. Biophys. Res. Comm. 99:700-706 (1981).
22. J. Elovson, Y. O. Huang, N. Baker, and R. Kannan, Apolipoprotein B is structurally and metabolically heterogeneous in the rat, Proc. Natl. Acad. Sci., USA, 78:157-161 (1981).
23. C. E. Sparks, D. J. Rader, and J. B. Marsh, Metabolism of two

forms of apolipoprotein B of VLDL by rat liver, J. Lipid Res. 24:156-166 (1983).

24. O. Faergeman, T. Sata, J. P. Kane, and R. J. Havel, Metabolism of apolipoprotein B of plasma very low density lipoproteins in the rat, J. Clin. Invest. 56:1396-1403 (1975).
25. C. E. Sparks, O. Hnatiuk, and J. B. Marsh, Hepatic and intestinal contribution of two forms of apolipoprotein B to plasma lipoprotein fractions in the rat, Canad. J. Biochem. 59: 693-699 (1981).
26. B. C. Sherrill, T. L. Innerarity, and R. W. Mahley, Rapid hepatic clearance of the canine lipoproteins containing only the E apoprotein by a high affinity receptor, J. Biol. Chem. 255: 1804-1807 (1980).
27. R. J. Havel, Y.-S. Chao, E. E. Windler, L. Kotite, and L. S. S. Guo, Isoprotein specificity in the hepatic uptake of apolipoprotein E and the pathogenesis of familial dysbetalipoproteinemia, Proc. Natl. Acad. Sci., USA, 77:4349-4353 (1980).
28. A. D. Cooper, S. K. Erickson, R. Nutik, and M. A. Shrewsbury, Characterization of chylomicron remnant binding to rat liver membranes, J. Lipid Res. 13:757-768 (1982).
29. S. H. Gianturco, A. M. Gotto, S.-L. C. Hwang, J. B. Karlin, A. H. Y. Lin, S. C. Prasad, and W. A. Bradley, Apolipoprotein E mediates uptake of S_f 100-400 hypertriglyceridemic very low density lipoproteins by the low density lipoprotein receptor pathway in normal human fibroblasts, J. Biol. Chem. 258: 4526-4533 (1983).
30. D. Y. Hui, T. L. Innerarity, and R. W. Mahley, Lipoprotein binding to canine hepatic membranes:metabolically distinct apo-E and apo-B-E receptors, J. Biol. Chem. 256:5646 (1981).
31. T. Kita, J. L. Goldstein, M. S. Brown, Y. Watanabe, C. A. Hornick, and R. J. Havel, Hepatic uptake of chylomicron remnants in WHHL rabbits: A mechanism genetically distinct from the low density lipoprotein receptor, Proc. Natl. Acad. Sci., USA, 79:3623-3627 (1982).
32. H. Jansen, A. van Tol, and W. C. Hulsmann, On the metabolic function of heparin-releasable liver lipase, Biochem. Biophys. Res. Commun. 92:53-59 (1980).
33. R. W. Mahley and K. S. Holcombe, Alterations of the plasma lipoproteins and apoproteins following cholesterol feeding in the rat, J. Lipid Res. 18:314-324 (1977).
34. J. B. Marsh, Apoproteins of lipoproteins in a nonrecirculating perfusate of rat liver, J. Lipid Res. 17:85-90 (1976).
35. R. L. Hamilton, M. C. Williams, C. J. Fielding, and R. J. Harvel, Discoidal bi-layer structure of nascent high density lipoproteins from perfused rat liver, J. Clin. Invest. 58: 667-680 (1976).
36. G. Utermann, H. J. Menzel, and K. H. Langer, On the polypeptide composition of an abnormal high density lipoprotein (LP-E) occurring in LCAT-deficient plasma, FEBS Letters 45:29-32 (1974).

37. J. B. Marsh and C. E. Sparks, The effect of fasting on the secretion of lipoproteins and two forms of apo B by perfused rat liver, Proc. Soc. Exp. Biol. Med. 170:178-181 (1982).
38. C. E. Sparks and J. B. Marsh, Metabolic heterogeneity of apolipoprotein B in the rat, J. Lipid Res. 22:519-527 (1981).
39. J. B. Marsh and C. E. Sparks, Lipoproteins in experimental nephrosis:plasma levels and composition, Metabolism 28:1040-1045 (1979).
40. J. B. Marsh and C. E. Sparks, Hepatic secretion of lipoproteins in the rat and the effect of experimental nephrosis, J. Clin. Invest. 64:1229-1237 (1979).

PROAPOLIPOPROTEIN A-I METABOLISM IN THE HUMAN AND THE RAT

Giancarlo Ghiselli and Bette C. Sherrill

Baylor College of Medicine
Department of Medicine, M/S A-601
6565 Fannin
Houston, Texas 77030

INTRODUCTION

Apolipoprotein A-I (apoA-I) is the major protein constituent of HDL and is polymorphic in plasma consisting of a series of isoforms denoted apoA-I_1 through apoA-I_5. Human apoA-I is secreted primarily by the liver and the small intestine.[1-5] Initial studies on the *in vitro* biosynthesis of human apoA-I by fetal and adult intestine, fetal liver and a hepatoma cell line indicated that newly secreted apoA-I was a more basic isoprotein than plasma apoA-I.[6-8] Thus it was suggested that the conversion of the newly secreted apoA-I to the circulating mature apoA-I takes place in the plasma; however, the nature of this conversion process, which resulted in a net change of two positive charges, was unknown. Recent advances in our understanding of the biosynthesis of human apoA-I have allowed a more definitive analysis of the processing and metabolism of plasma apoA-I. Initial studies have revealed that apoA-I is biosynthesized as a 267 amino acid precursor protein, preproapoA-I.[9-11] The presegment is 18 amino acids long and cotranslational cleavage of preproapoA-I to proapoA-I occurs intracellularly during vectoral translocation into the lumen of the rough endoplasmic reticulum. Human proapoA-I contains six amino acids, Arg-His-Phe-Trp-Gln-Gln, attached to the amino terminal end of the mature apoA-I. In more recent studies proapoA-I has been isolated from human plasma and lymph and correspond to the apoA-I_1 isoform on isoelectrofocusing.[12] In plasma, proapoA-I accounts for less than 5% of the total mass of circulating apoA-I.[12]

Further studies in a number of other animal species showed that secretion of apoA-I as a proform is a common process in mammals.[13-16] Rat proapoA-I also circulates in plasma.[16,17] The rat proapoA-I pro-

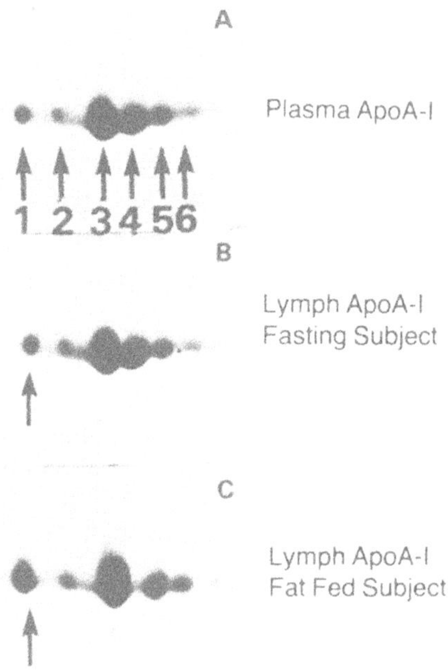

Fig. 1 Two dimensional gel electrophoresis of human apoA-I from d<1.21 g/ml plasma lipoproteins (panel A) and fasted and fat-fed thoracic duct lymph lipoproteins (panels B and C, respectively). Lymph samples were collected for approximately 2 hours before and during 4 hours following the fat meal (100 gr of cream). Only the area of the gel corresponding to apoA-I is presented. The arrow indicates the position of apoA-I_1 (proapoA-I) in panels B and C, and isoforms 3, 4, 5 and 6 are mature apoA-I forms.[12]

segment has been sequenced and, similar to human, contains six amino acids, Ser-Glu-Phe-Trp-Gln-Gln, attached to the amino terminal end of apoA-I.[16] The conversion of proapoA-I to mature apoA-I in human and rat will be reviewed in the discussion to follow.

ProApoA-I CONVERSION IN THE HUMAN

In order to elucidate the kinetics of the proapoA-I to mature apoA-I proteolitic conversion process, proapoA-I was isolated from human thoracic duct lymph chylomicrons collected after rat feeding. This lipoprotein fraction has been found to be particularly enriched with proapoA-I compared to chylomicrons from lymph collected during

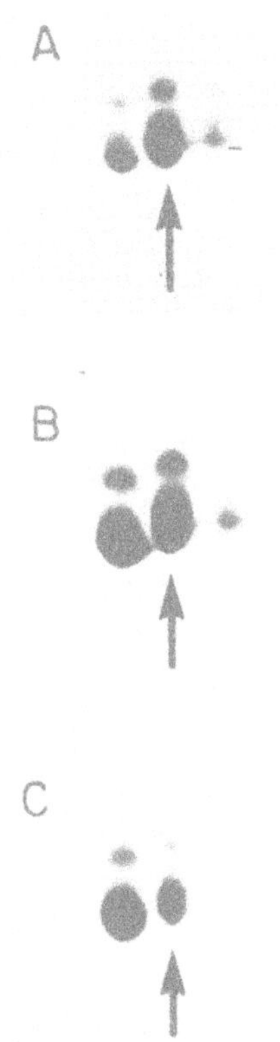

Fig. 2 Two dimensional gel electrophoresis of rat apoA-I from intestinal lymph chylomicrons (S_f>400; panel A), from chylomicron-depleted lymph lipoproteins (d<1.21 g/ml, panel B) and from plasma lipoproteins (d<1.21 g/ml, panel C). The arrow indicates the position of proapoA-I. The more basic apoA-I isoprotein on the right is mature apoA-I.[18]

a fasting period (Fig. 1). ProapoA-I was isolated by a combination of molecular sieve chromatography on a 6% agarose column (BioGel A-1.5m) equilibrated with buffer containing 0.1% sodium dodecylsulfate and of preparative isoelectrofocusing in 7.5% polyacrylamide gels. Mature apoA-I (apoA-I isoforms 3,4 and 5) were isolated by the same procedure.

ProapoA-I and mature apoA-I were radioiodinated, with ^{125}I and ^{131}I, respectively, and the tracers injected into normal volunteers as free proteins. Blood samples were collected sequentially beginning 10 min after the injection for 14 days and the radioactivity quantitated in plasma as well as in the HDL (d=1.063 to 1.210 g/ml) lipoprotein fraction. Analysis of the radioactivity distribution among the different apoA-I isoforms in HDL, including proapoA-I and

	PROSEGMENT	"MATURE" PROTEIN
RAT	H_2N-SER-GLU-PHE-TRP-GLN-GLN-	ASP-GLU-PRO-GLN-
HUMAN	H_2N-ARG-HIS-PHE-TRP-GLN-GLN-	ASP-GLU-PRO-PRO-
	-6 -5 -4 -3 -2 -1	1 2 3 4

Fig. 3 Amino acid sequence of the proapoA-I prosegment in human and in rat. The initial N-terminal segment (four amino acids) of the mature apoA-I are also given. Ser for Arg and Glu for His are substituted at residues -6 and -5 in rat proapoA-I peptide as compared to human. Rat and human peptides also have different net charges (see Figs. 1 and 2 for comparison). The electrophoretic mobility of rat proapoA-I is one charge unit more acidic than rat mature apoA-I and human proapoA-I is two charge units more basic than human major mature apoA-I; consistent with the difference in the hexapeptide sequences of the proproteins. A homology is, however, evident from residues -4 to 3, i.e., Phe-Trp-Gln-Gln-Asp-Gln-Pro in both species. This suggests that the apoA-I propeptidase responsible for cleavage of the propeptides has a high degree of specificity and that the mechanism of proapoA-I cleavage has been maintained during evolution.

the mature isoforms, revealed that proapoA-I was rapidly converted in the circulation into more acidic proteins corresponding to the mature apoA-I isoforms 3, 4 and 5, the process being virtually completed in 24 hours.[18] Analysis of the proapoA-I and mature apoA-I specific activity curves revealed that mature apoA-I was solely derived from proapoA-I in plasma, supporting the conclusion that proapoA-I is the only form of apoA-I secreted *in vivo* as had been previously shown *in vitro* by others.[6-8]

ProApoA-I CONVERSION IN THE RAT

In order to assess the general validity of the proapoA-I to mature apoA-I conversion process and to gain insight into the functional significance of proapoA-I secretion, the rat was utilized as an experimental model. In rat, as in man, apoA-I is polymorphic in plasma and the isoforms have similar molecular weight but different charge, as determined by two dimensional polyacrylamide gel electrophoresis (Fig. 2). Initial evidence that apoA-I secreted by the liver in rat did not correspond to the predominant form found in plasma was obtained by analyzing newly secreted proteins in liver perfusates during *in situ* liver perfusions with ^{3}H-leucine.[17] The data were consistent with the secretion of an apoA-I proform, requiring further processing in plasma to obtain the mature forms as had been suggested from the human studies.

Comparative analysis of the apoA-I isoform pattern of intestinal lymph and of plasma lipoproteins revealed that the newly secreted apoA-I form is particularly abundant in the lymph chylomicron fraction.[16] ProapoA-I and mature apoA-I were isolated by preparative isoelectrofocusing and the determined partial amino acid sequence indicated that the isoform initially secreted by the liver and abundant in the lymph chylomicrons was proapoA-I with an additional six amino acids at the terminal end of the mature form which was predominant in the plasma lipoproteins[16] (Fig. 3). However, in contrast to that observed in man, rat proapoA-I is quantitatively more important in plasma and accounts for approximately 25% of the total circulating apoA-I mass.

In vivo turnover experiments indicate that, in rat, conversion is complete in 6-12 hours depending on the alimentary status of the animal.[19] In man and in rat most of the injected radioiodinated proapoA-I is associated with HDL. In rat proapoA-I conversion was enhanced and occurred more rapidly if the animals were fed, thereby increasing the intestinal contribution of chylomicrons to plasma. These data suggested that although the majority of proapoA-I is associated with HDL, conversion is activated by or occurs on chylomicrons. In all of the experiments, proapoA-I production rate closely matched mature apoA-I production rate and proapoA-I conversion fully accounted for mature apoA-I synthesis. Conceivably, proapoA-I is the major, if not the sole, form of apoA-I secreted *in vivo* also in the rat.

Initial plasma clearance of proapoA-I and mature apoA-I was also investigated. For these experiments, ^{125}I-proapoA-I and ^{131}-mature apoA-I were reassociated with chylomicrons and HDL by incubation and reisolation of the lipoprotein-labeled apolipoprotein complex by ultracentrifugation. The tracers were then injected into fasted rats and blood samples collected every 90 seconds for 15 min. During this time no significant mass of proapoA-I converted to mature apoA-I allowing a careful monitoring of the catabolism of the two apoA-I forms in plasma. The results of these experiments are illustrated in Fig. 4. ProapoA-I and mature apoA-I disappeared from the plasma space virtually at the same rate. However, both proapoA-I and mature apoA-I disappeared faster when associated with chylomicrons relative to the rate when associated with HDL. ProapoA-I and mature apoA-I association to the different lipoprotein fractions isolated by ultracentrifugation was virtually identical. Thus these results support the conclusion that proapoA-I and mature apoA-I behave identically in plasma.

Further *in vivo* experiments suggested that proapoA-I, besides being converted to mature apoA-I, may also be directly catabolized. At 10 min after the injection of radioiodinated proapoA-I and mature apoA-I, associated either to HDL or to chylomicrons, radioactivity was determined in a series of tissues. The radioactivity was found chiefly in the liver and the kidney, possibly as internalized mate-

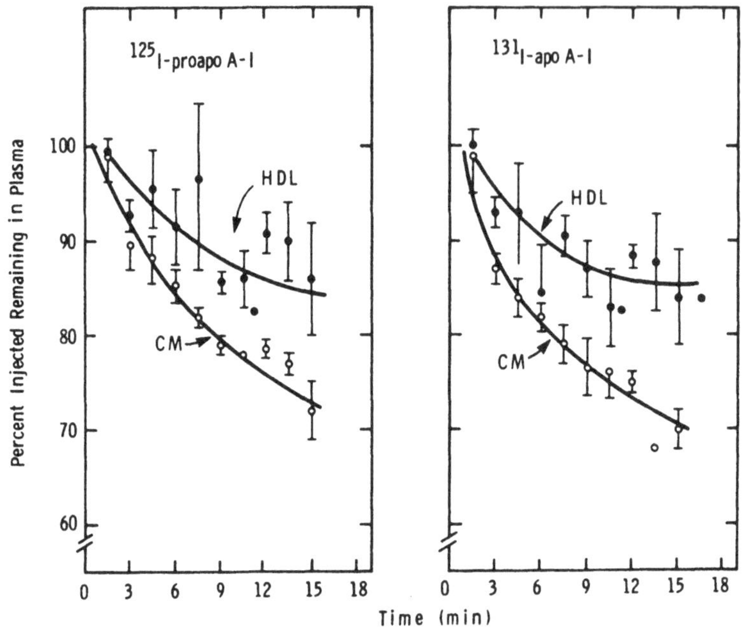

Fig. 4 Plasma disappearance of ^{125}I-proapoA-I and ^{131}I-mature apoA-I associated to HDL or to chylomicrons (CM). Animals were fasted 12 hours prior to the beginning of the experiments. Radioiodinated apolipoprotein-lipoprotein complexes were injected via a femoral vein and sequential 90 sec blood samples (0.05 to 0.1 ml) collected from the opposite femoral vein.

rial. Although this catabolic pathway does not appear to be of major quantitive importance as determined by input-output analysis of the plasma proapoA-I and mature apoA-I specific activity curves, it may become important in the case where proapoA-I conversion is inefficient. Perhaps direct proapoA-I catabolism accomplishes a specific function in lipid transport or there may be target tissues or organs for proapoA-I. This hypothesis remains to be tested, however.

FUNCTIONAL SIGNIFICANCE OF ProApoA-I CONVERSION

Little is known about the site of conversion, i.e., the site of action of the proapoA-I propeptidase. The process may occur while proapoA-I is associated with lipoproteins and the protease is present in plasma.[19,20] However, the conversion seen *in vitro* occurs at a limited rate and is incomplete only reaching 30% at most after 6 hours of incubation.[20] This would be consistent with several possibilities: a) that the protease is labile; b) that the protease-proapoA-I complex is destroyed *in vitro*; or alternatively, c) that the protease is only present in the circulation to a limited extent and is primarily tissue-bound as is lipoprotein lipase. The data obtained in the rat showing an increase in the conversion rate of proapoA-I when chylomicrons are circulating suggest that the chylomicron/proapoA-I complex may be a preferable substrate for proapoA-I propeptidase.[19] Others also have proposed that a proapoA-I protease activity is associated to this lipoprotein function.[20] Chylomicrons are enriched in proapoA-I both in man and in rat in comparison to plasma HDL.[12,16] Possibly the elevated concentration of proapoA-I in lymph chylomicrons just reflects the fact that these are newly secreted lipoproteins. Newly secreted HDL, according to the current conceptualization for apoA-I secretion, would also be enriched or perhaps only contain proapoA-I. Like the lymph chylomicrons, nascent HDL have a short lifetime in plasma. Newly secreted HDL and chylomicrons are rapidly acted upon by enzymes and their lipid and apolipoprotein content change dramatically during their pathway to mature circulating lipoproteins. The ability of these newly secreted particles to undergo such rapid catabolic changes may depend on the presence of the transient proapoA-I which stabilizes their structure at the time of secretion, directs their path of maturation in plasma and ultimately is eliminated through a specific proteolytic process. Perhaps full maturation of these newly secreted lipoproteins follow proapoA-I conversion. This conceptualization leads to the idea that the conversion of proapoA-I initiates and/or terminates specific metabolic function(s) of each of the two apoA-I forms.

A possible defect in proapoA-I processing to mature apoA-I is thought to be the underlying cause of Tangier disease.[10] The proapoA-I to mature apoA-I mass ratio is greatly increased in these subjects as compared to normal[21] and HDL levels are dramatically reduced. Thus defects in proapoA-I metabolism and conversion may profoundly affect HDL levels in plasma. Further research on proapoA-I metabolism will undoubtedly provide new insights into apoA-I and HDL metabolism and may suggest new mechanisms for the modulation of plasma HDL levels and the development of atherosclerosis.

REFERENCES

1. P. H. R. Green and R. M. Glickman, J. Lipid Res. 22:1153-1173 (1981).
2. T. E. Felker, M. Fainaru, R. L. Hamilton, and R. J. Havel, J. Lipid Res. 18:465-473 (1977).
3. R. M. Glickman and P. H. R. Green, Proc. Natl. Acad. Sci., U.S.A., 76:2569-2573 (1977).
4. A. L. Wu and H. G. Windmueller, J. Biol. Chem. 253:857-866 (1978).
5. D. S. W. Anderson, E. J. Schaefer, T. J. Bronzert, T. D. Lingren, T. Forte, T. E. Starzl, G. D. Niblack, L. A. Zech, and H. B. Brewer, Jr., J. Clin. Invest. 67:857-866 (1981).
6. V. I. Zannis, J. L. Breslow, and A. J. Katz, J. Biol. Chem. 255:8612-8617 (1980).

7. V. I. Zannis, J. L. Breslow, T. R. SanGiacomo, D. P. Aden, and B. B. Knowles, Biochemistry 20:7089-7096 (1981).
8. V. I. Zannis, D. M. Kurnit, and J. L. Breslow, Biochemistry, 257:536-544 (1982).
9. S. W. Law, G. Gray, and H. B. Brewer, Jr., Biochem. Biophsy. Res. Comm. 112:257-264 (1983).
10. J. I. Gordon, H. F. Sims, S. R. Lentz, C. Edelstein, A. M. Scanu, and A. W. Strauss, J. Biol. Chem. 258:4037-4044 (1983).
11. W. Stoffel, E. Kruger, and R. Dentmann, Hoppe-Seyler's Z. Physiol. Chem. 364:227-237 (1983).
12. G. Ghiselli, E. J. Schaefer, J. A. Light, and H. B. Brewer, Jr., J. Lipid Res. 24:731-736 (1983).
13. J. C. E. Miller, R. R. Barth, P. H. Shaw, R. W. Elliott, and N. D. Hastie, Proc. Natl. Acad. Sci., U.S.A., 80:1511-1515 (1983).
14. P. Cheun and L. Chan, Nucleic Acid Res. 11:3703-3715 (1983).
15. M. L. Blue, P. Ostapchuk, J. S. Gordon, and D. L. Williams, J. Biol. Chem. 257:1151-1159 (1982).
16. G. Ghiselli, W. A. Bradley, A. M. Gotto, Jr., and B. C. Sherrill, Biochem. Biophys. Res. Comm. 116:704-711 (1983).
17. G. Ghiselli, H. B. Brewer, Jr., and H. G. Windmueller, Biochem. Biosphy. Res. Comm. 107:144-149 (1982).
18. G. Ghiselli, E. J. Schaefer, S. Law, J. A. Light, and H. B. Brewer, Jr., Clin. Res. 31:500a (1982).
19. B. C. Sherrill, W. A. Bradley, A. M. Gotto, Jr., and G. Ghiselli, Arteriosclerosis 3:505a (1983).
20. C. Edelstein, J. J. Gordon, K. Toscas, H. F. Sims, A. W. Strauss, and A. M. Scanu, J. Biol. Chem. 258:11430-11433 (1983).
21. V. I. Zannis, D. M. Kurnit, and J. L. Breslow, J. Biol. Chem. 257:536-544 (1982).

ISOLATION AND CHARACTERIZATION OF THE APOLIPOPROTEIN GENES

Jan L. Breslow

The Rockefeller University
Biochemical Genetics and Metabolism
New York, New York 10021-6399

STRATEGY FOR ISOLATING AND CHARACTERIZING THE APOLIPOPROTEIN GENES

In our laboratory, we have isolated and are in the process of characterizing cDNA and genomic clones for four of the apolipoproteins: apo A-I, apo CII, apo CIII, and apo E. Our strategy has been to identify a region of the apolipoprotein primary amino acid sequence specified by relatively unambiguous codons. We have then synthesized cDNA oligomers corresponding to all possible mRNA's that could code for these amino acids. This mixture of oligomers is radiolabeled and used as a probe to screen a library of cDNA made from adult human liver mRNA and cloned in a plasmid vector. A cDNA clone is then radiolabeled and used as a probe to screen a library of human genomic DNA cloned in bacteriophage lambda. The selected cDNA and genomic clones were characterized by restriction endonuclease mapping, subcloning, and DNA sequencing. Chromosomal localization of the apolipoprotein genes was accomplished through the use of cDNA probes and somatic cell hybrids. In the latter technique, human cells and rodent cells were fused and then propagated in culture. During this process, the hybrids tend to lose human chromosomes. After a period of time, the hybrid cells contain the rodent genome and only a few human chromosomes. At that time, the hybrids are characterized as to which human chromosomes are still remaining, and DNA is prepared and probed for the apoprotein gene of interest. After looking at many hybrids, one observes which human chromosome is present whenever the apoprotein gene is present and which human chromosomes are absent whenever the apoprotein gene is absent. In this way, it is possible to deduce which human chromosome contains a particular apoprotein gene. Through these studies we have been able to determine that the apo A-I and apo CIII genes reside on human chromosome 11.[1] Another group has shown through family studies of the inheritance of protein polymorphisms that the apo A-IV and apo A-I

TABLE 1

APOLIPOPROTEIN GENES

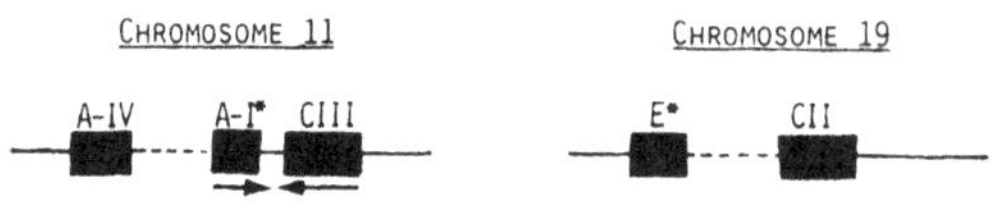

	DISORDER	GENE LESION
1)	APO A-I APO CIII DEFICIENCY	DNA INSERTION IN APO A-I GENE
2)	HYPERTRIGLYCERIDEMIA	ALTERED APO CIII ALLELE
3)	TYPE III HYPERLIPOPROTEINEMIA	APO E STRUCTURAL GENE MUTATIONS

*APO A-I AND APO E GENES STRUCTURALLY SIMILAR (INTRON LOCATION AND INTRAGENIC DUPLICATIONS).

genes are linked. Thus, three of the apolipoprotein genes are on human chromosome 11. In addition, we have also shown that the genes for apo E and apo CII reside on human chromosome 19.[2,3] I will summarize briefly our knowledge of the structure and mutations at each of these apoprotein chromosomal loci (see Table 1).

APO A-I/APO CIII GENE LOCUS

The gene for apo A-I has been characterized.[4] This gene is approximately 2,200 base pairs long and is interrupted by three intervening sequences or introns. In addition, the gene for apo CIII is very close to the gene for apo A-I. Studies indicate that apo A-I and apo CIII are coded for by opposite DNA strands.[5] This is a very unusual configuration and may have some functional significance. In clinical studies, we have examined DNA from individuals reported by Norum and collaborators who have very low plasma HDL levels, absence of apo A-I and apo CIII, as well as very severe premature atherosclerosis. We have shown that these individuals have an alteration in their apo A-I gene. This alteration is due to an insertion of DNA in the region of their apo A-I gene that codes for the apo A-I protein.[6,7] This is the first demonstration of a DNA insertion causing disease in humans and is also the first demonstration at the DNA level of a genetic lesion causing atherosclerosis. In another clinical study, Rees et al. have found that a specific DNA alteration near the apo A-I gene was present in 50% of individuals with elevated plasma triglyceride levels and in only 5% of normal individuals. Our investigations have shown that the DNA alteration associated with the apo A-I gene is actually an alteration in the apo CIII gene.[5] Our findings raise the question as to whether primary abnormalities in the apo CIII gene can cause elevated triglyceride levels in humans and by this mechanism be associated with human atherosclerosis.

APO E GENE LOCUS

We have also performed extensive studies of the apo E gene. Apo E

TABLE 2

APO E POLYMORPHIC SITES*

Position	A.A. (W.T.)	Codon	A.A. (Mutants)	Mutation
112	Cys	TGC	Arg	TGC→CGC
145	Arg	CGT	Cys	CGT→TGT
146	Lys	AAG	Gln	AAG→CAG
158	Arg	CGC	Cys	CGC→TGC

*Amino acid localization of polymorphic sites identified by Rall, Weisgraber and Mahley.

in normolipidemic humans is distributed equally between HDL and VLDL. This apolipoprotein is involved in receptor mediated lipoprotein recognition by cells. In addition, apo E appears to be important in the metabolism of dietary cholesterol, since it has been observed in both animals and humans that the ingestion of dietary cholesterol leads to the appearance of unusual lipoproteins that are rich in apo E. In the past, we have demonstrated that apo E occurs in different individuals in one of six phenotypes. Through family studies we showed that the apo E phenotypes were the result of three alleles at a single genetic locus and proposed that this variation in apo E was due to structural gene mutations.[8] This work has been confirmed and the actual amino acid residues at which genetic variation takes place have been identified. In other studies, we and others have shown that homozygosity for one of the apo E alleles, E2, resulting in the apo E phenotype E2/2, is the underlying biochemical defect in the disorder type III hyperlipoproteinemia.[9] This disorder is characterized by elevated plasma cholesterol and triglyceride levels, xanthomas, and premature coronary and peripheral vascular disease. An analysis of apo E phenotypes in the general population indicates that 1-2% are homozygous and 25% heterozygous for the E2 apo E allele. As a consequence, the apo E genetic locus can be considered a common atherosclerosis gene. Further studies have indicated that the actual expression of hyperlipidemia and atherosclerosis in this condition is dependent upon other environmental, endocrine, or genetic factors. In recent work, we have isolated the gene for apo E. This gene is approximately 4,000 base pairs long and is interrupted by three intervening sequences.[2] Our studies at the DNA level have indicated common features between the structures of the apo E and the apo A-I genes. Both genes have three introns in similar locations and in each case the fourth exon consists largely of tandemly repeated DNA sequences that presumably arose by intragenic duplications. These similarities imply a close phylogenetic relationship between these genes and indicate that they may have arisen from a common evolutionary precursor. In addition, we have identified the particular DNA base alterations responsible for the different apo E structural gene alleles (see Table 2). Through this work it is now possible to construct DNA probes that recognize the normal apo E allele as well as each of the mutant apo E alleles. Therefore, it is now possible to screen for mutant apo E alleles in the population with DNA probes.

SUMMARY

These types of studies lay the foundation for understanding the human apolipoproteins at the genetic level. In addition, through a few specific examples, we have already shown evidence at the DNA level that lesions in apolipoprotein genes can play a role in human atherosclerosis. This work is in its infancy but, in the future, we hope it will have a major impact on our ability to understand genetic susceptibility to atherosclerosis in the general population.

REFERENCES

1. G. A. P. Bruns, S. K. Karathanasis, and J. L. Breslow, The human apolipoprotein AI-CIII gene complex is located on chromosome 11, Arteriosclerosis, In Press (1983).
2. J. McPherson, G. A. P. Bruns, S. K. Karathanasis, and J. L. Breslow, Isolation, characterization and mapping to chromosome 19 of the human apolipoprotein E gene, J. Biol. Chem., submitted (1984).
3. C. Jackson, G. A. P. Bruns, and J. L. Breslow, Human apolipoprotein CII: Isolation and characterization of a cDNA clone and mapping of the gene to chromosome 19, Proc. Natl. Acad. Sci. U.S.A., In Press (1984).
4. S. Karathanasis, V. I. Zannis, and J. L. Breslow, Isolation and characterization of the human apolipoprotein A-I gene. Proc. Natl. Acad. Sci., U.S.A, 80:6147 (1983).
5. S. K. Karathanasis, J. McPherson, V. I. Zannis, and J. L. Breslow, Linkage of human apolipoprotein A-I and C-III genes, Nature 304:371 (1983).
6. S. K. Karathanasis, R. A. Norum, V. I. Zannis, and J. L. Breslow, An inherited polymorphism in the human apolipoprotein A-I gene locus related to the development of atherosclerosis, Nature 301:718 (1983).
7. S. Karathanasis, V. I. Zannis, and J. L. Breslow, A DNA insertion has occurred in the apolipoprotein A-I gene of patients with premature atherosclerosis, Nature 305:823 (1983).
8. V. I. Zannis and J. L. Breslow, Human VLDL apo E isoprotein polymorphism is explained by genetic variation and post translational modification, Biochemistry 20:1033 (1981).
9. J. L. Breslow, V. I. Zannis, T. R. SanGiacomo, J. L. H. C. Third, T. Tracy, and C. J. Glueck, Studies of familial type III hyperlipoproteinemia using as a genetic marker the apo E phenotype E2/2, J. Lipid Res. 23:1224 (1982).

APOPROTEIN MEASUREMENTS

John J. Albers

Northwest Lipid Research Clinic
University of Washington School of Medicine
465 Harborview Hall, Seattle, Washington 98104

INTRODUCTION - IMPACT OF APOPROTEIN MEASUREMENTS

The development and application of methods of measuring apoproteins have significantly increased our knowledge of apoprotein and lipoprotein structure and metabolism, resulting in a dramatic increase in our understanding of the physiology and pathophysiology of lipoproteins. The apoproteins are not only essential structural components of the lipoproteins but also play an important role in the regulation of lipoprotein metabolism through their function as ligands for cellular receptors and cofactors of lipolytic enzymes.

Apoprotein measurements are also useful for the differential diagnosis of the dyslipoproteinemic states. Normal and abnormal lipid transport can be characterized in terms of apoprotein profiles as well as in terms of lipid and lipoprotein profiles. Thus, dysapolipoproteinemic states can be described on the basis of a) the absence or deficiency of one or more apoproteins; b) an increase in the level of one or more apoproteins; c) an altered distribution of apoproteins among the lipoprotein classes or subclasses; d) the presence of altered structural forms or variants of an apoprotein and e) an altered distribution of different forms of a given apoprotein. For example, dysapolipoproteinemia characterized by the absence or near absence of apo A-I, apo B, apo C-II, or apo E, or a combied deficiency of apo A-I and C-III have been described. Two distinct genetic disorders, familial hypercholesterolemia and familial combined hyperlipidemia, are usually characterized by elevations in apo B, and dysbetalipoproteinemia is associated with elevations of apo E.[2] Altered structural forms of apo A-I such as that found in Tangier disease (apo $A\text{-}I_{Tangier}$) and apo $A\text{-}I_{Milano}$ can produce profound effects on the levels and distribution of the lipoproteins and apoproteins.[3,4] Also, altered distribution of the isoforms of apo E or the presence of variant forms of apo E is associated with dysbetalipoproteinemia.[5,6]

Apoprotein measurements are helpful in monitoring the progress of therapeutic interventions. My colleagues and I at the University of Washington have evaluated the effects of a number of drugs on apoproteins. For example, we have studied the effect of anabolic steroid therapy or stanozolol for post-menopausal osteoporosis on lipoprotein lipids and apoproteins.[7] Stanozolol significantly increases LDL cholesterol (30 $\pm$ 28 mg/dl) and decreases HDL cholesterol (33 $\pm$ 12 mg/dl). Within HDL, stanozolol caused a much greater drop in HDL_2 (85%) than HDL_3 (35%). Apoprotein A-I and A-II also dropped significantly (A-I by a mean of 41% and A-II by 24%).

Stanozolol also markedly decreased Lp(a) lipoprotein levels from an average of 5.7 mg/dl to a low of 1.4 mg/dl after only 2 weeks of therapy. In contrast to Lp(a) lipoprotein, apoprotein B increased slightly but nonsignificantly in response to steroid therapy. Similar to apo A-I and A-II, apo D and the enzyme lecithin-cholesterol acyltransferase (LCAT) decreased during stanozolol treatment (23 and 29%, respectively). It is clear that anabolic steroids can have profound effects on lipoprotein and apoprotein levels. The potential consequences of these changes must be taken into consideration when prescribing anabolic steroids.

Apoprotein measurements have also been used to monitor the drug regimens for subjects with familial combined hyperlipidemia and familial hypercholesterolemia.

EPIDEMIOLOGICAL CORRELATION OF APOPROTEINS WITH CARDIOVASCULAR DISEASE

Epidemiologic evidence suggests that measurement of apoproproteins will be used to predict risk of developing coronary heart disease (CHD). Many studies have examined the association between apoprotein levels and coronary heart disease (Table 1). Apoprotein B (Table 1) has consistently been found to be higher and apo A-I (Table 1) and A-II have generally been found to be lower in patients with coronary disease than in control subjects. Examination of seven studies taken from the literature shows that apo B values of control subjects averaged 108 mg/dl and patients with CHD averaged 141 mg/dl. For A-I, in eight studies, control values averaged 130 mg/dl while patients with CHD had lower A-I values, with an overall mean of 113 mg/dl. Limited case-control data are available on the other apoproteins.

Thus, studies in the literature suggest that there is a positive association between apo B and CHD and a negative association between apo A (A-I, A-II) and CHD. Most of these studies have been of the case-control design and few of these studies have reported other de-

TABLE 1

APOPROTEIN B (mg/dl)

Study	Control	CHD
1	104	149
2	83	118
3	125	179
4	113	126
5	119	150
6	113	143
7	102	125
Overall Mean	108	141

APOPROTEIN A-I (mg/dl)

Study	Control	CHD
1	119	107
2	120	112
3	126	109
4	117	100
5	175	156
6	140	105
7	125	111
8	114	106
Overall Mean	130	113

terminants of apoprotein levels such as lifestyle, environmental and and hereditary characteristics, and drugs or diseases which can significantly alter apoprotein levels and potentially account for the association found between apoproteins and CHD. Therefore, prospective studies of apoproteins and CHD employing a follow-up study design which adequately control for other risk factors of CHD are needed.

MOLECULAR CHARACTERISTICS OF APOPROTEINS

The unique molecular properties of apoproteins and their lipid-binding characteristics must be considered in the development and standardization of apoprotein immunoassays. Purified apoproteins undergo self-association to form discrete oligomeric complexes and also undergo mixed association between different apoproteins to form mixed oligomeric species. The amount of association varies with the apoprotein and specific experimental conditions such as temperature, pH, buffer, and protein concentration. Often, purified apoproteins also contain irreversible protein complexes or aggregates. The apoprotein monomers, the various oligomeric species, and the aggregates may differ significantly in immunoreactivity. During storage, purified apoproteins can undergo proteolytic degradation or fragmentation, absorb to glass or plastic, and alter the nature or degree of self-association and form irreversible aggregates. As a result, the immunoreactivity of purified apoproteins can change with time in storage.

In plasma or serum samples the apoproteins are generally associated with several different macromolecular lipoprotein species. The apoprotein conformation or type of association in the lipoprotein complex can vary significantly with the experimental conditions. A change in apoprotein conformation may change its immunoreactivity.

Lipids or other apoproteins can block or mask the antigenic site of a given apoprotein. Apoproteins in standards and test samples should be in the same physical state or conformation in order to ensure accurate and reproducible results. Thus, knowledge of inter- and intramolecular properties of apoproteins must be considered when preparing standards, samples, and reference materials for apoprotein quantitation.

ANTIBODIES: POLYCLONAL AND MONOCLONAL

Thus far, polyclonal antibodies produced by conventional immunization techniques have been used for apoprotein immunoassays. Because apoproteins contain multiple antigenic determinants, antiserum raised against apoproteins by conventional techniques usually react with multiple antigenic determinants. These polyclonal antisera are heterogeneous with respect to affinity and specificity to the various antigenic determinants or epitopes expressed on the apoproteins. Thus, differences in the absolute values of an apoprotein can vary, depending on the antiserum.

Apoprotein antibodies have been used for apoprotein quantitation as well as to probe lipoprotein structure. For example, in 1970, I performed quantitative precipitations of ^{125}I labeled HDL with anti-A-I, anti-A-II and both antisera.[8] Nearly all the lipoprotein associated radioactivity was precipitated with anti-A-I, whereas approximately 90% of the radioactivity was precipitated with anti-A-II. This relatively simple immunochemical experiment was the first evidence that suggested that HDL contains lipoprotein particles with both apo A-I and apo A-II and that some particles contain apo A-I without A-II, but HDL does not appear to contain particles with A-II but no A-I. After a gap of several years, these studies have been extended by Cheung and Albers.[9] After subfractionation of HDL by CsC1 gradient centrifugation we evaluated the content of A-I and A-II in HDL particles with specific anti-A-I or anti-A-II. The A-I/A-II ratio in particles precipitated with anti-A-I varied with hydrated density (Fig. 1), with the lighter density HDL having the highest ratio, and the heavier density HDL having a molar ratio of approximately 2:1. However, particles precipitated with anti-A-II had a nearly constant A-I/A-II molar ratio of approximately 2.0 (range 1.9-2.3) regardless of the density of the subfraction (Fig. 1). Thus, the proportion of HDL particles containing A-I without A-II varied with the hydrated density of the subfraction (Table 2). The lighter density subfraction had a much higher proportion of particles containing A-I without A-II than did the heavier density subfractions.

These studies illustrate the importance of absolute values for the apoproteins. Either lower values for A-I or higher values for A-II, or both, would suggest that the A-I/A-II molar ratio in particles containing both apoproteins is 1:1 rather than 2:1. Valid con-

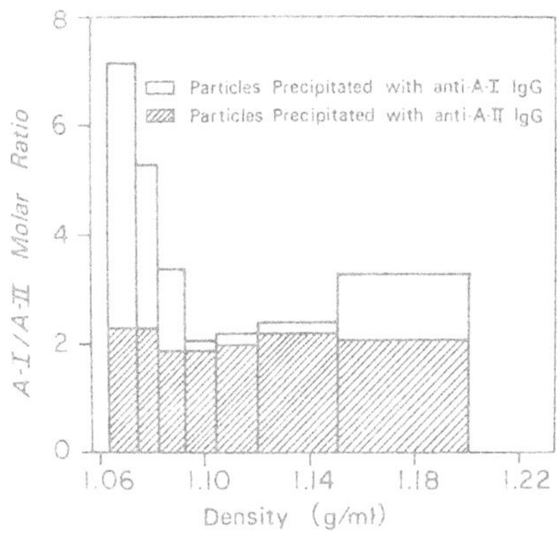

Fig. 1 Density subfractions of HDL after CsCl gradient ultracentrifugation. A-I/A-II molar ratio in HDL particles precipitated with anti-A-I or anti-A-II.

clusions regarding the molecular model of these particles rest on the validity of the absolute apoprotein vaules.

Numerous investigators have succeeded in producing monoclonal antibodies to apoproteins by hybridoma methodology. This technology makes it possible to produce large quantities of exquisitely specific antibody. The super-fine specificity of monoclonal antibodies makes them particularly suited as probes for lipoprotein structure. Schonfeld and colleages,[10] Marcel and coworkers,[11] and Tsao, Curtiss and Edgington,[12] have shown the usefulness of monoclonal antibodies in mapping the antigenic determinants of the B protein in lipoprotein particles. Such site-specific antibodies should permit the spe-

TABLE 2

PERCENTAGE OF A-I NOT PRECIPITATED WITH A-II IN HDL SUBFRACTIONS

Density Subfraction (g/ml)	Percentage of A-I not precipitated with anti-A-II
1.063-1.075	66
1.075-1.083	54
1.083-1.093	41
1.093-1.105	10
1.105-1.120	7
1.120-1.149	9
1.149-1.200	32
1.200-1.250	81

cific identification and quantification of polymorphic forms of the apoproteins. Also, monoclonal antibodies could facilitate the exploitation of the immunometric or antibody immunassays. Furthermore, the uniformity of these antibodies as well as the ability to produce large amounts of these reagents could facilitate immunoassay standardization. However, the superfine specificity of monoclonal antibodies makes them in general less suited for quantitation of total apoprotein mass in plasma lipoproteins. It should be possible, however, to select a monoclonal antibody directed to an epitope common to all the molecules of a given apoprotein and that would remain available to the antibody upon changes in apoprotein conformation. Alternatively, for apoprotein quantification, a mixture of monoclonal antibodies directed against different epitopes of a given apoprotein could be used.

IMMUNOASSAY METHODS

Many types of immunoassays are currently used for measurement of the apoproteins. Each methodological approach has its advantages and disadvantages. Although radial immunodiffusion (RID) and electroimmunoassay (EIA) are both relatively simple to perform and do not require expensive equipment, they both require relatively large amounts of antibody and cannot be automated. Radioimmunoassay (RIA) uses small amounts of antibody and has great sensitivity. Sensitive immunoassay methods are, however, generally not necessary for most apoprotein measurements. Because radiolabeled reagents have limited shelf life and radioisotopes are costly to dispose of and represent a biological hazzard, the nonisotope methods such as enzyme-linked immunoabsorbent assay (ELISA) and the nephelometric or turbidometric methods have gained popularity. Both the ELISA and nephelometric methods can be readily automated. The advantages of ELISA include high sample throughout, minimal maintenance of the system and elimination of radioactive isotopes. In nephelometric and turbidometric techniques the intensity of light depends upon the size and refractive index of the immunocomplex. If the distribution of lipoproteins containing a given apoprotein is not homogeneous in size or if the immunoxomplex is heterogeneous in morphology, errors in the absolute value of the apoprotein can arise.

Normal values for apoproteins vary from laboratory to laboratory, even among laboratories using the same method (Table 3). However, it is clear that some of this variation is method-dependent, e.g., with regard to normal values for apo B, the lowest values are obtained by the radial immunodiffusion method, which tends to underestimate the larger apo B-containing particles in plasma. The highest values are obtained by the nephelometric procedures, which can significantly overestimate apo B because of light scattering of the triglyceride-rich particles. Thus, the absolute values of the apoprotein will vary not only with the particular antibody used and the particular

TABLE 3

NORMAL VALUES FOR APOPROTEIN B

Method	No. of Laboratories	Overall Mean (mg/dl)	Range of Means (mg/dl)
RID	4	87	82- 97
RIA	8	90	83- 99
EIA	8	95	63-132
NIA	4	115	82-159

conditions of treatment of the sample, but they can also vary systematically with the nature of the particular method.

The best estimate of normal values of the apoproteins obtained from the literature and from the structural considerations are shown in Table 4.

STANDARDIZATION

Differences in apoprotein values among laboratories indicate the need for standardization, particularly the need for reliable standards and stable reference and control materials. The standardization of apoprotein immunoassays represent a difficult challenge in view of the multiplicity of methods and reagents and the instability of purified apoproteins. Because of the problems of the preparation and storage of primary standards and reference material, a serum pool is recommended for use as a reference pool and secondary standard. Comparison of antibody reagents among investigators is also encouraged to evaluate the degree to which different antibodies account for the differences in absolute apoprotein values among laboratories.

TABLE 4

NORMAL LEVELS OF APOPROTEINS (mg/dl)

Apoprotein	$\bar{x} \pm$ SD	Apoprotein	$\bar{x} \pm$ SD
A-I	120 ± 20 (male)	C-I	7 ± 2
	135 ± 25 (female)	C-II	4 ± 2
A-II	33 ± 5 (male)	C-III	13 ± 5
	36 ± 6 (female)	D	6 ± 1
B	98 ± 20	E	5 ± 2

CONCLUSIONS

Apoprotein measurements have become increasingly important in the lipoprotein field, not only for research studies of apoprotein structure and function, but also for their clinical application for the characterization of the dyslipoproteinemic states, for monitoring the progress of therapeutic intervention and as risk factors for CHD.

REFERENCES

1. J. D. Brunzell, J. J. Albers, Alan Chait, S. M. Grundy, E. Groszek, and G. B. McDonald, Plasma lipoproteins in familial combined hyperlipidemia and monogenic familial hypertriglyceridemia, J. Lipid Res. 24:147-155 (1983).
2. R. S. Kushwaha, W. R. Hazzard, P. W. Wahl, and J. J. Hover, Type 3 hyperlipoproteinemia - diagnosis on whole plasma by apolipoprotein-E immunoassay, Ann. Int. Med. 87:509-516 (1977).
3. E. J. Schaefer, L. L. Kay, L. A. Zech, and H. B. Brewer, Jr., Tangier Disease. High density lipoprotein deficiency due to defective metabolism of an abnormal apolipoprotein A-I (APOA-$I_{Tangier}$), J. Clin. Invest. 70:934-945 (1982).
4. K. H. Weisgraber, S. C. Rall, Jr., T. P. Bersot, R. W. Mahley, G. Franceschini, and C. R. Sirtori, Apolipoprotein A-I_{Milano}. Detection of normal A-I in affected subjects and evidence for a cysteine for arginine substitution in the variant A-I, J. Biol. Chem. 258:2508-2513 (1983).
5. G. Utermann, M. Jaeschke, and J. Mangel, Familial hyperlipoproteinemia type III: Deficiency of a specific apolipoprotein (apo E-III) in the very-low-density lipoproteins, FEBS Lett. 56:352-355 (1975).
6. K. H. Weisgraber, S. C. Rall, Jr., and R. W. Mahley, Human E apoprotein heterogeneity. Cysteine-arginine interchanges in the amino acid sequence of the amino acid sequence of the apo-E isoforms, J. Biol. Chem. 256:9077-9083 (1981).
7. H. M. Taggard, D. Applebaum-Bowden, S. Haffner, G. R. Warnick, M. C. Cheung, J. J. Albers, C. H. Chestnut, III, and W. R. Hazzard, Reduction in high density lipoproteins by anabolic steroid (Stanozolol) therapy for postmenopausal osteoporosis, Metabolism 31:1147-1152 (1982).
8. J. J. Albers and F. Aladjem, Precipitation of ^{125}I-labeled lipoproteins with specific polypeptide antisera. Evidence for two populations with differing polypeptide compositions in human high density lipoproteins, Biochemistry 10:3436-3442 (1971).
9. M. C. Cheung and J. J. Albers, Distribution of high density lipoprotein particles with different apoprotein composition: Particles with A-I and A-II and particles with A-I but no A-II, J. Lipid Res. 23:747-753 (1982).
10. M. J. Tikkanen, R. Dargar, B. Pfleger, B. Gonen, J. M. Davie, and G. Schonfeld, Antigenic mapping of human low density

lipoprotein with monoclonal antibodies, J. Lip. Res. 23:1032-1038 (1982).

11. Y. L. Marcel, M. Hogue, R. Theolis, Jr., and R. W. Milne, Mapping of antigenic determinants of human apolipoprotein B using monoclonal antibodies against low density lipoproteins, J. Biol. Chem. 257:13165-13168 (1982).
12. B. P. Tsao, L. K. Curtiss, and T. S. Edgington, Immunochemical heterogeneity of human plasma apolipoprotein B: II. Expression of apolipoprotein B epitopes on native lipoproteins, J. Biol. Chem. 257:15222-15228 (1982).

USE OF MONOCLONAL ANTIBODIES IN STUDIES OF LIPOPROTEIN STRUCTURE AND FUNCTION

Gustav Schonfeld, Matti J. Tikkanen*, and Kyung-soo Hahm

Lipid Research Center
Departments of Preventive Medicine and Medicine
Washington University School of Medicine
St. Louis, Missouri 63110

SUMMARY

In order to probe the structure and function of apoB, monoclonal antibodies directed against human LDL were produced. The seven antibodies tested were found to be directed against five individual antigenic determinants of apoB in holo-LDL. One of the antibodies inhibited the binding of ^{125}I-LDL to the apoB, E receptor of cultured human fibroblasts.

Limited proteolysis of LDL results in the production of relatively stable lipoprotein "core" particles that retain many physical, chemical and immunological properties of the native lipoprotein. Perturbations of the structure of apoB by limited proteolysis of LDL had selective effects on the expression of various epitopes in the resulting LDL "cores" - the expression of some was unaffected, others were abolished. In addition, the various epitopes could be localized by immunoblotting to different proteolytic fragments of apoB present in the LDL "cores". Limited proteolysis also provided water soluble cleavage peptides, some of which exhibited immunoreactivity. Digested LDL "core" particles and cleavage peptides both interacted with the LDL receptors of cultured human fibroblasts. These experiments suggest that apoB may consist of repeating subunits of similar structure.

The immunoreactivity of LDL may be determined not only by the structure of the protein moiety itself, but also by other lipoprotein constituents. Studies utilizing both polyclonal and monoclonal anti-apoB antibodies have shown that apoB reacts differently in different types of lipoprotein particles (i.e., VLDL, IDL and LDL). We studied the immunological reactivities of apoB within the LDL class. The results showed that the expression of epitopes in different LDL preparations indeed varied, and that the number of epitopes expressed, appeared to be influenced by the lipid composition of LDL.

INTRODUCTION

Lipoproteins are complex particles consisting of several types of lipids of varying hydrophobicity and of apoproteins. The amphipathic phospholipids and apoproteins form the surface regions of the particles, whereas the hydrophobic cholesterol esters and triglycerides fill the inner core regions. The association between apoproteins and lipids is thought to occur at the hydrophobic surfaces of amphipathic helical regions of apoproteins, whereas the hydrophilic faces of the helices probably interact with polar regions of phospholipids, other apoproteins or water.[1] The amino acid sequences of several apoproteins including apoAI, AII, and the apo's C are known and their lipid binding regions have been identified. This was possible because these apoproteins are of relatively small molecular weight and water soluble. Less is known about the interactions of apoB with lipids and with the surface regions of lipoproteins. Two major (B-100 and B-48) and two minor (B-74 and B-26) forms of apoB have been described.[2] All are large proteins which aggregate in aqueous solutions. Their amino acid sequences are unknown, but it has been suggested that they may be composed of repeating subunits of smaller molecular weight.[3]

Monoclonal antibodies, because they are directed against discrete epitopes, are powerful probes of the structures of proteins, even of proteins whose chemical structure is not defined. In order to study the structure and function of apoB, we have produced monoclonal antibodies against LDL.

METHODS

Production of Monoclonal Antibodies

Female Balb/cJ mice (Jackson Memorial Laboratories, Bar Harbor, Maine) were immunized with human LDL.[4] About 10^8 mouse splenic cells were fused with $\sim 10^7$ SP2/0-Ag14 mouse myeloma cells using polyethylene glycol.[5] Fusion products were grown in Dulbecco's modified Eagle's medium containing 5% newborn calf serum and 10% globulinemic horse serum (DME-S) containing 14 mg/l hypoxanthine, 0.176 mg/l aminopterin and 3 mg/l thymidine (DME-S-HAT) for 3 weeks. Media were tested for antibody activity. Cells were cloned by dilution in 0.2% agar (in DME-S), and those continuing to show antibody activity were expanded further as ascites tumors in Pristane (2-6-10-14 tetramethylpentadecane, Aldrich Chemical Co., Milwaukee, Wisconsin)-treated Balb/cJ mice.

Binding Assays Using Microtiter Plates

Testing of hybridoma fluids was done on 96-well microtiter plates (Dynatech Laboratories, Inc., Alexandria, Virginia). First 105 μl of rabbit antihuman LDL antiserum were added to each well. After 16 hrs at 23°C, wells were rinsed with PBS (0.16 M NaCl and 0.05 M phosphate, pH 7.4), filled with PBS-3% bovine serum albumin (PBS-BSA) for 4 hrs and rinsed again with PBS. Then each well received 130 μl of hybridoma culture media (sample), media from irrelevant fusion products ($blank_1$) or unspent DME-S ($blank_2$), plus 100,000 cpm of ^{125}I-LDL and incubation was carried out overnight. Microtiter wells were rinsed with PBS, sliced and counted in a Packard gamma spectrometer.

Competitive displacement of ^{125}I-labeled antibodies by non-labeled antibodies was studied on microtiter plates coated with 150 μl of LDL (20 μg/ml) overnight at 23°. After rinsing with PBS and blocking with PBS-BSA, wells received increasing amounts of non-labeled antibodies and a constant amount ($\sim$100,000 cpm) of one ^{125}I-labeled antibody. Each antibody was labeled and in turn tested against the other "cold" antibodies. Plates were then processed as above.

Immunoreactivity of different LDL preparations was assayed in competitive displacement assays: microtiter wells were coated with 150 μl of monoclonal antibody solution (5 μg/ml PBS) overnight as 4°C. Then wells were incubated with 3% BSA-PBS (3 hrs, 23°C) in order to saturate extra binding sites on the plastic. Wells then received serial dilutions (in 150 μl) of unknown LDL samples (highest dose 12.5 μg LDL protein/ml), and a constant amount of ^{125}I-LDL (100,000 cpm in 20 μl 3% BSA-PBS). All dilutions were carried out in 3% BSA-PBS. After incubation overnight at 4°C, wells were rinsed three times with PBS, sliced and counted in a gamma counter. The results were expressed as percent of the immunizing LDL which was used as a standard and also as label.

Purification of Antibodies

The antibodies were IgG by immunoassay using class-specific antisera. Following precipitation of IgG from ascites fluid in 50% saturated $(NH_4)_2SO_4$, antibodies were isolated on an immunosorbent column[6] prepared from the immunizing LDL and CNBr-activated Sepharose 4B (Pharmacia Fine Chemicals, Uppsala, Sweden). The coupling of LDL to Sepharose was carried out in 0.1 M $NaHCO_3$ buffer, pH 8.3, (2 hrs, 23°C) according to the directions of the manufacturer using 25 ml of swollen gel and 64 mg of LDL. Columns (8x40 mm) (Chromaflex Disposable Columns, Kontes Glass Co., Vineland, New Jersey) containing 3.5 ml gel were prepared, one for each antibody. Unbound protein was eluted with 0.9% NaCl (15 ml) and the specifically bound fraction was neutralized upon elution by adding 1.1 M Tris buffer, pH 8.6. Between

30-40 percent of sample protein was recovered in the bound fraction. Purified antibodies migrated as single sharp bands on cellulose acetate electrophoresis (Microzone Electrophoresis System, Beckman Intrument, Inc., Fullerton, California) and formed three bands on isoelectric focusing.[7]

Preparation of Fab Fragments

1-2 mg of affinity purified antibody was incubated at 37°C for 4 hrs in 6 ml 0.1 M phosphate buffer, pH 8.0, 2 mM Na_2EDTA, 10 mM 1-cysteine and papain 10 μg/mg antibody (Sigma Chemical Company, Inc., St. Louis, Missouri).[8] Separation of Fab from Fc fragments and partially digested antibody was by chromatography on DEAE cellulose (DE 52; Whatman, Ltd., Kent, England) linear gradient, starting buffer 0.005 M, phosphate pH 8.0; limiting buffer 0.3 M, phosphate pH 8.0). Fab fragments immobolized on microtiter wells bound ^{125}I-LDL, they migrated cathodically as a single arc on immunoelectrophoresis, and showed bands of ∿25,500 apparent molecular weight on SDS gel electrophoresis in the presence of 1% 2-mercaptoethanol (100°, for 2 min).[9]

Isolation of LDL's

Erythrocytes were immediately separated from plasma. Sodium azide (0.02%), EDTA (1 mM), chloramphenicol (50 mg/l) and gentamycon sulfate (100 mg/l) were added to the plasma. Isolation of LDL was carried out between densities 1.025-1.050 with two ultracentrifugations at each density. After dialysis against sodium chloride (0.15 M) and EDTA (1 mM, pH 8.2), the LDL was sterilized by filtration through a 0.2 μm filter (Acrodisc®, Gelman, Ann Arbor, Michigan) and stored in the EDTA-saline containing the above-mentioned concentrations of antibacterial agents at 4°C. On 3% polyacrylamide gel electrophoresis only three bands corresponding to B-100, B-74 and B-26 could be visualized. LDL preparations were analyzed for protein,[10,11] phospholipid[12], triglyceride and free and esterified cholesterol (Triglyceride and Cholesterol Kits, Biodynamics, Indianapolis, Indiana).

^{125}I-labeling of antibodies was carried out using chloramine-T[13] and that of LDL using lactoperoxidase.[14]

Enzymatic Proteolysis of Low Density Lipoprotein

Freshly isolated LDL was used for enzymatic digestions at a concentration of about 20 mg/ml in 1 mM EDTA - 0.16 M NaCl, pH 8.2. The digestions were performed at 37°C under a nitrogen atmosphere at an enzyme to substrate ratio of 1/40 (w/w) using the following enzymes: (a) trypsin-TPCK (Millipore Corp., Freehold, New Jersey) dissolved in 1.0 mM acetic acid-0.1 mM calcium chloride,[15] (b) <u>Staphylococcus</u>

aureus V8 protease (Miles Laboratories, Inc., Elkhart, Indiana) dissolved in 50 mM ammonium bicarbonate buffer, pH 8.4[16] and (c) pronase (protease from streptomyces griseus) (Sigma Chemical Co., St. Louis, Missouri) dissolved in 0.1 M Tris, pH 7.4.[17] The enzyme solutions were prepared fresh before digestion. Incubations were for periods of time indicated below. "Pseudodigestions" of LDL (P-LDL) were performed as described above but without including enzymes. Digestions were stopped by addition to 5 ml of digestion mixtures of 10 μl of 1% phenylmethyl sulfonyl fluoride (PMSF) in isopropyl alcohol.

Isolation of Proteolysis Cores

The enzyme digestion mixtures were cooled to 10°C and applied to a 2.5x95 cm column of Sephadex G-50 superfine previously equilibrated with 1 mM EDTA - 0.16 M NaCl, pH 7.4. Proteolysis cores were eluted at the void volume of the column and were separated from cleaved peptides of molecular weight smaller than 10,000. In preliminary tests some effluent fractions containing cleavage peptides exhibited binding to cultured fibroblasts or monoclonal antibodies. Effluent fractions containing binding activity were pooled and concentrated to ∿10 mg/ml in an Amicon ultrafiltration cell equipped with a PM-10 Diaflow membrane, filtered through 0.45 μm filters (Millipore) and stored at 4°C.

In some instances LDL cores were characterized further. Aliquots of ^{125}I-LDL (10^6 cpm, 10 ng protein) were added to each of the proteolysis cores, which then were subjected to rate zonal ultracentrifugation through a linear density gradient of 1.00 to 1.30 g/ml NaBr.[18] The rotor effluent was collected in 10 ml fractions and the positions of lipoproteins were established by the ultraviolet absorption, protein concentration, and radioactivity of each fraction.

Cell Studies

Cultures of normal human fibroblasts and the quantitation of cell associated and degraded ^{125}I-LDL were performed as described.[19,20] Cells were grown in Eagle's minimal essential medium (15% fetal calf serum) for 5 days and in 10% lipoprotein-deficient serum for 48 hrs. At the start of the experiments increasing amounts of antibodies purified by affinity chromatography, or their isolated Fab fragments, were added to the culture media, followed 5 minutes later by ^{125}I-LDL (5 g/ml). Incubations in triplicate were carried out at 37°C for 4 hrs. At the end of incubations cells were washed, dissolved in 0.1 M sodium hydroxide and aliquots were taken for determination of cell protein[11] and of counts. Results are expressed as ng ^{125}I-LDL bound/mg cell protein.

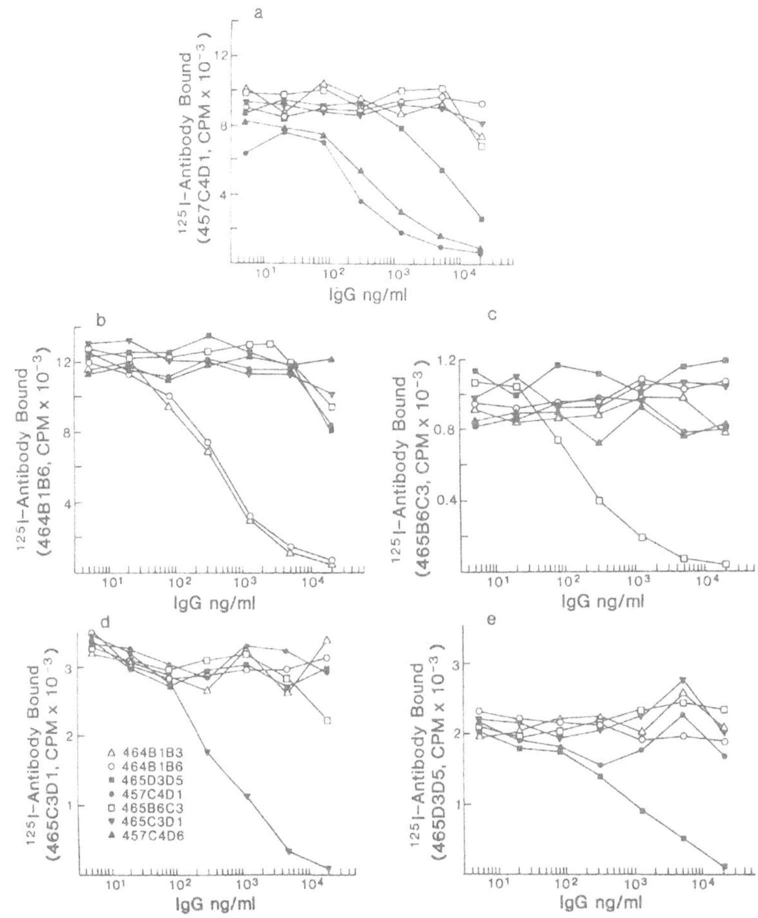

Fig. 1 Inhibition of binding of ^{125}I-antibodies to LDL by unlabeled antibodies. Microtiter wells were coated with 150 µl of LDL (20 µg/ml) overnight at 23°C, rinsed with PBS and blocked with PBS-BSA. Wells then received increasing amounts of unlabeled antibodies as indicated on the abscissae and a constant amount of ^{125}I-labeled antibodies (indicated on the ordinates). After incubation (16 hrs at 23°C) wells were rinsed again with PBS, sliced and counted in a gama counter.

Gel Electrophoresis and Immunoblotting

The peptides of proteolysis cores were separated in polyacrylamide slab gels containing 0.1% SDS, 3.5-15% linear gradient acrylamide and 0.4% bisacrylamide cross-linked with ammonium persulfate.[21] The electrode buffer was 0.025 M Tris, 0.195 M glycine in 0.1% SDS, pH 8.3. Sample solutions containing 20% sucrose, 2.5% SDS, 5 β-mercaptoethanol, 0.0075% bromophenol blue and 10-50 µg protein

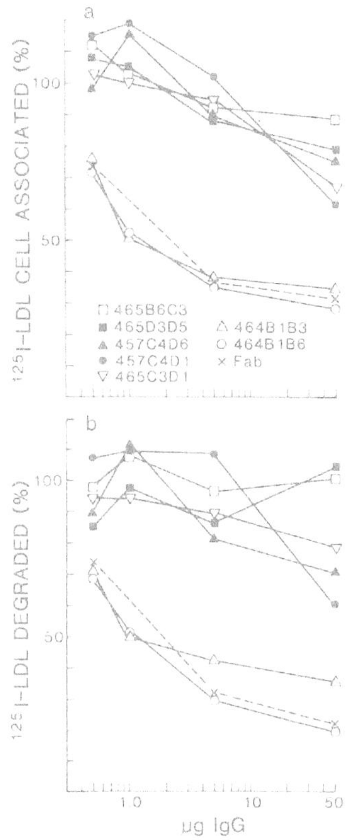

Fig. 2 The binding (a) and degradation (b) of ^{125}I-LDL by cultured normal human fibroblasts. Cells were grown in Eagle's minimal essential medium (15% fetal calf serum) for 5 days and in 10% lipoprotein-deficient serum for 48 hrs. At the start of experiments increasing amounts of affinity purified antibody were added to the culture media. 5 min later, 5 µg/ml of ^{125}I-LDL (∿ 100 cpm/ng) were added. At the end of incubations (4 hrs at 37°C), cell associated and degraded LDL counts were determined. In a separate experiment, equivalent amounts of antigen binding Fab fragments (2/3 of IgG mass) were used instead of whole antibodies. The results are expressed as percent of maximum binding obtained in the absence of antibodies.

per 40 µ l were heated for 2 min at 100°C before applying to the gels. Electrophoresis was performed at room temperature in the model 220 vertical slab electrophoresis cell (Bio-Rad Laboratories, Richmond, California) at a constant voltage of 32 V for 17-18 hrs. Gels were stained with Coomassie blue or were subjected to electrophoretic transfer of peptides (Western blotting).[22] Aminophenylthioether

(APT) paper was prepared from Whatman #50 paper by reacting the paper with 1, 4-butanediol diglycidyl ether and 2-aminothiophenol.[23] APT paper was diazotized to diazophenylthioether (DPT) paper using $NaNO_2$/HCl. Before transfer, polyacrylamide gels were cut longitudinally, one section was stained as above and the rest was mounted in a Trans-Blot cell (Bio-Rad Laboratories). Electrophoretic transfer was performed at 1.6 A for 2 hrs at 5°C. Coomassie blue stainable material was quantitatively transferred by the procedure. After transfer, the DPT paper was washed by gentle shaking in TEG buffer (0.4 M Tris(hydroxymethyl)aminomethane, pH 8.8/40% (v/v) ethanolamine/1% (w/v) gelatin) for 2 hrs at room temperature, rinsed in deionized water, blotted on paper and placed into heat-sealable freezer bags. ^{125}I-labeled monoclonal antibodies were diluted (0.5 ml per lane containing 0.7×10^6 cpm) in TENG-T buffer (50 mM Tris(hydroxymethyl)aminomethane, pH 7.4/4 mM Na_2 EDTA/150 mM NaCl/0.25% (w/v) gelatin/0.05% (v/v) Triton X-100) containing also nonimmune ascites fluid (10%, v/v), and added to the freezer bags containing the transferred proteins. In control incubations a ^{125}I-labeled non-related monoclonal antibody (antihuman C3 complement antibody) was used. The DPT papers were thoroughly wetted with antibody solution and excess solution was squeezed out. Bags were heat-sealed and incubated at room temperature for 18 hrs. DPT papers were rinsed and washed with TENG-T buffer for 2 hrs. The papers were then rinsed in deionized water, blotted, air-dried, and autoradiographed at -70°C with DuPont Cronex Lightning-Plus XL intensifying screens using Kodak X-Omat AR X-ray film.

RESULTS AND DISCUSSION

To assess whether antibodies bound at different antigenic sites on apoB in holo-LDL, the ability of each antibody to compete with the other antibodies for binding to LDL was assessed. LDL was immobilized on microtiter plates, increasing amounts of unlabeled antibody and a constant amount of labeled antibody were added to the wells (Fig. 1). The binding of ^{125}I-labeled antibody 457C4D1 was markedly inhibited by increasing amounts of non-labeled antibodies 457C4D1 and 457C4D6, but other antibodies did not inhibit at all or inhibited less effectively (Fig. 1a). The binding of ^{125}I-464B1B6 was inhibited by increasing amounts of non-labeled antibodies 464B1B3 and 464B1B6, but not by other antibodies (Fig. 1b). Similarly, the binding of ^{125}I-labeled antibodies 465B6C3, 465C3D1 and 465D3D5 was inhibited only by their respective non-labeled parent compounds (Figs. 1c-e). These antibodies appear to define at least five epitopes of apoB in holo-LDL.

Inhibition by Antibodies of Binding of ^{125}I-LDL To Fibroblasts

The effect of various antibodies on the cellular binding and degradation of ^{125}I-LDL was investigated by adding increasing amounts of purified antibody followed by a constant amount of the labeled

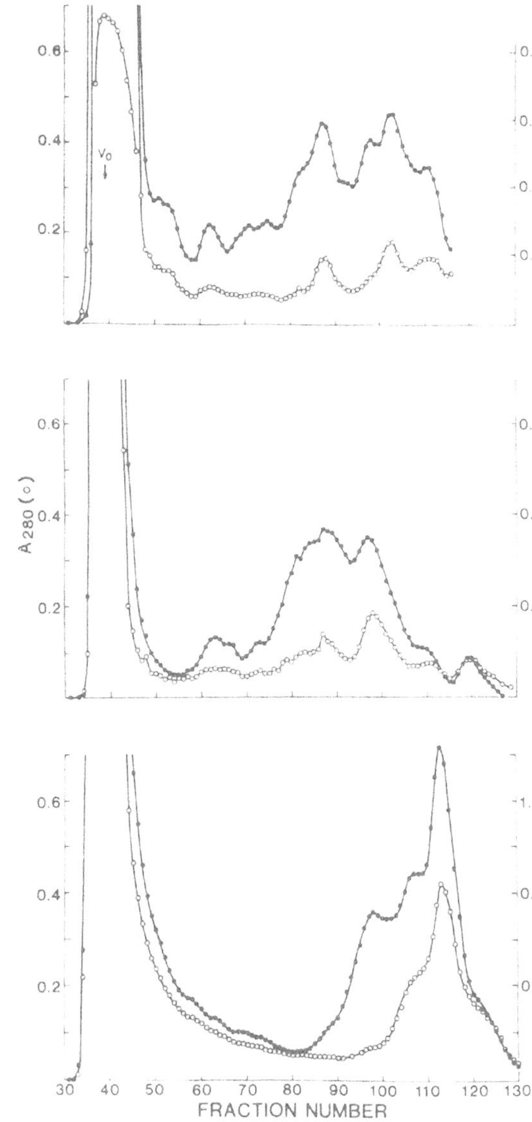

Fig. 3 Elution profiles of enzymatic proteolysis mixtures. Top: trypsin; Middle: staphylococcal protease; Bottom: pronase. After 24 hrs of incubation, mixtures were gel filtered on Sephadex G-50 (2.5x95 cm) at 10°C in 1 mM EDTA - 0.16 M NaCl and 2.3 ml fractions were collected. Fractions containing small cleavage peptides were pooled for further analysis as follows: staphylococcal protease treated peptides; SP-IV: fractions 91-99; SP-V: fractions 101-113. Trypsin-treated peptides; T-IV: fractions 73-77; T-V: fractions 78-83; T-VII: fractions 95-99; T-VIII: fractions 100-107. LDL-cores were fractions 35-45.

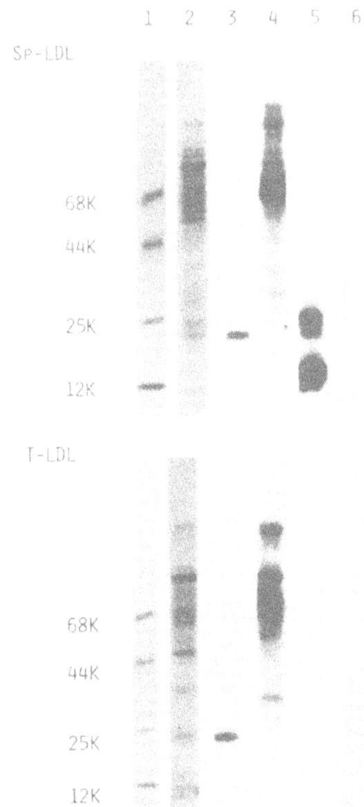

Fig. 4 Autoradiogram of ^{125}I-labeled monoclonal antibodies bound to electrophoretically transferred T core and SP core peptides. Following 3.5-15% gradient polyacrylamide gel electrophoresis of enzyme treated LDL cores isolated by Sephadex column chromatography and transfer of the core protein to diazophenylthioether paper, the paper was incubated with ^{125}I-labeled monoclonal anti-LDL antibodies, and sites of antibody localization were visualized by autoradiography. Lane 1: M.W. markers: 68 K bovine serum albumin, 44 K ovalbumin, 25 K α-chymotrypsinogen, 12 K cytochrome C. Coomassie stain. Lane 2 Top: SP-LDL core (Coomassie stain). Lane 2 Bottom: T-LDL core (Coomassie stain). Lane 3: ^{125}I-antibody 1a; Lane 4: ^{125}I-antibody 2a; Lane 5: ^{125}I-antibody 3; Lane 6: ^{125}I-antihuman C3 complement antibody (control). Antibody 3 bound to SP-LDL but not to T-LDL. Antibodies 4 and 5 (not shown) were not well visualized on several attempts. For antibody numbers see Table 2.

lipoprotein to the culture media of cultured normal human fibroblasts (Fig. 2). Antibodies 464B1B3 and 464B1B6 both inhibited the cellular binding and degration of ^{125}I-LDL, whereas the other antibodies inhibited only at 100-fold greater doses. The incubations with anti-

TABLE 1

CHEMICAL COMPOSITIONS OF LDL PROTEOLYSIS CORES ISOLATED BY GEL FILTRATION

	P	PL	TG	UC	CE
			Weight %		
T-LDL	14.6	21.9	4.2	15.0	44.3
SP-LDL	15.8	22.4	4.6	13.0	43.3
P-LDL	20.1	20.2	4.7	13.6	41.3

After 24 hours of proteolysis, the incubation mixtures were filtered on a 2.5x95 cm Sephadex G-50 column (See Fig. 3), and fractions 30-45 were pooled for analysis. Abbreviations: T-LDL, SP-LDL, and P-LDL indicate trypsin, staphylococcal protease and pseudodigested LDL, respectively. P = protein; PL - phospholipid; TG = triglyceride; UC = unesterified cholesterol; CE = cholesterol ester.

bodies were repeated on three other occasions with similar results. In a separate experiment, equivalent amounts of antigen-binding Fab fragments of antibody 464B1B6 were added to the system and they provided the same degree of inhibition. Thus, antibodies 464B1B3 and 464B1B6 define epitopes close to the cell receptor recognition domain of apoB in LDL.

Proteolysis of LDL

Proteolysis with trypsin and staphylococcal protease resulted in the loss of ∿20% of LDL protein from the lipoprotein particles during 24 hrs of treatment. Each enzyme also produced characteristic elution profiles of water soluble cleavage peptides (Fig. 3). SDS polyacrylamide gel electrophoresis (3.5-20% gradient) of the isolated T and SP cores indicated that each protease also produced a characteristic pattern of cleavage products (Fig. 4). On 3.5% polyacrylamide SDS gel electrophoresis, the protein moieties of the cores consisted solely of chains whose molecular weight appeared to be >100 K, whereas the smallest subspecies of apoB (B-26) had an apparent M.W. of >150 K (data not shown). Despite the major perturbations of their apoproteins, compositions of T cores and SP cores remained similar to that of pseudodigested LDL (Table 1). Pronase treatment over 24 hrs caused ∿60% losses of protein from LDL and on gel electrophoresis most of the core peptides were small (>44 K) (not shown). Cleavage peptides also were small, eluting near the salt volume of the column (Fig. 3). Solutions of pronase cores were turbid, indicating of a disruption of the structure of the lipoprotein.

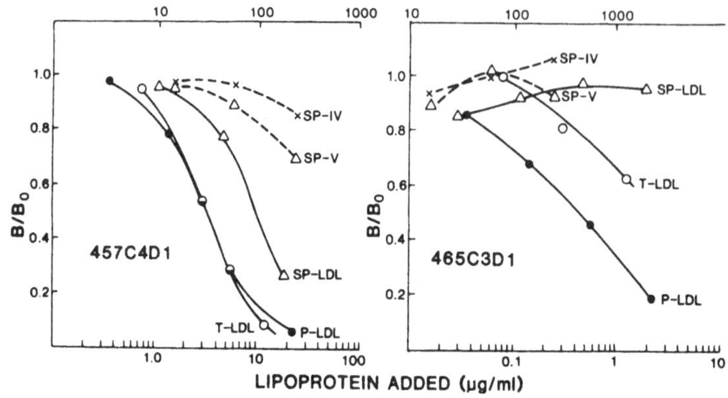

Fig. 5 Competitive displacement of ^{125}I-labeled LDL by trypsin and staphylococcal protease treated cores or peptides. Microtiter wells were coated with 5 μ l/ml of monoclonal antibody 1 or 4 (457C4D1 or 465C3D1) overnight at 23°C, rinsed with PBS, and blocked with PBS-BSA (3 hrs, 23°C). Wells then received increasing amounts of unlabeled enzyme treated LDL (T-LDL or SP-LDL), or pseudodigested LDL (P-LDL) isolated by gel permeation chromatography, or cleavage peptides (for definition of SP-IV and SP-V fractions see Legend to Fig. 2) as well as a constant amount (∿100,000 cpm) of ^{125}I-labeled LDL. After incubation (16 hrs, 23°C) wells were rinsed with PBS, sliced and counted in a gamma counter.

NOTE: Dashed line curves relate to abscissae <u>on the top</u>, continuous curves relate to abscissae <u>on the bottom</u> of the figure.

The isolated T cores and SP cores were characterized further by zonal ultracentrifugation. Some heterogeneity of the cores was observed but the flotation properties of the major peaks differed only to a minor degree from those of pseudodigested LDL and remained unchanged relative to the ^{125}I-labeled LDL used as internal standard. About 65% of the protein of T- and SP-LDL were recovered in peaks corresponding to native LDL; recovery for pseudo-LDL was 98%. The percentage chemical composition of the zonal peaks was very similar to those of P-LDL. Peptide profiles of zonal LDL cores on SDS gel electrophoresis were indistinguishable from those of the cores isolated by gel permeation chromatography.

Immunoreactivity of Proteolysis Cores and Cleavage Peptides with Monoclonal Anti-LDL Antibodies

Five monoclonal antibodies designated as antibodies 1-5 which are directed against at least five non-overlapping antigenic determinants

TABLE 2

EFFECTS OF LIMITED PROTEOLYSIS ON APPARENT ApoB CONTENTS OF LDL "CORES"

Antibody	Apparent Apo B Contents				
	T-LDL		SP-LDL		Pro-LDL
	Column	Zonal	Column	Zonal	Column
457C4D1 [1a]	107	98	68	75	0
457C4D6 [1b]	95	61	62	46	0
464B1B3 [2a]	140	126	115	154	32
464B1B6 [2b]	114	92	103	85	34
465B6C3 [3]	0	0	42	33	10
465C3D1 [4]	18	9	0	0	0
465D3D5 [5]	28	42	30	61	8

The results are means of two assays; two LDL samples were separately digested and LDL cores were isolated on Sephadex and subjected to zonal ultracentrifugation. The apparent apoB contents were determined by competition assays on microtiter plates. For each LDL preparation duplicate determinations at 3-5 doses were carried out with coefficients of variation of ∿8%. Data are expressed as percent of protein relative to the pseudodigested LDL protein standard. Column fractions represent LDL cores recovered after fractionation on Sephadex G-50.
Zonal fractions represent LDL-like peaks recovered after zonal ultracentrifugation of LDL cores.

on LDL-apoB were used in the immunoblotting analysis. All five antibodies have been shown to react with apoB-100 when Western blots of non-digested LDL were incubated with labeled antibodies (not shown). Three antibodies (1a, 2a and 3) each bound to at least one core peptide on Western blots (Fig. 4). Antibodies 4 and 5 did not bind to core peptides, although antibody 5 bound to transferred pseudo-digested LDL protein (not shown). The overall patterns of binding revealed that the epitopes detectable by immunoblotting could be separated from the others, confirming that the epitopes were distinct.

The effects of 24 hours of limited proteolysis on the expression of epitopes in holo-LDL were determined in competitive radioimmunoassays on microtiter plates. Representative displacement curves for 24-hour digested T- and SP-LDL cores with antibodies 1 and 4 are shown in Fig. 5. Digestion produced differential effects on the immunoreactivity of LDL with each of the antibodies, destroying some epitopes, leaving some decreased and others unaffected or even increased (Table 2). In general, the apparent apoB contents of the zonal peaks resembled those of the cores obtained from the Sephadex G-50 column effluents (Table 2). Pronase treatment caused the most marked de-

TABLE 3

APPARENT ApoB CONTENTS OF LDL PROTEOLYTIC CLEAVAGE PEPTIDE FRACTIONS SEPARATED FROM "CORES" BY GEL FILTRATION

	T V	T VII	T VIII	SP IV	SP V
457 C4D1 [1a]	0	0	0	0.4	0.7
457 C4D6 [1b]	0	0	0	0	<0.1
464 B1B3 [2a]	0	0	0	0.5	0.9
464 B1B6 [2b]	<0.1	0	<0.1	0.5	1.0
465 B6C3 [3]	0	0	0	0.3	0.9
465 C3D1 [4]	0	0	0	0	0
465 D3D5 [5]	0	0	0	<0.1	0

Results are expressed as percent of protein relative to LDL protein standard. Duplicate determinations of 2-3 doses were carried out with coefficients of variation of ∿8%.

creases in the apparent apoB content of LDL, including a nearly total loss of antigenicity toward five of the seven antibodies tested. Virtually all of the immunoreactivity of the T and SP cores was retained vis-a-vis antibody 2 which is known to inhibit the binding ^{125}I-LDL to fibroblasts (Fig. 2). By contrast, immunoreactivity of LDL with antibody 3 was almost totally lost after trypsin digestion and with antibody 4 after treatment with staphylococcal protease. The progessive destruction of one epitope (antibody 4) during digestion was monitored in a time-course experiment in which an LDL preparation was treated with staphylococcal protease for increasing periods of time and the ability of chromatographically isolated core LDL to compete with ^{125}I-LDL for binding to antibody 4 was tested. Pseudodigestions of LDL (P-LDL) were carried out in parallel. After incubations of 3 and 6 hours the apparent apoB contents per mass core LDL protein decreased to 82, 45, 0 and 0% of pseudodigested LDL, respectively.

The immunoreactivities of various water soluble peptide fractions also were determined in competitive microtiter plate radioimmunoassays (examples of displacement curves are shown in Fig. 5 and results for those cleaved peptides which showed detectable competitive activity are given in Table 3). Immunoreactivity was shown particularly in assays containing antibodies 1a, 2a, 2b and 3. The maximum apparent apoB content was one percent of the standard LDL-apoB. Note that in spite of the losses of epitope 2 from holo-LDL, the immunoreactivity of the LDL cores vs. antibody 2 was retained or increased, suggesting that apoB may be composed of repeating structures.

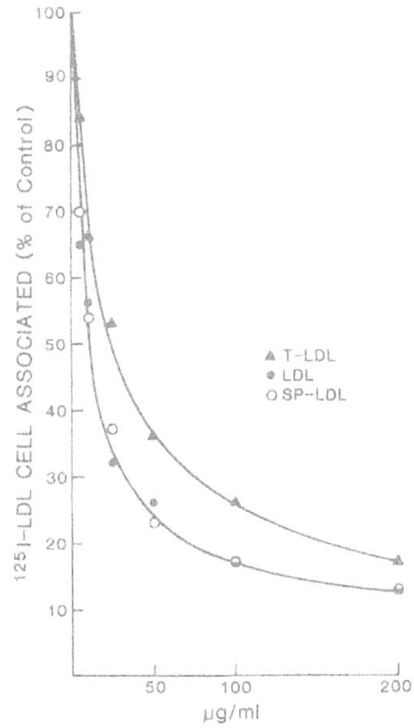

Fig. 6 Binding of ^{125}I-labeled LDL to cultured normal human fibroblasts in the presence of T-LDL or SP-LDL. Cells were grown in Eagle's minimal essential medium (15% fetal calf serum) for 5 days and in 10% lipoprotein deficient serum for 48 hours. At the start of the experiment, 5 μg/ml of ^{125}I-LDL (∿100 cpm/ng) and increasing amounts of T-LDL, SP-LDL or P-LDL were added to the culture media. At the end of incubations (4 hours at 37°C), cell associated LDL counts were determined. Similar results were obtained for ^{125}I-LDL degradation (not shown).

Interaction of Proteolysis Cores and Peptides with Cultured Human Fibroblasts

The competitive ability of the 24-hour SP cores vs. ^{125}I-LDL for binding to cells was identical with that of pseudodigested LDL, whereas the competitiveness of T cores was somewhat diminished (Fig. 6). The water soluble cleavage peptide fractions obtained from the gel filtration column effluents also were tested in cell assays (Table 4). The material in fractions T-IV, and SP-IV caused inhibition of binding of ^{125}I-LDL to cells. Acetylation of active peptides abolished their inhibiting capacity. Similar inhibiting activity was present in T-V and SP-V peptides; other peptides had no activity (not shown). These results also suggest that apoB may be composed of repeating structures.

TABLE 4

INHIBITION OF I^{125}-LDL BINDING TO CULTURED HUMAN FIBROBLASTS BY PROTEOLYTIC LDL PEPTIDES

Inhibitor Dose (μg/ml)	^{125}I-LDL Bound in the Presence and Absence of Inhibitors (% of control)			
	T IV	SP IV	Ac T IV	Ac SP IV
50	56	49	-	-
100	44	40	-	-
200	56	33	102	98
none	100	100	100	100

Cultured fibroblasts grown in 10% LPDS for 48 hrs before the experiment were exposed to the indicated peptide inhibitors at 4°C for 2 hrs at the indicated concentrations. Five μg of I^{125}-LDL were added and incubation was continued for another 2 hrs at 4°C. Dextran sulfate releasable I^{125}-LDL then was determined. Results are expressed as percent of control with no inhibitors present; 100% binding was 45±3 ng/mg cell protein. T=tryptic; SP=staphylococcal protease; Ac T=acetylated T peptides; Ac SP=acetylated SP peptides. For identification of fractions T-IV and SP-IV in the gel filtration column effluent, see fig. 3 & text. Determinations for T and SP peptides were carried out in duplicate and those for Ac peptides in triplicate.

Epitope Expression on Holo-LDL

Low density lipoproteins were isolated from blood samples of 17 consecutive patients visiting the Lipid Clinic, including subjects with various forms of hyperlipoproteinemia.

The average chemical composition of the LDL preparations is shown in Table 5. The percentage of triglyceride correlated positively with percent protein (r=0.72, Pearson correlation coefficient, p=0.0011) and inversely with percent total cholesterol (r=-0.89, p=0.0001), as well as with percent esterified cholesterol (r=-0.68, p=0.0023) but not with free cholesterol. In addition, the percentage of total cholesterol correlated negatively with percent protein (r=-0.84, p=0.0001) but percent phospholipid did not correlate significantly with any of the other LDL constituents.

Immunoreactivity of LDL Preparations

The reactivities of LDL samples were analyzed by comparing their

TABLE 5

COMPOSITION OF LDL

	N	Protein	Phospholipid	Cholesterol Ester	Free Cholesterol	Triglycerides
% of LDL mass	17	22.5 ± 1.6	22.5 ± 1.1	39.1 ± 4.9	8.9 ± 1.9	6.5 ± 2.0
(range)		(20.8 - 26.0)	(20.6 - 24.4)	(32.3 - 45.9)	(7.1 - 15.0)	(3.9 - 10.4)

Results are means ± SD

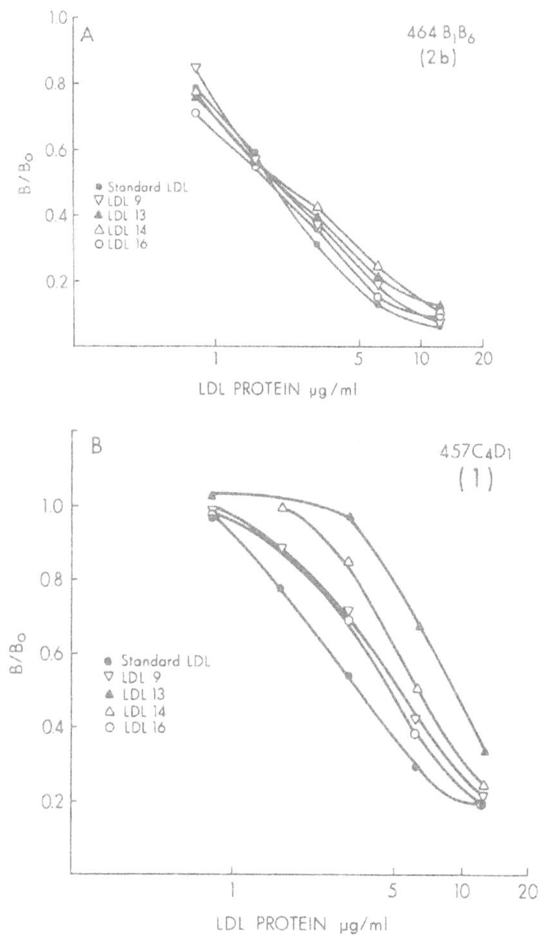

Fig. 7 Competitive displacement curves produced by different LDL preparations with antibodies [2b] 464B1B6 (A) and [1] 457C4D1 (B). The immunizing LDL preparation was used as LDL standard. The results (expressed as percent of LDL standard) were calculated from the curves using 3 or 4 points from the parallel parts of the curves.

capacities to displace ^{125}I-LDL from binding to different monoclonal antibodies. The displacement curves (examples shown in Fig. 7) were parallel with that produced by the LDL standard when antibodies 1, 2a, 2b, 3 or 4 were used, which allowed accurate quantitation of the apparent apoB content of LDL (expressed as percent of LDL standard). The calculated results of all assays are compiled in Fig. 8. Eight out of 17 displacement curves produced with antibody 5 were non-parallel as compared to the LDL standard curve. Therefore, the cor-

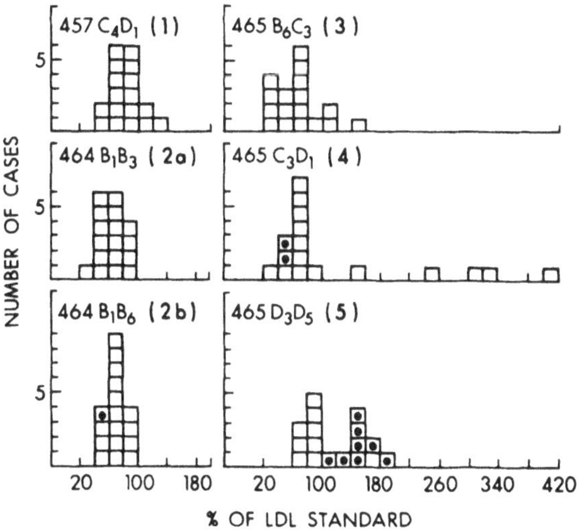

Fig. 8 Distribution of apparent apoB contents in 17 different LDL preparations. The apparent apoB contents were calculated from competitive displacement curves (see Fig. 1). The following means+SD values and ranges (in parentheses) of values were obtained [1] 457C4D1: 82.5+19.4 (50-127), [2a] 464B1B3: 64.7+16.3 (33-96), [2b] 464B1B6: 68.8+14.4 (44-95), [3] 465B6C3: 65.9+32.3 (29-143), [4] 465C3D1: 128.3+119.6 (35-413). The cases marked with black dots (antibody 465D3D5) indicate apparent apoB content values derived from displacement curves that were nonparallel with the curve produced by the LDL standard.

responding apparent apoB contents of the LDL preparations are not accurate. The results obtained with antibody 5 were excluded from subsequent calculations of correlation.

Relation of LDL Lipid Composition to Immunoreactivity

The immunoreactivities of LDL preparations as determined by antibodies 2a (Fig. 9B), 2b, 3 and 4 correlated significantly and positively with their percentages of phospholipids (Table 6). On the other hand, immunoreactivity as determined by antibody 1 correlated inversely with percent triglyceride (Fig. 9A) and positively with percent total cholesterol. Calculations of the Spearman coefficients of rank correlation preserved the above-mentioned significant correlations with the exception of the correlations between phospholipid percentages and immunoreactivities as determined by antibody 2b ($p=0.085$) and antibody 4 ($p=0.084$). The percentages of esterified or free cholesterol alone did not correlate significantly with immunoreactivity as determined by antibody 1. Other statistically signifi-

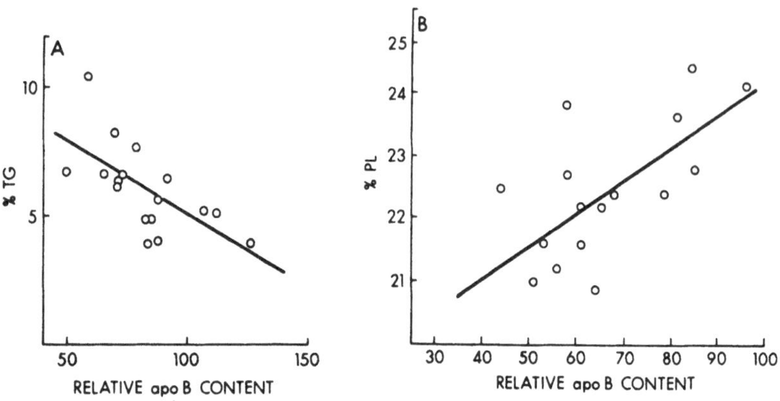

Fig. 9 Relations between relative apparent apoB content and percent composition in 17 LDL preparations. A. Apparent apoB content as determined by antibody 475C4D1 [1] vs. percentage of triglyceride: y=-0.056x +10.62. B. Apparent apoB content as determined by antibody 464B1B3 [2a] vs. percentage of phospholipid: y=0.049x +19.15. Correlation coefficients: see Table 3.

cant relationships between apparent apoB contents and percentage composition of lipids were not found.

TABLE 6

RELATION OF APPARENT ApoB CONTENT TO LIPID COMPOSITION IN 17 LDL PREPARATIONS

Code	Identifying Number	%PL	%CHOL	%TG
1	457C4D1	0.00	0.65***	-0.63**
2a	464B1B3	0.68***	0.01	-0.27
2b	464B1B6	0.51*	-0.16	0.02
3	465B6C3	0.71***	-0.25	-0.01
4	465C3D1	0.54*	0.05	0.15

Values are Pearson correlation coefficients. PL = phospholipid, CHOL = cholesterol, TG = triglyceride.

*p<0.05; **p<0.01; ***p<0.005.

Since LDL is a complex of apoB and various lipid constituents, it is not possible from the above experiments to differentiate between apoB heterogeneity due to differences in protein structure and heterogeneity secondary to the influence of the lipids associated with apoB, although the profound effects on LDL immunoreactivity produced by chemical modification of amino acid residues and proteolytic cleavage of peptides are consistent with a central role for the protein moiety in the formation of epitopes[4]. Nevertheless, it is clear that other constituents of LDL significantly affect the expression of some epitopes of apoB.

The experiments summarized in this report, as well as other work,[4,24-33] illustrate the usefulness of the immunologic approach, using monoclonal and polyclonal antibodies, for studies of lipoprotein structure and function.

ACKNOWLEDGMENTS

Supported by NIH Grant HL 15308, the Mallinckrodt Hybridoma Contract and a *Fogarty International Fellowship.

REFERENCES

1. A. M. Gotto, Jr., R. L. Jackson, J. D. Morrisett, H. J. Pownall, and J. T. Sparrow, Molecular association of lipids and proteins in plasma lipoproteins: A review, in: "Lipoprotein Metabolism," Heiner Greten, ed., Springer Verlag, Berlin, p. 152-157 (1976).
2. J. P. Kane, D. A. Hardman, and H. E. Paulus, Heterogeneity of apolipoprotein B: Isolation of a new species from human chylomicrons, PNAS 77(5):2465-2469 (1980).
3. D. G. Deutsch, R. L. Heinrikson, J. Foreman, and A. M. Scanu, Studies of the cyanogen bromide fragments of the apoprotein of human serum low density lipoproteins, Biochim. Biophys. Acta 529:342-350 (1978).
4. M. J. Tikkanen, R. Dargar, B. Pfleger, B. Gonen, J. M. Davie, and G. Schonfeld, Antigenic mapping of human low density lipoprotein with monoclonal antibodies, J. Lipid Res. 23:1032-1038 (1982).
5. G. Galfre, S. C. Howe, C. Milstein, G. W. Butcher, and J. C. Howard, Antibodies to major histocompatibility antigen produced by hybrid cell lines, Nature 266:550-552 (1977).
6. S. C. March, I. Parikh, and P. Cuatrecasas, A simplified method for cyanogen bromide activation of agarose for affinity chromatography, Anal. Biochem. 60:149-152 (1974).
7. D. E. Briles and J. M. Davie, Detection of isoelectric focused antibody by autoradiography and hemolysis of antigen-coated erythrocytes, J. Immunol. Methods 8:363-372 (1975).

8. J. L. Fahey and B. A. Askonas, Enzymatically produced subunits of proteins formed by plasma cells in mice, I-gamma globulin and gamma-myeloma proteins, J. Exp. Med. 115:623-639 (1962).
9. K. Weber and M. Osborne, The reliability of molecular weight determinations by dodecyl sulfate polyacrylamide gel electrophoresis, J. Biol. Chem. 244:4406-4412 (1969).
10. T. Sata, R. J. Havel, and A. L. Jones, Characterization of subfractions of triglyceride-rich lipoproteins separated by gel chromatography from blood plasma of normolipemic and hyperlipemic humans, J. Lipid Res. 13:757-768 (1972).
11. O. H. Lowry, N. J. Rosenbrough, A. L. Farr, and R. J. Randall, Protein measurement with the Folin phenol reagent, J. Biol. Chem. 193:265-275 (1951).
12. G. R. Bartlett, Phosphorus assay in column chromatography, J. Biol. Chem. 234:466 (1958).
13. F. G. Greenwood, W. M. Hunter, and J. S. Glover, The preparation of ^{136}I-labelled human growth hormone of high specific radioactivity, Biochem. J. 89:114-123 (1963)
14. J. J. Marchalonis, An enzymic method for the trace iodination of immunoglobulins and other proteins, Biochem. J. 113:209-305 (1969).
15. K.-S. Hahm, On the primary structure of pig heart aconitase, Ph.D. Dissertation, Duquesne University (1979).
16. G. R. Drapeau, Cleavage of glutamic acid with staphylococcal protease, in: "Methods in Enzymology, XLVII, Part E, C. H. W. Hirs and S. N. Timasheff, editors, Academic Press, New York pp. 189-191 (1977).
17. M. J. Levine, M. C. Herzberg, M. S. Levine, S. A. Ellison, M. W. Stinson, H. C. Li, and T. Van Dyke, Specificity of salivary-bacterial interactions: Role of terminal sialic acid residues in the interaction of salivary glycoproteins with streptococcus sanguis and streptococcus mutans, Infection and Immunity 19(1):107-115 (1978).
18. J. R. Patsch, W. Patsch, S. Sailer, and H. Braunsteiner, Isolation and partial characterization of two abnormal human plasma lipoproteins: LP-X_1 and LP-X_2, Biochim. Biophys. Acta 434: 419-427 (1976).
19. J. L. Goldstein and M. S. Brown, Binding and degradation of low density lipoproteins by cultured human fibroblasts, J. Biol. Chem. 249: 5153-5162 (1974).
20. R. E. Ostlund, Jr., B. Pfleger, and G. Schonfeld, Role of microtubules in low density lipoprotein processing by cultured cells, J. Clin. Invest. 63:75-84 (1979).
21. J. B. Swaney and K. S. Kuehl, Separation of apolipoproteins by an acrylamide-gradient sodium dodecyl sulfate gel electrophoresis system, Biochim. Biophys. Acta 446:561-565 (1976).
22. H. Towbin, T. Staehelin, and J. Gordon, Electrophoretic transfer of proteins from polyacrylamide gels to nitrocellulose sheets: Procedure and some applications, PNAS 76(9):4350-4354 (1979).
23. P. M. Kelley and M. J. Schlesinger, Antibodies to two major

chicken heat shock proteins cross-react with similar motions in widely divergent species, Mol. Cell Biol. 2:267-274 (1982).

24. G. Schonfeld, W. Patsch, B. Pfleger, J. L. Witztum, and S. W. Weidman, Lipolysis produces changes in the immunoreactivity and cell reactivity of very low density lipoproteins, J. Clin. Invest. 64:1288-1297 (1979).

25. G. Schonfeld and W. Patsch, The interactions of lipoproteins with cellular receptors, in: "Drugs Affecting Lipid Metabolism," R. Fumagalli, D. Kritchevsky, and R. Paoletti, eds., Elsevier/North Holland, Biomedical Press, pp. 37-52 (1980).

26. W. Patsch, J. L. Witztum, R. Ostlund, and G. Schonfeld, Structure, immunology, and cell reactivity at low density lipoprotein from unbilical vein at a newborn type II homozygote, J. Clin. Invest. 66:123-129 (1980).

27. S. Goldstein and M. J. Chapman, Radioimmunological study of the surface protein of the human serum low-density lipoprotein: Comparison of the native particle and the products obtained by tryptic treatment, Biochem. Biophys. Res. Commun. 87(1): 121-127 (1979).

28. B. P. Tsao, L. K. Curtiss, and T. S. Edgington, Immunochemical heterogeneity of human plasma apoliprotein B II. Expression of apolipoprotein B epitopes on native lipoproteins, J. Biol. Chem. 257:15222-15228 (1982).

29. L. K. Curtiss and T. S. Edgington, Immunochemical heterogeneity of human plasma apolipoprotein B. 1. Apolipoprotein B binding of mouse hybridoma antibodies, J. Biol. Chem. 257:15213-15221 (1982).

30. S. J. T. Mao, R. E. Katzmar, J. C. Silverfield, M. C. Alley, K. Kluge, and C. G. Fathman, Immunochemical properties of human low density lipoproteins as explored by monoclonal antibodies, Biochim. Biophys. Acta 713:365-374 (1982).

31. R. W. Milne, R. Theolis, Jr., R. B. Verdery, and Y. Marcel, Characterization of monoclonal antibodies against human low density lipoprotein, Arteriosclerosis 3:23-30 (1983).

32. T. S. Watt and R. M. Watt, Detection of unique antigenic determinants on human plasma low density lipoprotein and on delipidated apolipoprotein B, Proc. Natl. Acad. Sci., U.S.A., 80: 124-128 (1983).

33. K.-S. Hahm, M. J. Tikkanen, R. Dargar, T. C. Cole, J. M. Davie, and G. Schonfeld, Limited proteolysis detecting destroys epitopes on apolipoprotein B in low density lipoproteins, J. Lipid Res. 24:877-885 (1983).

APOLIPOPROTEIN E: RECEPTOR BINDING PROPERTIES

K. H. Weisgraber, T. L. Innerarity, S. C. Rall, Jr., and R. W. Mahley

The Gladstone Foundation Laboratories and the Departments of Pathology and Medicine, University of California San Francisco, California 94140

INTRODUCTION

Apolipoprotein E (apo-E) was first described in human very low density lipoproteins (VLDL)[1,2] and has now been demonstrated in several lipoprotein classes in a variety of species.[3] It occurs in chylomicrons and their remnants, VLDL, and a subfraction of high density lipoproteins (HDL) referred to as HDL_1, HDL_c, or HDL-with apo-E.[3,4] The amino acid sequence of apo-E has been determined.[5] The protein consists of a single polypeptide chain of 299 residues with a molecular weight of ~34,000.

As demonstrated by Utermann and associates[6] and Zannis and Breslow,[7] apo-E exhibits a genetically determined polymorphism that is expressed at the level of the structural gene.[8] On isoelectric focusing gels, three major isoforms (E4, E3, and E2) and six phenotypes (E4/4, E3/3, E2/2, E4/3, E4/2, and E3/2) are commonly observed.[9]

An important property of apo-E is its ability to interact with lipoprotein receptors.[10,11] As a result of this interaction, apo-E plays a central role in lipoprotein metabolism. Sherrill et al. have shown that apo-E on chylomicron remnants binds to hepatic receptors and therefore is responsible for the hepatic clearance of chylomicron remnants.[12] It has also been postulated that apo-E is involved in the transport of excess cholesterol from peripheral cells back to the liver for elimination, with the HDL-with apo-E subclasses participating in the so-called reverse cholesterol transport process.[13,14] Recent experimental evidence supports this concept and demonstrates that lecithin:cholesterol acyltransferase plays an integral part in this process.[15]

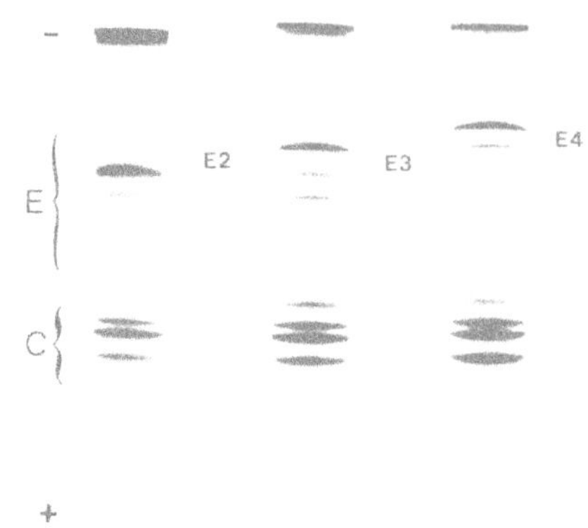

	E2/2	E3/3	E4/4
Relative Charge	0	+1	+2
Residue 112	Cys	Cys	Arg
Residue 158	Cys	Arg	Arg

Fig. 1 Isoelectric focusing gels of VLDL from three subjects homozygous for apo-E phenotypes E2/2, E3/3, or E4/4. The charge differences between E2, E3, and E4 are explained on the basis of cysteine-arginine interchanges at residues 112 and 158 in the protein. Permission granted from Mahley and Angelin.[17]

Because of the ability of apo-E to interact with receptors, a dysfunction in the receptor binding properties of apo-E could potentially lead to abnormalities associated with the lipoproteins, such as accumulation in the plasma of remnants or other lipoprotein classes that are normally cleared through an apo-E-mediated process. Abnormal tissue accumulation of cholesterol is another possibility. In this review, the structure-function relationships of apo-E will be explored with particular emphasis on receptor binding. In addition, the role of apo-E in the expression of type III hyperlipoproteinemia will be briefly discussed.

APOLIPOPROTEIN E: STRUCTURE, RECEPTOR BINDING, AND TYPE III HYPERLIPOPROTEINEMIA

Three homozygous apo-E phenotypes have been identified and are depicted in Fig. 1, which shows the isoelectric focusing gels of VLDL from three subjects. An apo-E homozygous pattern is characterized by one major isoform band, either E4, E3, or E2, and a series of more acidic isoform bands. These minor bands have been demonstrated to arise from posttranslational addition of sialic acid to the major isoform.[7] As shown in Fig. 1, E2, E3, and E4 progressively differ from each other by one charge, with E4 being the most basic. The structural basis for this charge heterogeneity has been determined to involve cysteine-arginine substitutions at two sites in the protein, residues 112 and 158.[8] This structural information is summarized in the lower portion of Fig. 1. As will be shown later, other structural variants of E2 exist with amino acid substitutions at different sites in the protein. The most common form of E2 is the one shown in Fig. 1, the form that contains cysteine at residues 112 and 158.

As first demonstrated by Utermann and associates,[16] the lipid disorder type III hyperlipoproteinemia or familial dysbetalipoproteinemia is frequently associated with the E2/2 phenotype (for a review of type III hyperlipoproteinemia.[17] Briefly, the disorder is characterized by elevated plasma levels of cholesterol and triglyceride, typically each greater than 300 mg/dl. Subjects are frequently prone to premature atherosclerosis. The dyslipoproteinemia in these pa-

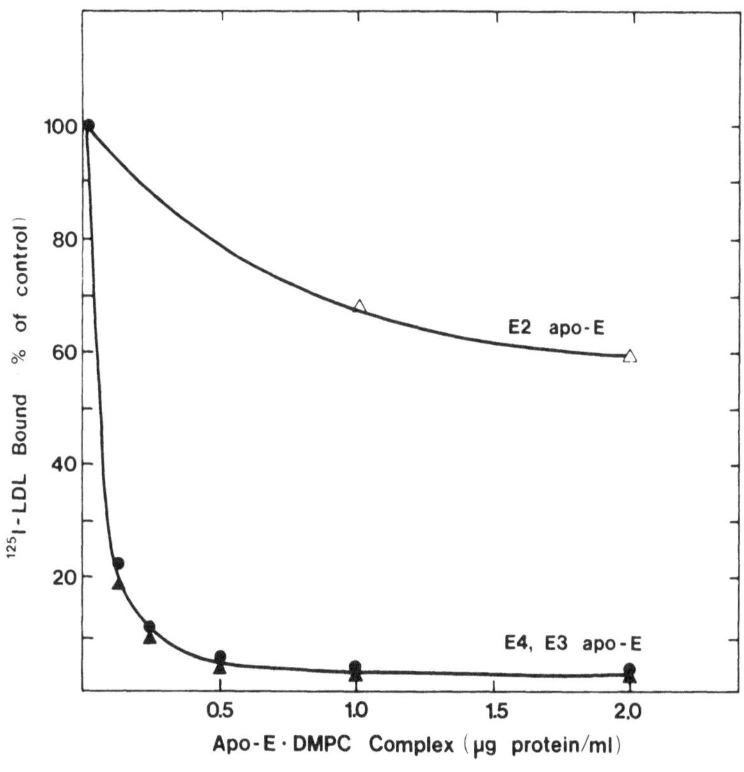

Fig. 2 Ability of various apo-E • DMPC recombinants to compete with ^{125}I-human LDL for binding to normal human fibroblasts at 4°C: apo-E2 (Δ), apo-E3 (▲), and apo-E4 (●). Permission granted from Weisgraber et al.[22]

tients is characterized by a plasma accumulation of β-VLDL, which are cholesterol-rich remnants of chylomicrons and hepatic VLDL.[18] A significant property of β-VLDL is their capability to cause massive cholesteryl ester accumulation in macrophages, which causes the macrophages to take on the appearance of foam cells.[19] Type III patients have lipid accumulation in a variety of tissues; most commonly, they display tubero-eruptive and planar xanthomas.[17]

The studies of Havel and associates using perfused rat livers[20] and Gregg and associates using in vivo experiments[21] suggested that the metabolism of apo-E2-containing lipoproteins was impaired relative to those containing apo-E3 and apo-E4. The implication was that a defect existed in the type III apo-E2, accounting for its retarded clearance, and that this dysfunction in E2 was responsible for the accumulation of lipoprotein remnants in these subjects. In a direct test of this hypothesis, advantage was taken of the structural information that was available concerning the apo-E isoforms; specifically, the effect that the cysteine-arginine interchanges had on receptor binding activity was studied.[22] The test system was fibroblast LDL receptors (apo-B,E receptors) and phospholipid recombinants of the three apo-E isoforms. As shown in Fig. 2, both apo-E3 and apo-E4 are equal and effective competitors against ^{125}I-human LDL for fibroblast binding sites. In marked contrast, the receptor binding activity of apo-E2 from a type III patient was significantly reduced (~1% of apo-E3 activity). These results demonstrated that the apo-E2 from a type III patient did have impaired receptor interaction and established that the cysteine-arginine interchange at residue 158 was the cause of this impaired activity. The cysteine-arginine interchange at residue 112, which occurs in E3 and E4 isoforms, does not affect receptor binding activity.

Schneider et al.[23] have demonstrated that there is a heterogeneity in the binding activity of apo-E2 from different type III subjects. The activities range from relatively inactive to moderately active. The structural basis for this binding heterogeneity has been determined to be the existence of additional apo-E structural variants, involving other sites and types of amino acid interchanges in the protein.[24-26] A summary of the current knowledge of structural variants and their receptor binding activities is presented in Table 1. The nomenclature used relates the variant structure to the structure of apo-E3, which is the most common or parent form of apo-E in human populations.[25] With this nomenclature, the focusing position on isoelectric focusing gels and the site and nature of the amino acid substitution are given. It is important to note that in all patients with type III hyperlipoproteinemia in which apo-E receptor binding activity has been determined, it has been established that the apo-E binding to fibroblast receptors was defective relative to normal binding activity.[22-26] Similar results have been obtained in studies examining the binding activity of the various structural forms of apo-E with hepatic apo-E receptors.[27]

TABLE 1

STRUCTURAL VARIANTS OF HUMAN Apo-E

AND THEIR BINDING ACTIVITY TO Apo-B,E RECEPTORS

Apo-E Variant		Binding Activity
Parent form:	apo-E3	normal
Variants:	apo-E4($Cys_{112} \rightarrow Arg$)	normal
	apo-E2($Arg_{158} \rightarrow Cys$)	severely defective
	apo-E2($Arg_{145} \rightarrow Cys$)	slightly defective
	apo-E2($Lys_{146} \rightarrow Gln$)	slightly defective
	apo-E3($Cys_{112} \rightarrow Arg$, $Arg_{142} \rightarrow Cys$)	moderately defective

The results from several screening studies of human populations show that frequency of the E2/2 phenotype is about 1%.[7,28-30] Yet, not all E2/2 subjects express clinical features of type III hyperlipoproteinemia. In fact, many E2/2 subjects have relatively low levels of plasma cholesterol. In light of the known heterogeneity in the E2/2 phenotype, the apparent question to be answered was: Do E2/2 subjects without hyperlipidemia have an apo-E2 that is different from previously determined structures, and is that apo-E functionally normal? When the apo-E2 from two hypocholesterolemic and two normocholesterolemic subjects were studied, they were found to have a severe binding defect suggesting that they were E2($Arg_{158} \rightarrow Cys$) forms. Sequence studies established that this was in fact the case.[31]

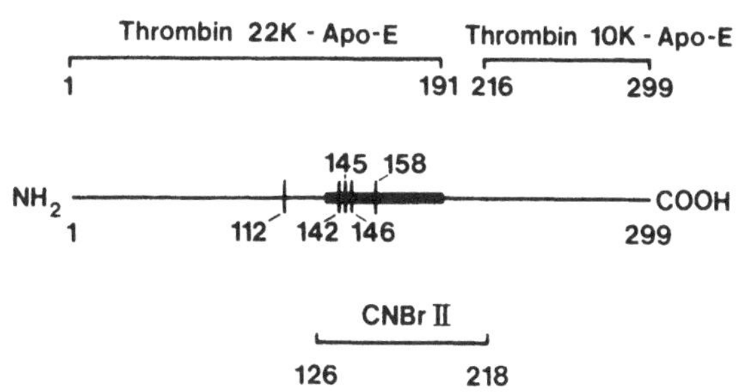

Fig. 3 Schematic representation of human apo-E3 and the major fragments of thrombin and cyanogen bromide digestion. Indicated on the center line are the known sites of amino acid substitution.

In summary, the molecular defect underlying type III hyperlipoproteinemia is the presence of a form of apo-E with defective receptor binding activity. This is consistent with the observation by Ghiselli and associates that apo-E deficient subjects express type III hyperlipoproteinemia.[32] However, the presence of a defective apo-E, while necessary, in itself is not sufficient for type III expression, at least in some cases. To explain the normo- and hypocholesterolemic subjects, one would have to conclude, as has been suggested by Utermann,[33] that other factors modulate the protein defect. These factors may be genetic in nature and may involve metabolic or hormonal influences. It is well known that type III subjects are very responsive to diet and drug therapy, and that obesity, hypothyroidism, diabetes, and age exacerbate the disease.

APOLIPOPROTEIN E RECEPTOR BINDING DOMAIN

Because of the importance of the interaction of apo-E with lipoprotein receptors,[11] it was of interest to determine the region of the molecule responsible for receptor binding. The results from the studies of the various structural forms of apo-E and their respective receptor binding activities provided some important clues.[22,24,25] A linear representation of the apo-E molecule is presented in the center of Fig. 3. Indicated on the diagram are known sites of amino acid substitution. As determined in Table 1, all but the substitution at residue 112 adversely affect receptor binding activity. These results would then indicate that the central portion of the apo-E molecule in the vicinity of residues 142 to 158 is involved in receptor binding.

A second approach that was used to determine the receptor binding site was to study the receptor binding activity of a series of apo-E3 fragments.[34] Two sets of fragments were used. The first set was generated by enzymatic digestion of apo-E with thrombin. As shown in Fig. 3, thrombin has a limited ability to digest apo-E, producing an NH_2-terminal fragment with an M_r of 22,000 (residues 1-191) and a COOH-terminal fragment with an M_r of 10,000 (residues 216-299).[34] When the fragments were combined with dimyristoylphosphatidylcholine (DMPC) and tested for receptor activity, only the NH_2-terminal fragment had activity. It possessed receptor binding activity equal to that of intact apo-E3 (Fig. 4).[34]

Cyanogen bromide fragments were the second series of apo-E3 fragments studied.[34] The four largest of the eight cyanogen bromide fragments of apo-E3 were combined with phospholipid and tested. The largest fragment, CNBrII (spanning residues 126-218), is depicted in Fig. 4. Only this fragment demonstrated significant receptor binding activity.[34] The results of the fragment binding studies indicated that the area highlighted in Fig. 3, which encompasses residues 126-191, contains the receptor binding region of apo-E. Note that this region includes the amino acid substitution sites known to affect receptor binding activity.

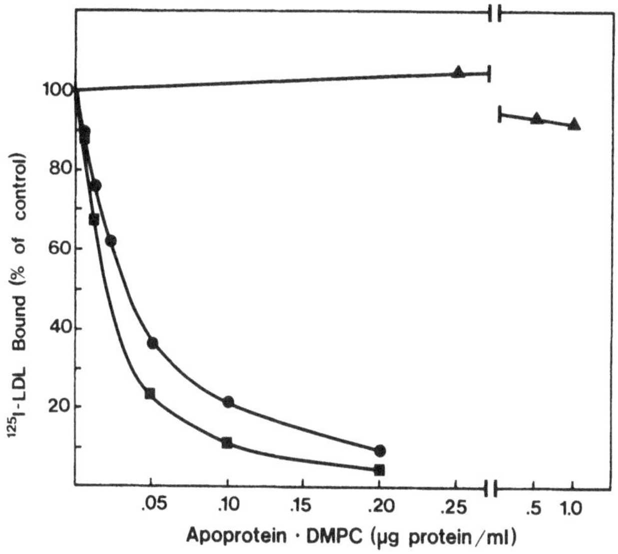

Fig. 4 Ability of intact apo-E3 and the two thrombolytic fragments to compete with ^{125}I-LDL for fibroblast receptors: apo-E3 (●), 22,000 M_r NH_2-terminal fragment (■), and 10,000 M_r COOH-terminal fragment (▲). Permission granted from Innerarity et al.[34]

A third approach used to delineate the binding region was the identification of an apo-E monoclonal antibody that inhibited receptor binding activity.[35] A basic assumption of this approach is that antibody binding in close proximity to or at the receptor recognition site will inhibit apo-E binding to the receptor, but binding to a noncritical region distant from the recognition site will not interfere with binding.

The five antibodies 1D7, 6C5, 3B7, 6H7, and 7C9 were preincubated with ^{125}I-apo-E•DMPC recombinants and their effect on apo-E receptor activity was tested with cultured fibroblasts.[35] As shown in Fig. 5, only one antibody, 1D7, had a significant inhibitory effect, blocking greater than 95% of the apo-E•DMPC binding activity.

The epitopes of the monoclonal antibodies were determined, using the apo-E3 fragments shown in Fig. 3 and a series of four synthetic fragments spanning various lengths of the apo-E sequence, beginning at residue 169 and ending at 148, 144, 139, and 129, respectively. The results from solid-phase radioimmunoassays are summarized in Table 2. The results from these binding assays narrowed the location of the 1D7 epitope to between residues 139-169. The other four monoclonal antibodies bound to the NH_2-terminal region of the pro-

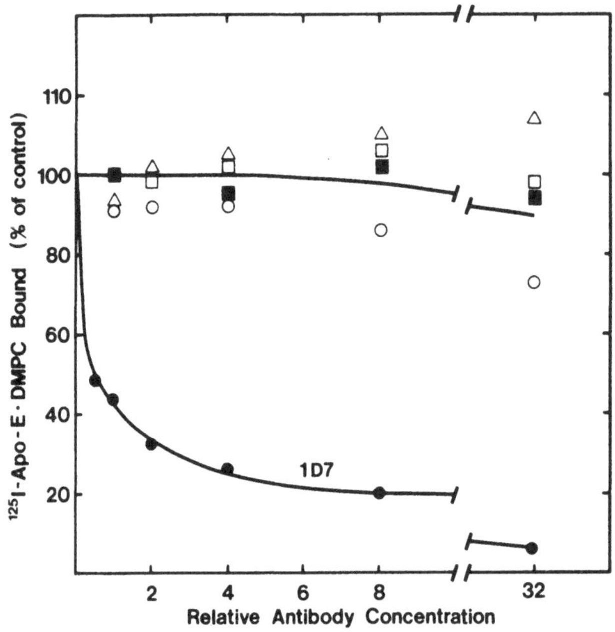

Fig. 5 Effect of apo-E monoclonal antibodies on ^{125}I-apo-E3 DMPC binding to normal human fibroblasts: 1D7 (●), 6C5 (O), 3B7 (■), 7C9 (□), and 6H7 (Δ). Permission granted from Weisgraber et al.[35]

tein between residues 1-126. The 1D7 epitope was further defined in solid-phase competition studies with several of the apo-E variants listed in Table 1. In these studies, the ability of the variants to compete with apo-E3 for binding to 1D7 was determined.[35] The results indicated that the amino acid substitutions at residues 142, 145 or 146 affected 1D7 interaction with apo-E3, but that the substitution at residue 158 did not. Taken together, the results of the fragment and competition studies indicate that the 1D7 epitope is in the vicinity of residues 140-150.

In conclusion, the results from three independent approaches that were used to determine the receptor binding domain of apo-E essentially give the same answer: The central region of the molecule is involved. A schematic representation of the predicted secondary structure of this region with the sites of amino acid interchange indicated by double amino acids is shown in Fig. 6. Beginning at residue 136 and extending to residue 158, the sequence is particularly enriched in basic amino acids. Previous results from chemical modification studies have suggested the importance of arginine and lysine residues in the receptor binding of apo-E.[36,37] In this regard, it is important to note that all of the substitutions that affect receptor binding activity involve lysine or arginine.

TABLE 2

BINDING OF Apo-E MONOCLONAL ANTIBODIES TO VARIOUS Apo-E3 FRAGMENTS

Apo-E3 Fragments	Antibodies				
	1D7	6C5	3B7	6H7	7C9
M_r-22K (residues 1-191)	+	+	+	+	+
M_r-10K (residues 216-299)	-	-	-	-	-
CNBrII (residues 126-218)	+	-	-	-	-
Residues 129-169	+				
Residues 139-169	+				
Residues 144-169	-				
Residues 148-169	-				

Figure 6 also illustrates that three of the interchange sites (residues 142, 145, and 146) occur in a predicted alpha helix and the fourth (residue 158) follows a beta turn that terminates the helix.

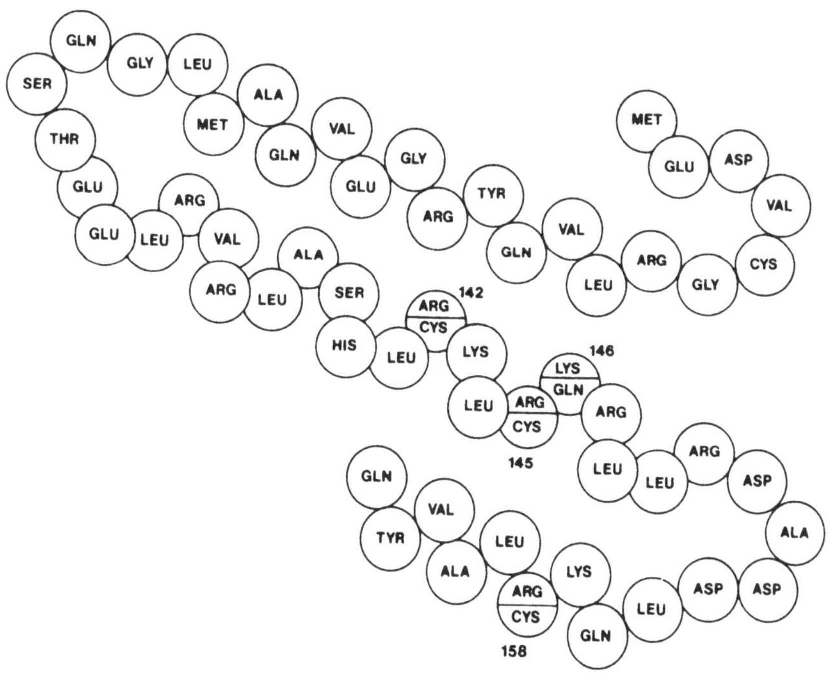

Fig. 6 Schematic representation of the predicted secondary structure of the receptor binding domain of apo-E.

SUMMARY

The E apoprotein plays a central role in lipoprotein metabolism. It is a key protein determinant responsible for the recognition of lipoproteins by specific lipoprotein receptors.[11] Structure-function studies are providing insights into the normal function of this apoprotein in cholesterol homeostasis and into the clinical abnormalities resulting from the occurrence of specific mutants.[17,38]

ABBREVIATIONS

Apolipoprotein E, apo-E; very low density lipoproteins, VLDL; high density lipoproteins, HDL; dimyristoylphosphatidycholine, DMPC.

ACKNOWLEDGMENTS

The authors wish to thank Barbara Allen and Russell Levine for editorial assistance, James Warger and Mark Sterne for the graphic arts, and Kerry Humphrey for manuscript preparation.

REFERENCES

1. V. G. Shore and B. Shore, Heterogeneity of human plasma very low density lipoproteins, Separation of species differing in protein components, Biochemistry 12:502-507 (1973).
2. F. A. Shelburne and S. H. Quarfordt, A new apoprotein of human plasma very low density lipoproteins, J. Biol. Chem. 249: 1428-1433 (1974).
3. R. W. Mahley, Alterations in plasma lipoproteins induced by cholesterol feeding in animals including man, in: "Disturbances in Lipid and Lipoprotein Metabolism," J. M. Dietschy, A. M. Gotto, Jr., and J. A. Ontko, eds., American Physiological Society, Bethesda, pp. 181-197 (1978).
4. K. H. Weisgraber and R. W. Mahley, Subfractionation of human high density lipoproteins by heparin-Sepharose affinity chromatography, J. Lipid Res. 21:316-325 (1980).
5. S. C. Rall, Jr., K. H. Weisgraber. and R. W. Mahley, Human apolipoprotein E, The complete amino acid sequence, J. Biol. Chem. 257:4171-4178 (1982).
6. G. Utermann, M. Hees, and A. Steinmetz, Polymorphism of apolipoprotein E and occurrence of dysbetalipoproteinemia in man, Nature 269:604-607 (1977).
7. V. I. Zannis and J. L. Breslow, Human very low density lipoprotein apolipoprotein E isoprotein polymorphism is explained by genetic variation and post-translational modification, Biochemistry 20:1033-1041 (1981).
8. K. H. Weisgraber, S. C. Rall, Jr., and R. W. Mahley, Human E

apoprotein heterogeneity, Cysteine-arginine interchanges in the amino acid sequence of the apo-E isoforms, J. Biol. Chem. 256:9077-9083 (1981).

9. V. I. Zannis, J. L. Breslow, G. Utermann, R. W. Mahley, K. H. Weisgraber, R. J. Havel, J. L. Goldstein, M. S. Brown, G. Schonfeld, W. R. Hazzard, and C. Blum, Proposed nomenclature of apo-E isoproteins, apo-E genotypes, and phenotypes, J. Lipid Res. 23:911-914 (1982).
10. T. L. Innerarity and R. W. Mahley, Enhanced binding by cultured human fibroblasts of apo-E-containing lipoproteins as compared with low density lipoproteins, Biochemistry 17:1440-1447 (1978).
11. R. W. Mahley and T. L. Innerarity, Lipoprotein receptors and cholesterol homeostasis, Biochim. Biophys. Acta 737:197-222 (1983).
12. B. C. Sherrill, T. L. Innerarity, and R. W. Mahley, Rapid hepatic clearance of the canine lipoproteins containing only the E apoprotein by a high affinity receptor, Identity with the chylomicron remnant transport process, J. Biol. Chem. 255: 1804-1807 (1980).
13. R. W. Mahley, Atherogenic hyperlipoproteinemia: the cellular and molecular biology of plasma lipoproteins altered by dietary fat and cholesterol, Med. Clin. North Am. 66:375-402 (1982).
14. R. W. Mahley, Development of accelerated atherosclerosis: concepts derived from cell biology and animal model studies, Arch. Pathol. Lab. Med. 107:393-399 (1983).
15. V. Gordon, T. L. Innerarity, and R. W. Mahley, Formation of cholesterol- and apo-E-enriched high density lipoproteins in vitro, J. Biol. Chem. 258:6202-6212 (1983).
16. G. Utermann, M. Jaeschke, and J. Menzel, Familial hyperlipoproteinemia type III: deficiency of a specific apolipoprotein (apo E-III) in the very low density lipoproteins, FEBS Lett. 56:352-355 (1975).
17. R. W. Mahley and B. Angelin, Type III hyperlipoproteinemia: recent insights into the genetic defect of familial dysbetalipoproteinemia, Adv. Intern. Med. 29:385-411 (1984).
18. M. Fainaru, R. W. Mahley, R. L. Hamilton, and T. L. Innerarity, Structural and metabolic heterogeneity of β-very low density lipoproteins from cholesterol-fed dogs and from humans with type III hyperlipoproteinemia, J. Lipid Res. 23:702-714 (1982).
19. J. L. Goldstein, Y. K. Ho, M. S. Brown, T. L. Innerarity, and R. W. Mahley, Cholesteryl ester accumulation in macrophages resulting from receptor-mediated uptake and degradation of hypercholesterolemic canine β-very low density lipoproteins, J. Biol. Chem. 255:1839-1848 (1980).
20. R. J. Havel, Y.-S. Chao, E. E. Windler, L. Kotite, and L. S. S. Guo, Isoprotein specificity in the hepatic uptake of apolipoprotein E and the pathogenesis of familial dysbetalipoproteinemia, Proc. Natl. Acad. Sci., U.S.A., 77:4349-4353 (1980).

21. R. E. Gregg, L. A. Zech, E. J. Schaefer, and H. B. Brewer, Jr., Type III hyperlipoproteinemia: defective metabolism of an abnormal apolipoprotein E, Science 211:584-585 (1981).
22. K. H. Weisgraber, T. L. Innerarity, and R. W. Mahley, Abnormal lipoprotein receptor-binding activity of the human E apoprotein due to cysteine-arginine interchange at a single site, J. Biol. Chem. 257:2518-2521 (1982).
23. W. J. Schneider, P. T. Kovanen, M. S. Brown, J. L. Goldstein, G. Utermann, W. Weber, R. J. Havel, L. Kotite, J. P. Kane, T. L. Innerarity, and R. W. Mahley, Familial dysbetalipoproteinemia, Abnormal binding of mutuant apoprotein E to low density lipoprotein receptors of human fibroblasts and membranes from liver and adrenal of rats, rabbits, and cows, J. Clin. Invest. 68:1075-1085 (1981).
24. S. C. Rall, Jr., K. H. Weisgraber, T. L. Innerarity, and R. W. Mahley, Structural basis for receptor binding heterogeneity of apolipoprotein E from type III hyperlipoproteinemic subjects, Proc. Natl. Acad. Sci., U.S.A., 79:4696-4700 (1982).
25. S. C. Rall, Jr., K. H. Weisgraber, T. L. Innerarity, T. P. Bersot, R. W. Mahley, and C. B. Blum, Identification of a new structural variant of human apolipoprotein E - E2(Lys$_{146}$ $\rightarrow$ Glyn) - in a type III hyperlipoproteinemic subject with the E3/2 phenotype, J. Clin. Invest. 72:1288-1297 (1983).
26. S. C. Rall, Jr., unpublished observation.
27. D. Y. Hui, T. L. Innerarity, and R. W. Mahley, Defective hepatic lipoprotein receptor binding of beta-very low density lipoproteins from type III hyperlipoproteinemic patients: importance of apolipoprotein E, J. Biol. Chem. 259:860-869 (1983).
28. G. Utermann, A. Steinmetz, and W. Weber, Genetic control of human apolipoprotein E polymorphism: comparison of one- and two-dimensional techniques of isoprotein analysis, Hum. Genet. 60:344-351 (1982).
29. R. J. Havel, Familial dysbetalipoproteinemia, Med. Clin. North Am. 66:441-454 (1982).
30. H.-J. Menzel, R.-G. Kladetzky, and G. Assmann, Apolipoprotein E polymorphism and coronary artery disease, Arterioscleroisis 3:310-315 (1983).
31. S. C. Rall, Jr., K. H. Weisgraber, T. L. Innerarity, R. W. Mahley, and G. Assmann, Identical structural and receptor binding defects in apolipoprotein E2 in hypo-, normo-, and hypercholesterolemic dysbetalipoproteinemia, J. Clin. Invest. 71:1023-1031 (1983).
32. G. Ghiselli, E. J. Schaefer, P. Gascon, and H. B. Brewer, Jr., Type III hyperlipoproteinemia associated with apolipoprotein E deficiency, Science 214:1239-1241 (1981).
33. G. Utermann, Apolipoprotein E: role in lipoprotein metabolism and pathophysiology of hyperlipoproteinemia type III, La Ricerca Clin. Lab. 12:23-33 (1982).
34. T. L. Innerarity, E. J. Friedlander, S. C. Rall, Jr., K. H. Weisgraber, and R. W. Mahley, The receptor binding domain of

human apolipoprotein E: binding of apolipoprotein E fragments, J. Biol. Chem. 258:12341-12347 (1983).

35. K. H. Weisgraber, T. L. Innerarity, K. J. Harder, R. W. Mahley, R. W. Milne, Y. L. Marcel, and J. T. Sparrow, The receptor binding domain of human apolipoprotein E: monoclonal antibody inhibition of binding, J. Biol. Chem. 258:12348-12354 (1983).

36. R. W. Mahley, T. L. Innerarity, R. E. Pitas, K. H. Weisgraber, J. H. Brown, and E. Gross, Inhibition of lipoprotein binding to cell surface receptors of fibroblasts following selective modification of arginyl residues in arginine-rich and B apoproteins, J. Biol. Chem. 252:7279-7287 (1977).

37. K. H. Weisgraber, T. L. Innerarity, and R. W. Mahley, Role of the lysine residues of plasma lipoproteins in high affinity binding to cell surface receptors on human fibroblasts, J. Biol. Chem. 253:9053-9062 (1978).

38. R. W. Mahley, Apolipoprotein E and cholesterol metabolism, Klin. Wochenschr. 61:225-232 (1983).

APOLIPOPROTEIN E MUTANTS, HYPERLIPIDEMIA AND ARTERIOSCLEROSIS

Gerd Utermann

Institut fuer Humangenetik und Genetische Poliklinik
der Philipps-Unversitaet
Marburg, Federal Republic of Germany

INTRODUCTION

A genetic polymorphism of apolipoprotein E was first described in 1977 and it was shown at that time that one phenotype in this genetic system is associated with primary dysbetalipoproteinemia.[1] It is now well established that genetic apo E polymorphism is under the control of 3 common alleles ($\Sigma 2$, $\Sigma 3$, $\Sigma 4$) at the apo E structural gene locus, that specify for isoforms E2, E3, and E4 and have frequencies of 0.077 ($\Sigma 2$), 0.773 ($\Sigma 3$) and 0.150 ($\Sigma 4$) in the German population.[2,3] Apo E2 and apo E4 differ from the parent apo E3 isoform by single cysteine for arginine interchanges at one of two positions in the primary structure: apo E2 ($Arg_{158} \longrightarrow Cys$) and apo E4 ($Cys_{112} \longrightarrow Arg$).[4,5] Examination of a DNA sequence that included the known apo E polymorphic sites showed that the mutant apo E phenotypes can be explained on the basis of a single base substitution in the first position of each of the respective codons.[6]

Recently additional rare apo E mutants have been identified that were designated E2* ($Arg_{145} \longrightarrow Cys$), E2** ($Lys_{146} \longrightarrow Gln$), E3-Leiden and E2-Damascus[7-9], G. Utermann, unpublished observations. The aminoacid interchanges in position 145($Arg \longrightarrow Cys$), 146($Lys \longrightarrow Gln$) and 158($Arg \longrightarrow Cys$) all result in E2 mutants that are functionally defective in that they display reduced binding activity to LDL(B/E)-receptors.[7,10,11] The most common E2 ($Arg_{158} \longrightarrow Cys$) mutant is however more severely defective (<2% of E3 control) in binding to the receptor than the other two E2 variants (about 40-50% of control E3). Homozygotes and compound heterozygotes for the E2 mutants accumulate remnants of triglyceride-rich lipoproteins in plasma, apparently due to the failure to catabolize these lipoproteins efficiently through receptor mediated endocytosis in the liver.[12,13] Despite the accumulation of cholesterol-rich remnants (beta-VLDL) in plasma, however, cholesterol levels are not increased in most E2 homozygotes but, on the contrary, are subnormal and especially LDL-cholesterol is greatly reduced in E-2/2 subjects.[1,14,15] Some E2 homozygotes do, however, develop severe type III hyperlipoproteinemia and there is evidence from the genetic and biochemical studies that additional independent factor(s) (genetic and/or environmental) operate in such patients.[14,16,17] Heterozygotes for the E2 isoform (phenotypes E-3/2 and -4/2) that comprise about 16% of the population on the average have plasma cholesterol, triglyceride, apo B and apo E levels that are intermediate between E2 homozygotes and individuals that lack an Σ2 allele[15,18], Utermann, unpublished results.

The higher frequency of a beta-VLDL subfraction in fasting plasma from E2 heterozygotes that is indicative for the presence of remnants in the postabsorptive state suggests that heterozygotes tend to a milder form of dysbetalipoproteinemia.[15] Since about half of the apo E in heterozygotes is a defective protein, they may be more prone to develop hyperlipidemia under certain circumstances.

The observations that apo E genes contribute to the normal variance of plasma lipid and apolipoprotein concentrations in the population and are associated with a specific form of hyperlipidemia suggests that they may also contribute to the genetic risk for arteriosclerosis.

RARE APO E MUTANTS

The presumably rare apo E2* ($Arg_{145} \longrightarrow Cys$) and apo E2** ($Lys_{146} \longrightarrow Gln$) isoforms are identical in charge with the common E2 ($Arg_{158} \longrightarrow Cys$) mutant. E3-Leiden has the same charge as the parent apo E3 isoform. Hence the common and rare isoforms cannot be distinguished by IEF or 2D-electrophoresis. All of the rare isoforms were distinguished from their common counterparts only by sequence analysis and/or binding properties to LDL(B/E)-receptors. These proteins were investigated in detail because they were found in patients with classical features of type III disease and it therefore was anticipated that the proteins might be abnormal. In population studies or in asymptomatic patients such mutants will however not be detected by present day screening methods. Therefore, the assumption that these mutants are rare is based on limited evidence and there are no data on their actual frequency in different populations.

We have recently shown that apo E2 ($Arg_{158} \longrightarrow Cys$) but not apo E2* ($Arg_{145} \longrightarrow Cys$) and apo E2** ($Lys_{146} \longrightarrow Gln$) exhibits anomalously slow mobility on SDS-polyacrylamide gels[19] resulting in an apparent M_r of apo E2 ($Arg_{158} \longrightarrow Cys$) that is about 1500 Daltons higher than that of the other isoforms (Fig. 1A). The defective binding of apo E2 ($Arg_{158} \longrightarrow Cys$) to LDL(B/E)-receptors and the anomalous behaviour in

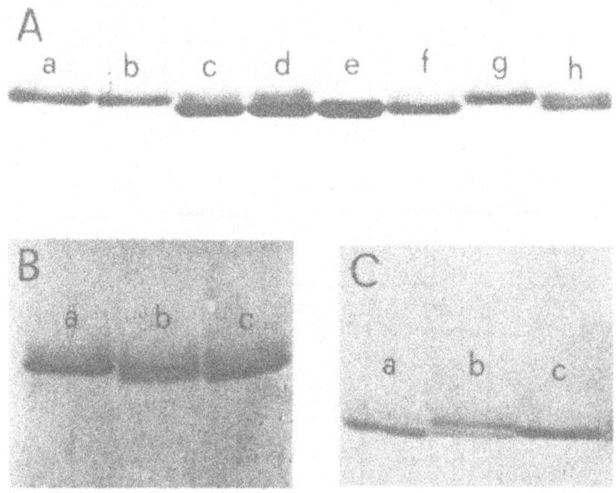

Fig. 1 SDS-polyacrylamide gels of the apo E from different patients with type III hyperlipoproteinemia and control subjects.

A: Lanes a and b: apo E-2/2 (Marburg), lane c: apo E-3/3 (San Francisco); lane d: apo E3 and E2 ($Lys_{146} \rightarrow Gln$) from patient D.F., who is heterozygous (E-3/2); lane e: isolated apo E2 from patient D.F.; lane f: apo E2 ($Arg_{145} \rightarrow Cys$) from patient W.M.; lane g: apo E2 ($Arg_{158} \rightarrow Cys$) from patient D.R.; lane h: apo E2 from patient J.T., who is heterozygous for E2 ($Arg_{158} \rightarrow Cys$) and E2 ($Arg_{145} \rightarrow Cys$).

B: Lane a: apo VLDL from an apo E2 ($Arg_{158} \rightarrow Cys$) homozygote; lane b: apo VLDL from apo E-3/2 heterozygote; lane c: apo VLDL from the E-2/2 subject (lane a) after treatment with (2-bromoethyl)-trimethyl-ammoniumbromide. Only the region of the gel in the vicinity of the apo E bands is shown.

C: Lane a: apo E-3/3; lane b: apo E-3/2; lane c: apo E-3/3 from patient C.V. (apo E3-Leiden).

SDS-polyacrylamide electrophoresis both can be partially or totally corrected by modification of the proteins cysteine residues to lysine analogues with cysteamine or to arginine analogues with (2-bromoethyl)-trimethylammoniumbromide (Fig. 1B)[11,19], U. Beisiegel, W. Weber, G. Utermann, unpublished results. Apo E3-Leiden, a mutant recently detected in a Dutch family with type III hyperlipoproteinemia also exhibits anomalous mobility in SDS-polyacrylamide gel electrophoresis. The mobility of this protein is intermediate between apo E2 ($Arg_{158} \rightarrow Cys$) and the other apo E isoforms (Fig. 1C). Notably the two apo E mutants that are most severely defective in binding to LDL (B/E)-receptors (E2 ($Arg_{158} \rightarrow Cys$) and E3-Leiden) at the same time exhibit anomalous mobility in SDS-polyacrylamide gel electrophoresis (Table 1).

TABLE 1

Apolipoprotein E Mutants[1]

Designation	Structure	Receptor binding	Migration im SDS	Association with HLP
E4	E 112 cys→arg	normal	normal	a) Type V b) Hypercholesterol-emia
E3	wild type	normal	normal	no
E3-Leiden	0 cys	severely reduced	abnormal	Type III
E2	E 158 arg→cys	severely reduced	abnormal	a) Type III b) Hypertriglycerid-emia
E2*	E 145 arg→cys	reduced	normal	Type III
E2**	E 146 lys→gln	reduced	normal	Type III
E2-Damascus-I	2 cys	reduced	normal	Type III
E2-Damascus-II	0 cys			

Data from Ref. 4,5,7-11,19 and U.Beisiegel, L.Havekes, G.Utermann, K.H.Weisgraber, unpublished results

Our observations have two implications: 1. The defective binding and abnormal behaviour in SDS of apo E isoforms E2 ($Arg_{158}\rightarrow Cys$) and E3-Leiden may be due to mutations at residues that critically influence the conformation of the apo E molecule. Physicochemical investigations are needed to test this hypothesis. 2. Our preliminary data on several further apo E mutants indicate that the altered mobility in SDS is limited to apo E2 ($Arg_{158}\rightarrow Cys$) and apo E3-Leiden[19], G. Utermann, K. H. Weisgraber, W. Weber, R. W. Mahley, unpublished results. Hence, SDS-polyacrylamide gel electrophoresis permits discrimination of the common E2 ($Arg_{158}\rightarrow Cys$) from other apo E2 variants by a simple technique.

SCREENING FOR APO E SUBTYPES AND FREQUENCIES OF RARE ISOFORMS

The mobility differences in SDS-polyacrylamide gel electrophoresis of apo E isoforms may be demonstrated with purified apo E, apo VLDL or apolipoproteins precipitated with heparin/Mg^{++}.[1] Hence, heparin/Mg^{++} precipitation of lipoproteins followed by electrophoresis in SDS may be used in addition to IEF as a complementary screening method for apo E isoforms (Fig. 2). The simultaneous application of both techniques permits distinction of 5 genetic apo E isoforms:

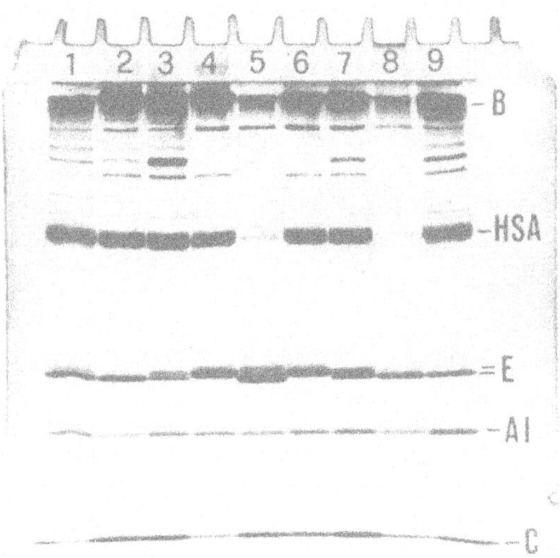

Fig. 2 SDS-polyacrylamide gel of apolipoproteins precipitated from individual human sera with heparin/Mg^{++}.[1] Lanes 1,2,8,9: apo E-3/3; lanes 3,7: apo E-3/2; lanes 4,5,6: apo E-2/2. Sample in lane 5 is from a Syrian patient (Y.N.) with type III HLP. Note that samples in lanes 4-6 were indistinguishable by electrofocusing.

TABLE 2

Apo E subtyping of 56 "E2 homozygotes"[1]

Group	N	Apo E-Subtype F/F	F/S	S/S
Hyperlipoproteinemia type III	39	3	-	36
Primary Dysbetalipoproteinemia	17	-	-	17

[1]Patients with type III HLP were it was known from sequence studies that an abnormal E2 isoform is present were not included

2-S (apo E $Arg_{158} \longrightarrow Cys$), 2-F (apo E $Arg_{145} \longrightarrow Cys$; apo E $Lys_{146} \longrightarrow Gln$), 3-F (the parent form), 3-I (E3-Leiden) and 4-F (E $Cys_{112} \longrightarrow Arg$)† and theoretically of 15 different apo E phenotypes. An important aspect of the SDS-PAGE method is that it permits detection of uncommon apo E phenotypes (see below).

The simultaneous determination of apo E phenotypes by IEF and SDS-PAGE in 472 unrelated German blood donors revealed that isoform E2-F is rare (frequency $\sim$ 0.001) and that isoform E3-I is very rare or absent in the German population (G. Utermann, unpublished).

RARE APO E MUTANTS AND GENETICS OF HYPERLIPOPROTEINEMIA TYPE III

A study of 56 individuals with the "homozygous" E-2/2 phenotype as defined by IEF supports the conclusion that isoforms E2* ($Arg_{145} \longrightarrow Cys$) and E2** ($Lys_{146} \longrightarrow Gln$) are rare in the German population. Fifty-three of these subjects exhibited the E2-S isoform upon SDS-PAGE and presumably are homozygous for the E2 ($Arg_{158} \longrightarrow Cys$) mutation (Table 2). These subjects included 36 with hyperlipoproteinemia type III and 17 with primary dysbetalipoproteinemia (normal or subnormal cholesterol levels). This suggests that structural differences between apo E2 and isoforms are not responsible for the differences in lipid levels and clinical symptoms

†We will use the preliminary phenotypic designations: S = slow mobility, F = fast mobility and I = intermediate mobility.

between these groups. This conclusion is in agreement with our previous genetic studies on type III hyperlipoproteinemia and emphasizes the importance of factors that are not related to the functional abnormality of apo E2 in the pathogenesis of the type III disorder.[14] Recently Rall et al.[17] obtained direct proof for the structural and functional identity of apo E in some homozygous E-2/2 subjects with different lipid levels, thus confirming our original genetic two-factor concept of type III HLP inheritance.[14,20,21]

APO E2-DAMASCUS

Three of the type III patients investigated were "homozygous" for the fast form of apo E2 (Table 2). A more detailed analysis of the E protein from one of these patients demonstrated an important aspect of the SDS-PAGE method: it permits detection of new unusual apo E phenotypes. This patient was of Syrian ancestry and had classcal features of HLP type III, including tuberous xanthomas at both elbows. Electrofocusing and 2D-electrophoresis both demonstrated the E-2/2 phenotype, but only the fast mobility form of apo E was seen on SDS-PAGE (Figs. 2,3).

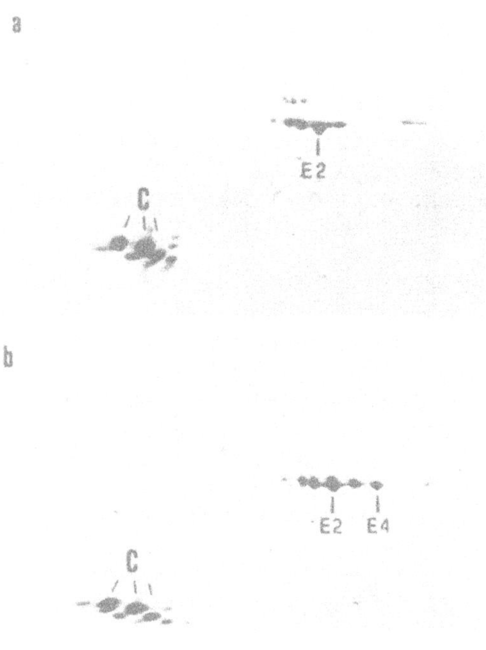

Fig. 3 2D-electrophoresis of apo VLDL from patient Y.N. with type III hyperlipoproteinemia (a) and of apo VLDL from the same patient after cysteamine modification (b).

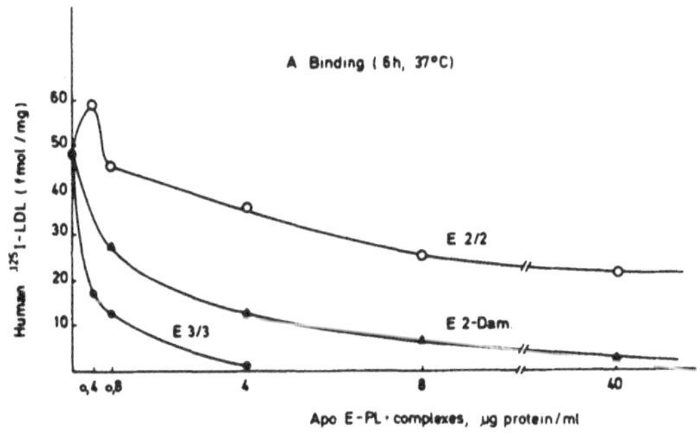

Fig. 4 Ability of apo E/phospholipid complexes from a control and patients with type III hyperlipoproteinemia to compete for binding of human ^{125}I-LDL to monolayers of HeLa cells. Apo E/egg lecithin complexes were prepared by a detergent dialysis method[10] (method A). The ^{125}I-LDL (62 cpm/mg protein) concentration was 10 µg/ml and the experiment was carried out for 6 hours at 37° C in 5% CO_2 atmosphere. The HeLa cells were grown in 10% human lipoprotein deficient serum for 48 hours in 24-well tissue culture plates. ●——● control apo E-3/3, O——O E-2/2 (slow mobility type in SDS-PAGE, compare Fig. 3, lanes 4,6) from patient B.K.; ▲——▲E-2/2 (fast mobility type in SDS-PAGE, compare Fig. 3, lane 5) from patient Y.N. (from U. Beisiegel, W. Weber, G. Utermann, in preparation).

The binding of the purified apo E from this patient to LDL(B/E)-receptors was reduced to about 50% of control apo E3. It was however not as severely defective as the common apo E2-S isoform from a patient with type III HLP (Fig. 4).

Treatment of the patients VLDL with the sulfhydryl reagent cysteamin[11] resulted in a shift of about half of the apo E2 to the E4 position (Fig. 3). This is consistent with the presence of 2 cysteine residues in this form of apo E2 that are converted to lysine analogues by the modification reaction. Another half of the patients apo E was however unaffected by the modification and presumably does not contain cysteine. Essentially identical results were obtained when the patients VLDL was modified with the sulfhydryl reagent (2-bromoethyl)-trimethylammoniumbromide (data not shown).

We conclude that the patient is a compound for two rare functionally defective apo E2 isoforms: one isoform containing 2 cys residues, that is however not identical with the E2 ($Arg_{158}\longrightarrow$Cys) mutant and one other isoform that does not contain cysteine and represents a novel rare apo E2 subtype.

APO E POLYMORPHISM AND HYPERLIPIDEMIA

An intriguing aspect of apo E polymorphism is its potential involvement in hyperlipidemia and atherosclerosis in the sense of a genetic risk factor. It is well established now from the investigations in several laboratories that most patients with type III hyperlipidemia have the homozygous E-2/2 phenotype as defined by IEF or 2D-electrophoresis.[22-28] As a consequence this phenotype can be utilized as a diagnostic marker for the type III disorder in patients with hyperlipidemia. Much less is known on the possible risk of heterozygotes for apo E2 or for homo- and heterozygotes for the E4 isoform to develop atherogenic forms of hyperlipidemia.

Ghiselli et al.[28] recently reported on a strong association of the apo E4 isoform with type V hyperlipidemia, but their findings were not confirmed by another group.[29] Apo E4 apparently is not deficient in binding to LDL(B/E)-receptors, and no other functional abnormalities of this isoform are known to date[11], U. Beisiegel and G. Utermann, unpublished results. Heterozygotes for the E2 isoform however have half of their apo E molecules in plasma lipoproteins in the form of a defective protein, and this may make them more prone to develop hyperlipidemia. In order to test this hypothesis we have determined the frequencies of the common apo E isoforms in 361 patients with hyperlipidemia (cholesterol > 280 mg/dl and/or triglyceride > 250 mg/dl) and compared to those in controls.[30] All available hyperlipidemic outpatients that were under the continuous care of the lipid ambulatory of the Department for Internal Medicine at the University of Marburg were included in this study. No selection according to lipoprotein phenotypes was performed.

This comparison demonstrated that the E2 isoform was significantly more frequent in the group of hyperlipidemics ($p < 0.0005$; Woolf procedure). This was however not due to a higher frequency of E2 homozygotes with type III HLP, but rather due to a significantly higher frequency of E2 heterozygotes in the patient groups ($p < 0.0005$, Tables 3,4).

Subgrouping of the hyperlipidemic patients into groups with pure hypertriglyceridemia, mixed hyperlipidemia (cholesterol and triglyceride elevated), and pure hypercholesterolemia revealed that (1.) isoform E2 was significantly more frequent in patients with hypertriglyceridemia ($0.001 > p > 0.005$), (2.) isoform E4 was significantly more frequent in patients with hypercholesterolemia ($0.01 > p > 0.005$) and (3.) isoforms E2 ($p < 0.005$) and E4 ($0.05 > p > 0.025$) were both more frequent in patients with mixed hyperlipidemia. Roughly 20% of patients with mixed hyperlipidemia had one of the rare phenotypes E-4/4, -4/2, or -2/2 and almost 50% of patients with pure hypercholesterolemia were homozygous or heterozygous for the allele $\Sigma 4$ (Table 3).

TABLE 3

Frequencies (%) of apo E phenotypes and genes in Hyperlipidemia

Apo E phenotype	HLP n=361	H-TG n=191	Mixed HLP n=130	H-CH n=40	B.D. n=1031
4/4	5.3	3.1	7.7	10.0	2.8
4/3	21.9	18.3	22.3	37.5	22.9
4/2	3.9	2.6	6.2	0	1.5
3/3	50.1	56.5	40.8	50.0	59.8
3/2	16.9	18.8	18.5	2.5	12.0
2/2	1.9	0.5	4.6	0	1.0
gene					
$\varepsilon 4$	0.181	0.136	0.219	0.288	0.150
$\varepsilon 3$	0.695	0.751	0.612	0.700	0.773
$\varepsilon 2$	0.123	0.113	0.169	0.013	0.077

HLP = total group of hyperlipidemics; H-TG = patients with pure hypertriglyceridemia; Mixed HLP = patients with elevation of cholesterol and triglyceride; H-CH = patients with pure hypercholesterolemia; B.D. = blood donors

TABLE 4

Relative risk for carriers of different apo E isoforms to develop hyperlipidemia

Isoform	HLP	H-TG	Mixed-HLP	H-CH
E 4	1.206	0.851	1.519***	2.427**
E 3	0.444*	0.825	0.244	0.498
E 2	1.740*	1.669**	2.445*	0.152

* $p < 0.0005$; ** $0.01 > p > 0.005$; *** $0.05 > p > 0.025$

As in our previous studies[14,22,23] all apo E2 homozygotes detected among hyperlipidemic subjects had features of hyperlipoproteinemia type III as defined by (1.) presence of beta-VLDL, (2.) a ratio of cholesterol/triglyceride in VLDL of > 0.42 and (3.) a density gradient ultracentrifugation profile of lipoproteins characterized by the presence of IDL and/or low LDL levels.

On the contrary E4 homozygous subjects did not present with a specific form of hyperlipidemia but exhibited phenotypes IIa, IIb, IV or V.

Previous studies have shown, that apo E-2/2 homozygotes invariably have primary dysbetalipoproteinemia and that some develop severe hyperlipoproteinemia type III. We now have obtained clear evidence for an association of apo E genes with hyperlipidemic states beyond the association of E2 homozygosity with the type III disorder. We conclude that alleles $\Sigma 2$ and $\Sigma 4$ both contribute to the susceptibility for and/or phenotypic expression of hyperlipidemia. Whereas the gene $\Sigma 2$ seems to exert its influence on plasma lipoproteins by an abnormal gene product (E2) that has reduced binding activity to lipoprotein receptors, the mechanism underlying the association of the $\Sigma 4$ gene with hyperlipidemia is presently unclear. Whatever the mechanism behind this association might be, it seems worth to be studied further by a combination of biochemical, metabolic, genetic, and epidemiological investigations.

APO E POLYMORPHISM AND ATHEROSCLEROSIS

The genetic polymorphism of apo E is the first example for a human gene locus that has a major effect on the normal variance of plasma lipid and apolipoprotein concentrations in human plasma and that moreover is associated with hyperlipidemic states. This suggests that this genetic system does also contribute to the genetic risk for atherosclerosis. We have attempted to prove this hypothesis by studying the apo E phenotype frequencies in 523 patients with myocardial infarction[31] (Table 5). This study however failed to support our hypothesis. No differences in the frequencies of E2 and E3 isoforms were observed between patients and controls. Surprisingly there was a lower frequency of the E4 isoform in the patients ($0.5 > p > 0.025$). This finding is opposite from what was expected and at present is unexplained. Notably there was no significant difference between patients and controls in the frequency of E2 homozygotes.

However, all 5 E2 homozygous survivors of myocardial infarction that were available for detailed analysis of plasma lipids and lipoproteins had hyperlipoproteinemia type III. One of the patients was always under drug therapy during this study but still had elevated triglyceride concentrations (cholesterol 229 mg/dl; triglyceride 283 mg/dl). In the four patients that were not under lipid lowering

TABLE 5

Apo E Phenotype and Gene Frequencies in Patients with Myocardial Infarction (M.I.) and Controls

Phenotype	Patients with M.I. n	%	Blood Donors n	%	
Apo E-4/4	12	2,3	29	2,8	
4/3	92	17,6	236	22,9	
4/2	11	2,1	15	1,5	χ^2_5 = 7,3731
3/3	333	63,7	617	59,8	0.2 > P > 0.1
3/2	68	13,0	124	12,0	
2/2	7	1,3	10	1,0	
Total	523		1031		
	$\varepsilon 4$ = 0.121 $\varepsilon 3$ = 0.790 $\varepsilon 2$ = 0.089		$\varepsilon 4$ = 0.150 $\varepsilon 3$ = 0.773 $\varepsilon 2$ = 0.077		

therapy, cholesterol levels ranged from 253-304 mg/dl and triglyceride from 311-587 mg/dl. All 5 E2 homozygous patients had beta-VLDL in fasting plasma, and density gradient ultracentrifugation revealed dysbetalipoproteinemia with elevated VLDL and IDL and low LDL concentrations. However none of the patients had xanthomas. The findings in the E2 homozygous survivors are in clear contrast to those in E-2/2 controls (Table 6). All E-2/2 controls of age > 40 years detected in proceeding studies had normal or subnormal plasma

TABLE 6

Plasma lipids (mg/dl) in E2/2 homozygous survivors of myocardial infarction and in E2/2 controls

	Myocardial Infarction N = 5	Control N = 11
Cholesterol	269 ± 29*	184 ± 28*
Triglyceride	419 ± 150*	151 ± 52*
Age (years)	54 ± 14	56 ± 13

* 0.005 > p > 0.002 by rank sum test

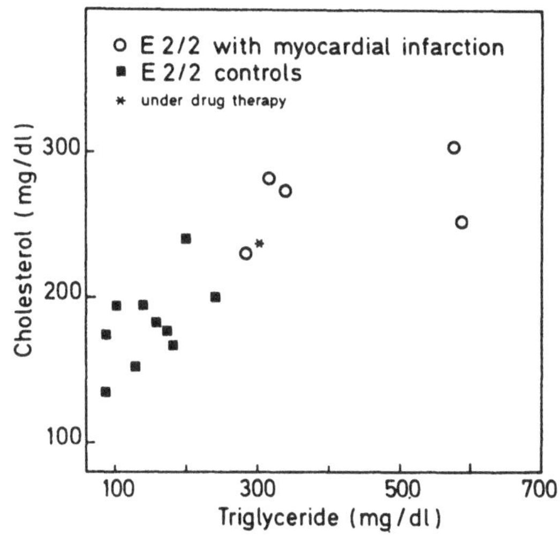

Fig. 5 Plasma lipid concentrations in E-2/2 homozygotes. For explanation see text.

cholesterol and only some had a mild elevation of plasma triglyceride.[31]

Thus, even though the frequency of E2 homozygotes in the group of myocardial infarction patients is not significantly higher than in controls, the E2 homozygous survivors are clearly different from the E-2/2 controls by means of their higher lipid levels. In fact, there was no overlap between these groups when both cholesterol and triglycerides were considered (Fig. 5). We conclude from these results that E2 homozygotes with hyperlipoproteinemia type III which are rare in the population are overrepresented in patients with myocardial infarction (frequency about 1/100). On the contrary, normolipidemic E2 homozygotes that have a frequency of 1% in the population were not observed in the patient groups. This suggests that uncomplicated E2 homozygosity may be a benefit rather than a risk for premature atherosclerosis. Hence it may be too simplistic an approach to determine apo E phenotype or gene frequencies in patients with coronary atherosclerosis in order to establish the postulated contribution of apo E genes to the risk for coronary artery disease. Considering the situation in the population one would expect that E-3/3, E-4/3 and E-4/4 subjects are overrepresented in the myocardial infarction patients due to their higher mean plasma cholesterol and apo E levels. From the association of the genes Σ2 and Σ4 with hyperlipidemia one would however predict a higher frequency of phenotypes E-2/2, -3/2, -4/2 and -4/4 in the patient groups. Such effects could partially counteract each other and result in an isoform frequency distribution that is not different from controls. Large studies on patients with atherosclerosis and unselected control groups that include determination of apo E phenotypes and lipid levels in all individuals are needed to test the hypothesis on the postulated contribution of apo E genes to the risk for atherosclerosis.

ABBREVIATIONS

IEF = Isoelectric focusing
SDS = Sodium dodecylsulfate
PAGE = Polyacrylamide gel electrophoresis
VLDL = Very low density lipoproteins
HLP = Hyperlipoproteinemia

REFERENCES

1. G. Utermann, M. Hees, and A. Steinmetz, Polymorphism of apolipoprotein E and occurrence of dysbetalipoproteinemia in man, Nature 269:604-607 (1977).
2. V. I. Zannis, P. W. Just, and J. L. Breslow, Human apolipoprotein E isoprotein subclasses are genetically determined, Am. J. Hum. Genet. 33:11-24 (1981).
3. G. Utermann, A. Steinmetz, and W. Weber, Genetic control of human apolipoprotein E polymorphism: Comparison of one- and two-dimensional techniques of isoprotein analysis, Hum. Genet. 60:344-351 (1982).
4. K. H. Weisgraber, S. C. Rall, Jr., and R. W. Mahley, Human E apolipoprotein heterogeneity: cysteine-arginine interchanges in the aminoacid sequence of the apo E isoforms, J. Biol. Chem. 256:9077-9081 (1981).
5. S. C. Rall, Jr., K. H. Weisgraber, and R. W. Mahley, Human apolipoprotein E: The complete amino acid sequence, J. Biol. Chem. 257:4171-4178 (1982).
6. J. L. Breslow, J. McPherson, A. L. Nussbaum, H. W. Williams, R. Lofquist-Kahl, S. K. Karathanasis, and V. I. Zannis, Identification and DNA sequence of a human apolipoprotein E cDNA clone, J. Biol. Chem. 257:14639-14641 (1982).
7. S. C. Rall, Jr., K. H. Weisgraber, T. L. Innerarity, and R. W. Mahley, Structural basis for receptor binding heterogeneity of apolipoprotein E from type III hyperlipoproteinemic subjects, Proc. Natl. Acad. Sci., U.S.A., 79:4696-4700 (1982).
8. S. C. Rall, Jr., K. H. Weisgraber, T. L. Innerarity, and R. Mahley, Structure and function of apolipoprotein E: Existence of multiple E2 alleles in type III hyperlipoproteinemia, in: "Proceedings from the International Symposium on Latent Dysbetalipoproteinemias and Atherosclerosis," J. L. de Gennes and R. Paoletti, ed., Raven Press, New York, In Press (1983).
9. L. M. Havekes, J. A. Gevers Leuven, E. van Corven, E. de Wit, and J. J. Emeis, Functionally inactive apolipoprotein E3 in

a type III hyperlipoproteinemic patient, Eur. J. Clin. Invest., In Press (1983).

10. W. J. Schneider, P. T. Kovanen, M. S. Brown, J. L. Goldstein, G. Utermannn, W. Weber, R. J. Havel, L. Kotite, J. P. Kane, T. L. Innerarity, and R. W. Mahley, Familial dysbetalipoproteinemia: Abnormal binding of mutant apolipoprotein E to LDL receptors of human fibroblasts and membranes from liver and adrenal of rats, rabbits, and cows, J. Clin. Invest. 68:1075-1085 (1981).
11. K. H. Weisgraber, T. L. Innerarity, and R. W. Mahley, Abnormal lipoprotein receptor-binding activity of the human E apoprotein due to cysteine-arginine interchange at a single site, J. Biol. Chem. 257:2518-2521 (1982).
12. R. J. Havel, Y. S. Chao, E. E. Windler, L. Kotite, and S. Guo, Isoprotein specifity in the hepatic uptake of apolipoprotein E and the pathogenesis of familial dysbetalipoproteinemia, Proc. Natl. Acad. Sci. USA 77:4349-4353 (1980).
13. R. E. Gregg, L. A. Zech, E. J. Schaefer, and H. B. Brewer, Jr., Type III hyperlipoproteinemia: Defective metabolism of an abnormal apolipoprotein E, Science 211:584-586 (1981).
14. G. Utermann, K. H. Vogelberg, A. Steinmetz, W. Schoenborn, N. Pruin, M. Jaeschke, M. Hees, and H. Canzler, Polymorphism of apolipoprotein E. II. Genetics of hyperlipoproteinemia type III, Clin. Genet. 15:37-62 (1977).
15. G. Utermann, N. Pruin, and A. Steinmetz, Polymorphism of apolipoprotein E. III. Effect of a single polymorphic gene locus on plasma lipid levels in man, Clin. Genet. 15:63-72 (1979).
16. W. R. Hazzard, G. R. Warnick, G. Utermann, and J. J. Albers, Genetic transmission of isoapolipoprotein E phenotypes in a large kindred: Relationship to dysbetalipoproteinemia and hyperlipidemia, Metabolism 30:79-88 (1981).
17. S. C. Rall, K. H. Weisgraber, T. L. Innerarity, R. W. Mahley, and G. Assmann, Identical structural and receptor binding defects in apolipoprotein E2 in hypo-, normo-, hypercholesterolemic dysbetalipoproteinemia, J. Clin. Invest. 71:1023-1031 (1983).
18. M. R. Wardell, P. A. Suckling, and E. D. Janus, Genetic variation in human apolipoprotein E., J. Lipid Res. 23:1174-1182 (1982).
19. G. Utermann, K. H. Weisgraber, W. Weber, and R. W. Mahley, Genetic polymorphism of apoliprotein E: Variable forms of apolipoprotein E2 distinguished on sodium dodecyl sulfate-polyacrylamide electrophoresis, manuscript submitted (1983).
20. G. Utermann, Apolipoprotein E: Role in lipoprotein metabolism and pathophysiology of hyperlipoproteinemia type III, La Ricerca in Clinica e in Laboratorio 12:23-33 (1982).
21. G. Utermann, Coronary heart disease, in: "Principles and Practice of Medical Genetics," A. E. H. Emery and D. L. Rimoin, eds., Churchill Livingstone Publ., Edinburgh, N.Y. (1983).
22. G. Utermann, M. Jaeschke, and J. Menzel, Familial hyperlipoproteinemia type III. Deficiency of a specific apolipoprotein

(Apo E-III) in the very low-density lipoproteins, FEBS-Letters 56:352-355 (1975).

23. G. Utermann, H. Canzler, M. Hees, M. Jaeschke, G. Muehlfellner, W. Schoenborn, K. H. Vogelberg, Studies on the metabolic defect in Broad- -disease (hyperlipoproteinemia type III), Clin. Genet. 12:139-154 (1977).

24. A. Pagnan, R. J. Havel, P. Kane, and L. Kotite, Characterization of human very low-density lipoproteins containing two electrophoretic populations: double pre-beta lipoproteinemia and primary dysbetalipoproteinemia, J. Lipid Res. 18:613-622 (1977).

25. J. L. Breslow, V. I. Zannis, T. R. San Giacomo, J. L. H. C. Thirs, T. Tracy, and C. J. Glueck, Studies of familial type III hyperlipoproteinemia using as a genetic marker the apo E phenotype E-2/2, J. Lipid Res. 23:1224-1235 (1982).

26. G. R. Warnick, C. Mayfield, J. J. Albers, and W. R. Hazzard, Gel isoelectric focusing method for specific diagnosis of familial hyperlipoproteinemia type III, Clin. Chem. 25:279-284 (1979).

27. W. S. Weidman, B. Suarez, J. M. Falko, J. L. Witzum, J. Kolar, M. Roben, and G. Schonfeld, Type III hyperlipoproteinemia: Development of a VLDL apo E gel isoelectric focusing technique and application in family studies, J. Lab. Clin. Med. 13:549-569 (1979).

28. G. Ghiselli, R. E. Gregg, L. A. Zech, E. J. Schaefer, and H. B. J. Brewer, Phenotype study of apolipoprotein E isoforms in hyperlipoproteinemic patients, Lancet I:405-407 (1982).

29. P. M. Stuyt, A. F. H. Stalenhoef, P. N. M. Demacker, and A. van't Laar, Hyperlipoproteinemia type V and apolipoprotein E4, Lancet, p. 934 (1982).

30. G. Utermann, H. Kaffarnik, and A. Steinmetz, Apolipoprotein E phenotypes in hyperlipidemia, Hum. Genet., In Press (1983).

31. G. Utermann, A. Hardewig, and F. Zimmer, Apo E phenotypes in patients with myocardial infarction, Hum. Genet., In Press (1983).

NONINVASIVE ASSESSMENT OF ATHEROSCLEROSIS IN NONHUMAN PRIMATES

M. Gene Bond, Sharon K. Wilmoth, Jean F. Gardin, Ralph W. Barnes, and Janet K. Sawyer

Departments of Comparative Medicine and Neurology
Bowman Gray School of Medicine of Wake Forest University
Winston-Salem, North Carolina 27103

ABSTRACT

Atherosclerosis is a progressive and degenerative disease of the artery wall which begins relatively early in life, years if not decades prior to the onset of clinical signs and symptoms. One of the major challenges which face investigators in this field of research is to establish the validity and reliability of noninvasive methods which can detect atherosclerotic plaques before they become severe enough to result in tissue ischemia, and to determine whether or not atherosclerotic lesions can be monitored both in terms of rate and direction over time. Although several methods of direct arterial visualization are available currently, high-resolution B-mode ultrasound imaging appears to have the most advantages. This technique is noninvasive, relatively inexpensive, and can visualize not only lumen contour and configuration, but also the atherosclerotic plaque in the underlying wall. Preliminary experiments in animal models suggest that lesions as small as 0.5 mm in the carotid arteries can be detected using this method. Whether or not atherosclerotic plaques can be monitored over time, however, has not been demonstrated.

INTRODUCTION

Atherosclerosis is a degenerative disease of the artery wall which has a predilection to occur at certain anatomic sites in the cardiovascular system. These sites include, but are not restricted to, the proximal segments of the three major coronary arteries, the distal common carotid artery, carotid artery bifurcation and proximal internal carotid artery, the abdominal aorta, and the iliac-femoral vessels of the lower extremity.

Large geographic based autopsy studies[1-3] have demonstrated clearly that focal accumulations of cholesterol, i.e., fatty dots and streaks, are present in the aorta and coronary arteries of some individuals by the end of the first decade of life, and further, these early changes become more diffuse through later decades. Atherosclerotic plaques are present in many individuals by the end of the third decade, and increase in extent, size, and complexity through subsequent decades. Unfortunately, a data base is not available currently which allows investigators insight into the development and natural history of atherosclerotic progression in the extracranial carotid arteries, or in the arteries supplying the lower extremity.

Although there is a general consensus among investigators that atherosclerotic plaques begin to evolve, at least in certain subjects, by the end of the third decade, these individuals are not generally recognized until the fifth and subsequent decades when the lesions become so severe that they result in clinically apparent signs or symptoms. At this time, based on examination of both autopsy and surgical specimens, the lesions may be considered end stage in terms of both size and tissue complications, such as necrosis, ulceration, mineralization, high-grade stenosis, etc.

There is an interval of years if not decades between atherogenesis and the occurrence of signs and symptoms. During this interval, plaques progress silently in terms of extent and severity. The identification of subjects with asymptomatic, preclinical stages of atherosclerosis, and the monitoring of the rate of change in the plaques of these individuals, remain one of the most important challenges which face investigators today. Arteriography, although an excellent method to detect atherosclerotic plaques which result in decreased lumen caliber, is not indicated in individuals who are without signs or symptoms of the disease, for the procedure is invasive, relatively expensive, requires hospitalization, involves dye injection and exposure to radiation, and also has a small but significant risk of mortality and morbidity. Digital intravenous subtraction angiography has several advantages when compared to routine arteriography, i.e., it is "relatively" less invasive, can be performed on an outpatient basis, etc. However, this method is not one at this time which can be used to scan large populations.

The method used most frequently during the past several decades to identify subjects who may have plaques has been to determine who is "at risk" for the disease. These traditional risk factors include a positive family history, hyperlipemia, hypertension, obesity, cigarette smoking, etc. "At risk," however, means that a subject with one or more of these characteristics has an increased <u>chance</u> of developing the clinical sequelae of atherosclerosis, e.g., angina, myocardial infarct, transient cerebral ischemic attacks, or stroke, but on an individual basis cannot define the stage of atherosclerosis development, the location of plaques nor whether these lesions are stable or are increasing in size or complexity.

Methods have been developed during the last two decades which allow for noninvasive arterial imaging of selected sites within the cardiovascular system.[4-10] Particularly, B-mode ultrasound imaging has been used to characterize advanced atherosclerotic lesions in the extracranial carotid arteries and in the abdominal aorta. B-mode ultrasound imaging has many advantages and some disadvantages when compared to traditional arteriographic procedures. The technique is noninvasive, relatively inexpensive, safe and can be used on an outpatient basis. The disadvantages are that it is a method which is best used for examining superficial vessels, such as common carotid arteries, carotid bifurcations, internal and external carotid arteries, abdominal aorta and the superficial arteries of the lower extremity. Deeper lying vessels, such as the coronary arteries, at present cannot be visualized because of their depth, intervening bone, and motion of the heart during the cardiac cycle. In addition, tortuous vessels and lesions that contain large amounts of mineral cannot, in general, be adequately visualized.

The majority of reported studies using B-mode ultrasound imaging procedures have been used almost exclusively in individuals who have severe and advanced atherosclerotic plaques.

Many previous studies have reported on the ability of B-mode ultrasound imaging techniques to visualize the extracranial carotid arteries in human subjects. Comerota[11,12] has reported on a comparative study of 884 vessels examined with B-mode ultrasound and arteriography. Accuracy of ultrasound when compared to arteriography was over 90% when scan quality was considered either good or excellent. The majority of discrepancies between the two methods were due to B-mode arteriogram mismatches, technically poor scans resulting from severe disease, interpretation errors, and plaques in the internal carotid artery that were too far distal to the carotid bifurcation to be visualized.

The sensitivity, specificity, accuracy, validity and reliability of B-mode ultrasound imaging of extracranial carotid arteries and vessels of the lower extremities is also being studied in a large United States Multicenter Trial for the Assessment of B-mode Ultrasound Imaging.[13] This study includes five clinical centers (Bowman Gray School of Medicine, New England Deaconess Hospital, Jefferson Medical Center, Miami Heart Institute and the University of Rochester), one animal ultrasound center (Bowman Gray School of Medicine) and a coordination center (Research Triangle Institute). Both blinded and randomized prospective studies are being done which compare data generated from B-mode ultrasound imaging with similar information from arteriograms, digital intravenous subtraction angiography, and from direct evaluation of carotid endarterectomy specimens. The human and animal ultrasound studies in this trial will be completed in 1984.

In a separate study, investigators at the Bowman Gray School of

Medicine have completed preliminary experiments on the ability of B-mode ultrasound techniques to detect very small lesions in the carotid arteries of nonhuman primates. The reasons for selecting nonhuman primate models for this research endeavor were twofold. First, nonhuman primates, when fed diets containing cholesterol, develop atherosclerotic plaques similar to those observed in human beings.[14-18] Second, these atherosclerotic plaques are small and are distributed in a way similar to those observed in human subjects. For these studies, we used a modified experimental 10 MHz ultrasound system (Horizons Research Laboratories, Inc., Fort Lauderdale, Florida) that was designed specifically to evaluate very small arterial structures. Adult male cynomolgus macaques (*Macaca fascicularis*) were fed an atherogenic diet which contained 1 mg cholesterol/Kcal with approximately 40% of calories from fat for 24 months. Prior to sacrifice, animals were anesthetized with Ketamine, positioned on a water-filled heating blanket, and the extracranial carotid arteries evaluated from multiple angles of interrogation. Instrument control settings were carefully monitored during the procedure and all measurements were made from freeze-frame video displays which were captured at peak systole. Total arterial wall thickness and plaque thickness were measured from near and far walls on longitudinal scans. In addition, lumen diameter was measured, using the same technique. Within three weeks of the ultrasound interrogation, the extracranial carotid arteries were evaluated with arteriography, and the animals killed immediately after that procedure. The cardiovascular system was flushed with phosphate buffer and pressure fixed *in situ* for 1 hour at each animal's systolic blood pressure. The arteriograms and pathology specimens are being evaluated, and therefore comparative data are not available at this time. Atherosclerotic plaques could be visualized in the common carotid arteries of many of these animals, using high-resolution, B-mode imaging. An example of a typical atherosclerotic plaque is presented in Fig. 1. This particular lesion was found in the distal left common carotid artery immediately proximal to the carotid bifurcation. The plaque, as expected, was circumferential and eccentric, being thicker on the far wall of the artery when compared to the near wall. The lesion on the far wall measured 0.5 mm in thickness, and gross examination of the fixed arterial tissue indicated a plaque was present at this site.

SUMMARY

Preliminary experiments on animal models of atherosclerosis indicate that very small arteries, similar in size to those found in newborn human infants, can be visualized, using high-resolution, B-mode ultrasound techniques. In addition, atherosclerotic plaques about 0.5 mm thick can be detected noninvasively in these arteries.

B-mode ultrasound imaging may well provide an important tool for recognizing specific individuals who are not only "at risk" for the

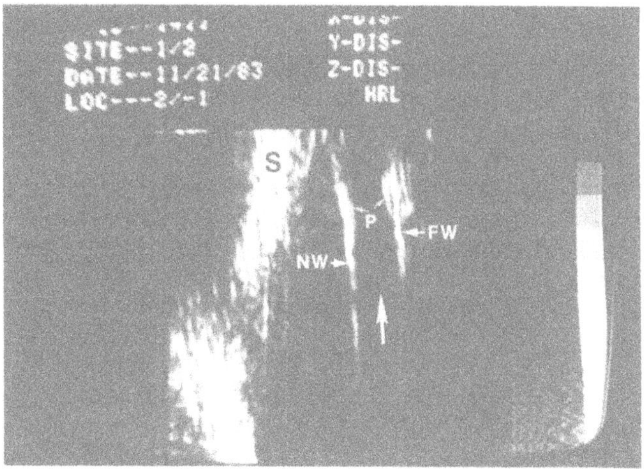

Fig. 1 Carotid artery atherosclerosis. Left distal common carotid artery, longitudinal anterior-oblique view. Skin surface (S) is on the left. Near wall (NW) and far wall (FW) are seen clearly. Arrow (↑) indicates direction of blood flow. A circumferential plaque (p) is present just proximal to the carotid bifurcation, and is thickest on the far wall. (Original magnification 8X).

disease, but more importantly, in recognizing subjects who have plaques at specific sites in the extracranial carotid arteries. In addition, this method may also provide a way in which both lesion thickness and lumen diameter changes can be monitored over time. The reliability and validity of ultrasound measurements, especially for the preclinical stages of atherosclerosis, as yet remains to be defined.

ACKNOWLEDGMENTS

The authors wish to acknowledge the encouragement of Thomas B. Clarkson, D.V.M., Director, Arteriosclerosis Research Center, Bowman Gray School of Medicine; James Martin, M.D., Director, Center for Medical Ultrasound, Bowman Gray School of Medicine; and James F. Toole, M.D., and William F. McKinney, M.D., Department of Neurology, Bowman Gray School of Medicine.

Financial support for these studies was provided by contracts through the National Heart, Lung, and Blood Institute HV-12902 and HV-12916. Additional support for the nonhuman primate studies was also generously provided by the Upjohn Company, Kalamazoo, Michigan.

REFERENCES

1. "The Geographic Pathology of Atherosclerosis," H. C. McGill, Jr., ed., Williams and Wilkins, Baltimore, Maryland (1968).
2. H. C. McGill, Jr., The geographic pathology of atherosclerosis, Lab. Invest. 18:463-467 (1968).
3. C. Tejada, J. P. Strong, M. R. Montenegro, C. Restrepo, L. A. Solberg, Distribution of coronary and aortic atherosclerosis by geographic location, race, and sex, Lab. Invest. 18:509-526 (1968).
4. C. P. Olinger, Ultrasonic carotid echoarteriography, Am. J. Roentgenol. Radium Ther. Nucl. Med. 106:282-295 (1969).
5. S. K. Blue, W. M. McKinney, R. W. Barnes, and J. F. Toole, Ultrasonic B-mode scanning for study of extracanial vascular disease, Neurology 22:1079-1085 (1969).
6. P. L. Cooperberg, W. D. Robertson, P. Fry, and V. Sweeney, High-resolution, real-time ultrasound of the carotid bifurcation, J. Clin. Ultrasound 7:13-17 (1979).
7. P. S. Green, Real-time, high-resolution ultrasonic carotid arteriography system, in: "Noninvasive Diagnostic Techniques in Vascular Disease," E. F. Bernstein, ed., C. V. Mosby Co., St. Louis, Missouri, pp. 29-39 (1978).
8. R. W. Hobson, M. D. Silvia, A. S. Katocs, J. A. O'Donnell, Z. Jamil, and P. Savitsky, Pulsed Doppler and real-time B-mode echo arteriography for noninvasive imaging of the extracranial arteries, Surgery 87:286-293 (1980).
9. P. R. Humber, G. R. Leopold, I. G. Wickbom, and E. F. Bernstein, Ultrasonic imaging of the carotid arterial system, Am. J. Surg. 140:199-202 (1980).
10. W. M. McKinney and G. J. Harpold, B-mode ultrasound interrogation of arteries, in: "Clinical Diagnosis of Atherosclerosis," G. M. Bond, W. Insull, S. Glagov, A. B. Chandler, and J. F. Cornhill, eds., Springer-Verlag, New York, pp. 173-188 (1983).
11. A. J. Comerota, J. J. Cranley, and S. E. Cooke, Real-time B-mode carotid imaging and diagnosis of cerebral vascular disease, Surgery 89:718-729 (1981).
12. A. J. Comerota, Correlation of B-mode ultrasound of the carotid artery with arteriography and pathology, in: "Clinical Diagnosis of Atherosclerosis," M. G. Bond, W. Insull, S. Glagov, A. B. Chandler, and J. F. Cornhill, eds., Springer-Verlag, New York, pp. 351-367 (1983).
13. J. F. Toole and A. Berson, Multicenter trial for assessment of B-mode ultrasound imaging, in: "Clinical Diagnosis of Atherosclerosis," M. G. Bond, W. Insull, S. Glagov, A. B. Chandler, and J. F. Cornhill, eds., Springer-Verlag, New York, pp. 389-397 (1983).

14. M. L. Armstrong and M. B. Megan, Responses of two macaque species to atherogenic diet and its withdrawal, in: "Atherosclerosis III. Proceedings of the Third International Symposium on Atherosclerosis," G. Schettler and A. Weizel, eds., Springer-Verlag, New York, pp. 336-338 (1974).
15. M. L. Armstrong and M. B. Megan, Arterial fibrous proteins in cynomolgus monkeys after atherogenic and regression diets, Circ. Res. 36:256-261 (1975).
16. W. Hollander, B. Kirkpatrick, and J. Paddock, Studies on the progression and regression of coronary and peripheral atherosclerosis in the cynomolgus monkey, 1. Effects of dipyridamole and aspirin, Exp. Mol. Pathol. 30:55-73 (1979).
17. D. Vesselinovitch and R. W. Wissler, Reversal of atherosclerosis: Comparison of nonhuman primate models, in: "Atherosclerosis V. Proceedings of the Fifth International Symposium on Atherosclerosis," A. M. Gotto, Jr., L. C. Smith, and B. Allen, eds., Springer-Verlag, New York, pp. 369-374 (1980).
18. D. M. Kramsch and W. Hollander, Occlusive atherosclerotic disease of the coronary arteries in monkey (Macaca irus) induced by diet, Exp. Mol. Pathol. 9:1-22 (1968).

NONINVASIVE ASSESSMENT OF ATHEROSCLEROSIS: STUDIES IN MAN

Robert J. Lusby

Department of Surgery, Clinical Sciences Building
Concord Hospital
Concord, New South Wales, Australia 2139

INTRODUCTION

Assessment of atherosclerosis using noninvasive techniques is performed in man in two main circumstances. Firstly, in the acutely symptomatic patient where the techniques enable diagnostic images and indices to be obtained. These provide objective data relating to the site and severity of disease and guide the physician in the choice of management. The second and perhaps more important application of these techniques is in the long-term assessment of patients. Most prospective trials of treatments aimed at retarding, preventing, bypassing or reversing disease progression have been conducted, using history and physical examination as the method of determining outcome. Noninvasive techniques now offer a means of quantitating the state of selected vessels and provide a safe and reliable means of repeating the studies and obtaining objective end points.

The morphology of lesions seen in atherosclerosis does not always correlate with symptoms.[1] The physiological data obtained from noninvasive testing has added new knowledge and raised many questions about our understanding of symptomatology and the significance of lesions. This paper outlines various applications of noninvasive testing with particular reference to cerebrovascular disease.

APPLICATIONS IN CEREBROVASCULAR DISEASE

In cerebrovascular disease where noninvasive tests have been intensively applied, the definition of what constitutes a clinically significant lesion remains to be determined. This is because the

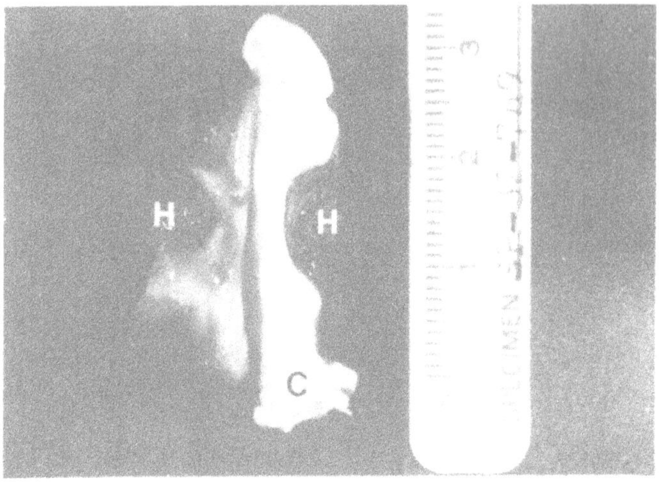

Fig. 1 Operative specimen obtained at carotid endarterectomy. A cast (C) made prior to opening shows the stenosis produced by the plaque haemorrhage (H).

mechanism whereby cerebral ischaemia is produced is incompletely understood. However a result of the widespread use of ultrasound and plethysmoraphic techniques has lead to a shift of emphasis from studies centered on highly stenotic lesions to the characterization of lesser lesions capable of producing emboli. The majority of patients with transient cerebral ischaemia have only moderate degrees of stenosis lying between 50 and 75% diameter reduction, and many have lesions of less than 50% stenosis.[2] There appears to be little difference if any between the type of neurological deficit and the degree of stenosis, adding weight to the embolic theory of symptom production. While these lesions may not be haemodynamically significant in terms of flow reduction, pressure drops or their ability to stimulate collateral flow, there are local pathological changes that may contribute to the production of symptoms. The development of hemorrhage within carotid atheromatous plaques (Fig. 1) with subsequent intimal thrombus formation and breakdown of the intimal surface is a prominent feature of these lesions.[2] Furthermore, embolic events associated with platelet, fibrin and thrombus deposits on the luminal surface are often seen in conjunction with recent intraplaque hemorrhage.[3-5]

The ability of ultrasound to image the tissues in the neck has become an important, noninvasive test. Currently, studies are being undertaken to determine the ability of ultrasound to detect the presence of intraplaque hemorrhage.

PERIORBITAL TESTS

The initial use of ultrasound in the detection of extracranial disease was in studies of periorbital blood flow changes based on the Doppler principle. The development of a directional Doppler ultrasound flow meter that displayed forward flow as an upward deflection and reverse flow as a downward deflection from the zero line allowed the display of flow direction in the collateral arteries to the brain. An unpredictable but definite redistribution of blood flow occurs in the presence of severe stenosis or occlusion in the carotid arteries.

The normal direction of flow is out of the orbit and onto the forehead. In the presence of disease in the internal carotid artery flow to the orbit may be reduced or reversed. This test of collateral flow is improved by the addition of compression manouvres[6,7] (Fig. 2). The test, while it detects up to 98% of lesions of greater than 50% diameter reduction, rarely detects more than 9% of lesser lesions. The highly specific test lacks the sensitivity for studies of lesser lesions. However in longitudinal studies it may serve as a marker for disease progression.

DOPPLER IMAGING

Hand-held Doppler flow meters can readily detect the movement of red blood cells in vessels. It is, however, often difficult to be certain which vessel is being examined in studies of the carotid

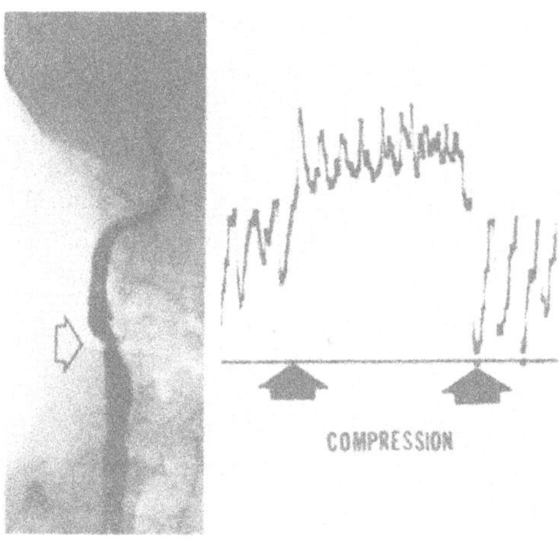

Fig. 2 Carotid angiogram showing high grade stenosis (open arrow). Tracing of suppraorbital Doppler signal shows reversal of direction on compression of the superficial temporal artery.

artery. Two-dimensional mapping of the moving column of blood has been developed to overcome this problem. Both continuous wave and pulsed Doppler systems may be used. In its simplest form, a Doppler imaging system consists of a continuous wave transducer, a storage monitor, and a probe position resolver. When a Doppler shift signal is detected, a bright spot, corresponding to the probe position at which the signal was detected, is stored on an oscilloscope. As the

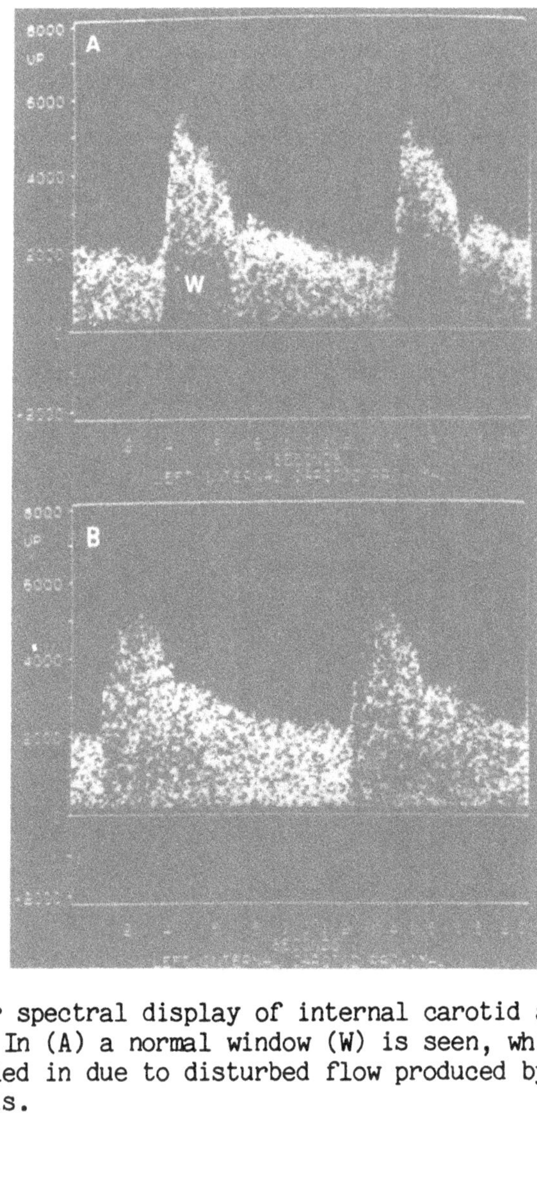

Fig. 3 Doppler spectral display of internal carotid artery blood flow. In (A) a normal window (W) is seen, while in (B) this is filled in due to disturbed flow produced by an arterial stenosis.

probe is moved back and forth across the skin and advanced up the neck, an image of the moving column of blood is generated. Errors in Doppler imaging have related to the single plane views obtained in many systems.[11,13] Computerized Doppler imaging has been developed to overcome some of these problems by simultaneously producing lateral and antero posterior images together with a histogram depicting cross-sectional area of the lumen at 1mm points along the vessel.[13]

DOPPLER FLOW STUDIES

Blood flow in the carotid artery can be detected with the Doppler probe and thus direct information can be obtained about changes in blood flow characteristics. Initial attempts at Doppler signal analysis looked at changes in the shape of the analog wave form obtained at sites proximal to, within and distal to bifurcation lesions. These tests proved impractical due to their inability to detect lesions of less than 50% diameter.

In the presence of stenosis the velocity of blood passing through the narrowed segment increases. This increase in velocity is detected by a change in the frequency of the Doppler shift signal. In addition energy changes occur as blood passes through the stenosis and encounters a segment of the vessel of wider diameter. Stored kinetic energy is dissipated in the form of disturbed blood flow or turbulance. Eddy currents and vorticles are produced which contain red blood cells moving in various directions with respect to the Doppler flow probe. The result is a broadening of the spectrum of frequencies detected as well as changes in the amplitude of the frequencies.

The changes outlined can be identified with the use of real time spectral analysers. The normal display (Fig. 3) shows a window of greater than 40% of the peak frequency. A window of less than 50% is consistent with mild disease, while complete filling in of the window is associated with severe stenosis. The severity of the stenosis is generally related to the peak frequency. An overall sensitivity of up to 98% has been reported for haemodynamically signinificant lesions with a sensitivty of 20% for those of less than 50% diameter reduction.[14,15]

DUPLEX SCANNING

Duplex scanning which combines real time B mode ultrasound imaging with Doppler signal analysis is the most advanced form of noninvasive testing used in the study of the carotid vessels. It is capable of producing information about the degree of luminal narrowing, changes in the velocity patterns and vessel wall composition. It can correctly identify the presence of disease in up to 97% of vessels, irrespective of the degree of luminal stenosis[15] (Fig. 4).

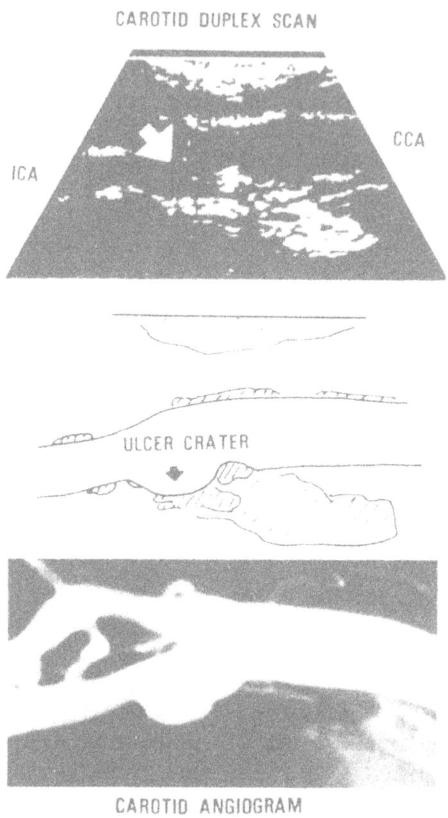

Fig. 4 Carotid duplex scan and angiography showing a non stenotic ulcerative lesion at the carotid bifurcation.

The ability of ultrasound imaging to determine plaque composition has only recently been determined.[16] The early results though encouraging have shown the need to obtain optimal imaging for proper assessment of lesions. The basic distinction is between two sonographic patterns of lesions - Heterogenous (Fig. 5) and Homogenous (Figs. 6 and 7). The heterogenous lesions demonstrate mixed high medium and low level echoes, often having areas within the lesion of the same echo genicity as blood. Pathological studies of these specimens show a close correlation between the heterogenous lesions and the presence of intraplaque haemorrhage. Up to 86% of such lesions contain intraplaque haemorrhage with the remainder being composed of mainly lipid and cholesterol. All ulcerated lesions in the study were found in the heterogenous group. Homogenous lesions are characterized by uniformly high or medium level echoes. High amplitude echoes with areas of acoustic shadowing correspond to calcifications.

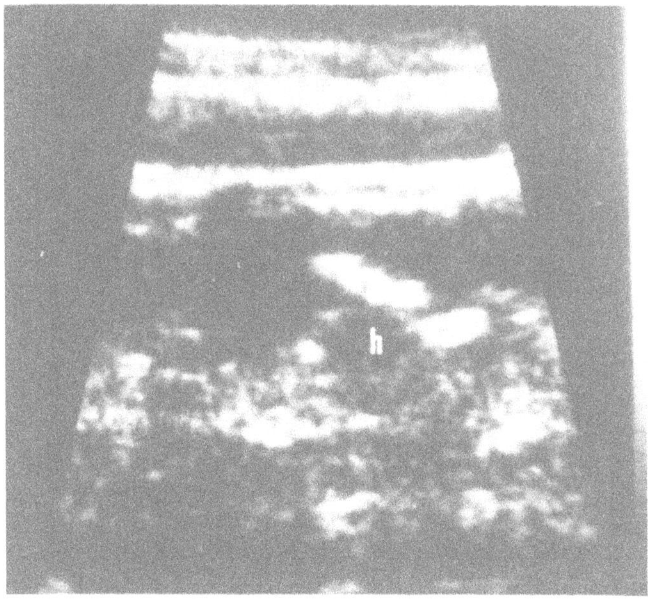

Fig. 5 Ultrasound image with a heterogenous lesion of the carotid artery showing various echogenic densities. Histopathology of the specimen revealed an intraplaque haemorrhage at site (H).

Pathologic studies of these lesions show a close correlation between homogenous ultrasound patterns and fibrous lesions, with no evidence of intraplaque haemorrhage.[16]

The clinical value of being able to distinguish between heterogenous and homogenous lesions lies in the fact that 91% of plaque haemorrhages and 100% of ulcerated lesions were in the heterogenous group. The increasing evidence linking plaque haemorrhage and symptomatic cerebral disease[2] and between ulceration and stroke[17] leads to the conclusion that the ultrasound characterization of plaque structure may be a significant step in determining clinically significantly disease.

OCULOPLETHYSMOGRAPHY

The first branch of the internal carotid artery is the opthalmic artery. A reduction in flow in the internal carotid artery due to stenosis is reflected in the pressure wave reaching the orbit. Two types of oculoplethysmographic (OPG) equipment to measure the orbital changes are currently in clinical use. The OPG-GEE[18] combines the principles of suction opthalodynamometry and oculoplethysmography.

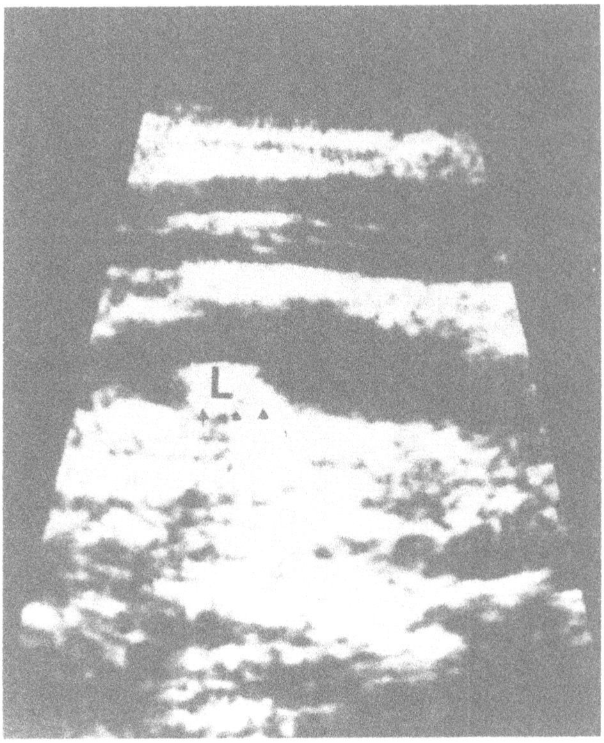

Fig. 6 Ultrasound image with a homogenous lesion of the carotid artery (L) protruding into the lumen.

It provides an objective method for simultaneous recording of the left and right opthalmic artery pressures. Air or fluid plethysmography cups can also be used to measure the delay in occular pulses relative to each other or to the ear pulses.[19] Up to 17% of asymptomatic patients with an abnormal OPG study will develop a stroke and 33% will have an episode of transient cerebral ischaemia. The presence of a normal OPG study carries a low 2% risk of stroke, indicating the value of this test as a predictor of stroke risk.[19,20] However, it is evident that many patients with stenotic lesions detected by OPG do not progress to stroke. Ultrasound imaging which can determine tissue characteristics of the plaques may play an important role in determining the at-risk subgroup of stenotic lesions. Studies are currently underway, evaluating the long-term clinical outcome of patients and the ability of both OPG and ultrasound imaging to predict stroke.

ARTERIAL DISEASE OF THE LIMBS

The early development of Doppler ultrasound techniques to deter-

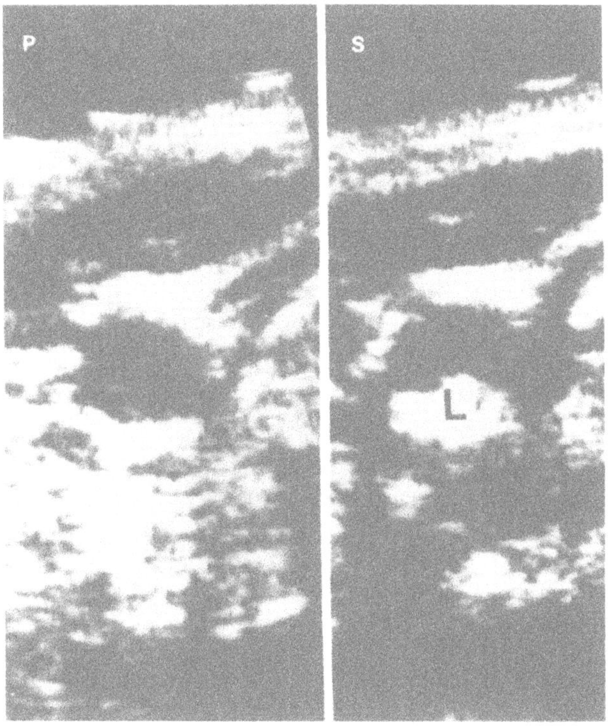

Fig. 7 Cross-sectional ultrasound images of the lesion in Fig. 6 image (P) is proximal to the stenosis, and image (S) is within the stenosis, and the lesion (L) is seen as a homogeneous lesion.

mine the arterial pressure in the lower limb at rest and following exercise, established the concept that the severity of haemodynamic disturbance produced by occlusive disease in the lower limbs correlates well with the severity of symptoms. The Doppler tests provide an accurate, objective method of evaluating symptoms beyond the morphological data provided by arteriography. The measurement of ankle blood pressure using the Doppler principle is perhaps the most widely used noninvasive test. It is simple, reliable, reproducible, accurate and available in most laboratories at low cost. The ankle brachial systolic index is perhaps the best known measure of functional impairment[21] with patients who claudicate having a mean index of 0.5 and those with rest pain generally having an index of less than 0.2. Normals have a resting index of greater than 0.95 and a post exercise index of greater than 0.8. Segmental limb Doppler pressures, when combined with segmental limb air plethysmography studies have been shown to improve this functional assessment, particularly in the diabetic patient, and both are now routinely performed in many vascular

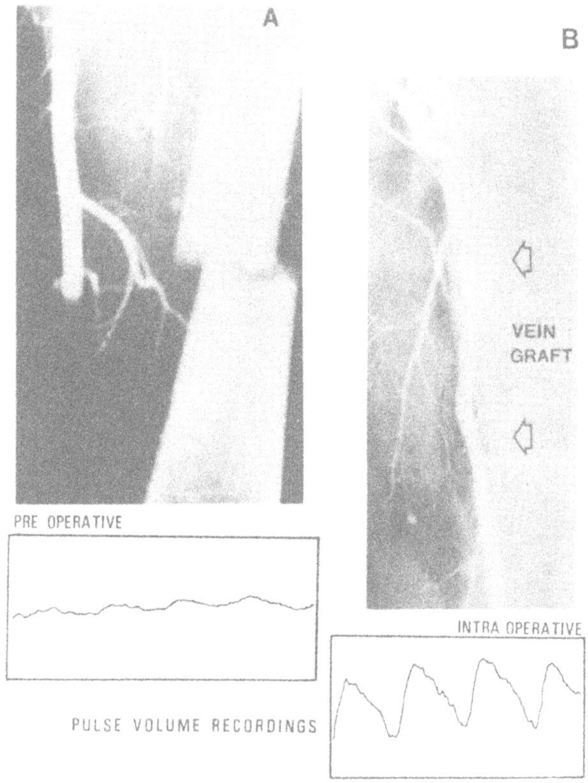

Fig. 8 (a) Angiogram showing occlusion of superficial femoral artery adjacent to a fracture of the femur. The pulse volume recorder (segmental air plethysmograph) shows reduced pressure/flow wave. This has improved in (b) following vein graft repair of damaged vessel.

laboratories. Knowledge of the location of functional stenosis is important in planning operative treatment. For example, in patients with altered penile function or impotence, Doppler pressure measurement may indicate the need to revascularize the pelvic vessels which would otherwise go untouched.[22]

Intraoperative monitoring of vascular reconstructions has played an important role in reducing the 6-20% incidence of early failure following arterial surgery. Segmental air plethysmography is a practical means of intraoperative monitoring providing a measure of limb perfusion distal to the level of the reconstruction (Fig. 8). It will reliably record, without delay, the improvement resulting from a reconstruction or the presence of a technical defect, allowing correction before the wound is closed. Postoperatively the response to surgery can be monitored frequently, accurately and objectively, both in the recovery room and upon return to the ward. Careful follow up after discharge from hospital using noninvasive tests can detect evidence of collateral development, disease progression or graft failure. Successful graft salvage can follow the early detection of graft stenosis or disease progression proximal or distal to a reconstruction.

More complex forms of noninvasive testing of limb blood flow are currently under development. Techniques include laplace waveform analysis of the femoral and distal vessel Doppler signal which offers information that relates to factors such as vessel stiffness, peripheral resistance and luminal stenosis.[24] Refinements of imaging techniques and Doppler signal analysis will help in obtaining the elusive goal of determining significance in a disease which affects various parts of the vasculature and appears by chance to manifest itself in any or all regions.

REFERENCES

1. R. J. Lusby, H. I. Machleder, W. Jeans, L. Ferrel, R. Skidmore, J. P. Woodcock, J. Sneeden, and R. N. Baird, Transient Ischemic Attacks: Characterization of Carotid Artery Morphology, Br. J. Surg. 69 (Suppl.) S41-44 (1982).
2. R. J. Lusby, L. D. Ferrell, W. K. Ehrenfeld, R. J. Stoney, and E. J. Wylie, Carotid plaque haemorrhage. Its Role in Production of Cerebral Ischaemia, Arch. Surg. 117:1479-8 (1982).
3. J. H. Edwards, I. I. Kricheff, F. Gorstein, T. S. Riles, and A. Imparato, Atherosclerotic Subintimal Haematoma of the Carotid Artery, Radiology 13:123-29 (1979).
4. A. Imparato, T. S. Riles, and F. Gorstein, The Carotid Bifurcation Plaque: Pathologic Findings Associated with Cerebral Ischaemia, Stroke 10:238-45 (1979).
5. T. S. Riles, F. G. Baumann, R. Mintzer, and A. M. Imparato, The Significance of Intramural Haemorrhage in the Carotid Bifurcation Plaque, Stroke 13:124 (1982).
6. E. C. Brockenbrough, Screening for the Prevention of Stroke: Use of a Doppler Flow Meter Information and Education Research Support Unit of Washington - Alaska RMP (monograph) (1969).
7. R. W. Barnes, H. E. Russel, G. E. Bone, and E. E. Slaymaker, Doppler Cerebrovascular Examination: Improved Results with Refinements in Technique, Stroke 8:468 (1977).
8. J. M. Reid and M. P. Spencer, Ultrasonic Doppler Technique for Imaging Blood Vessels, Science 176:1235-1236 (1972).
9. D. N. White and G. R. Curry, A Comparison of 424 Carotid Bifurcations Examined by Angiography and the Doppler Echoflow, Ultrasound in Medicine 4:363-376 (1978).
10. R. W. Barnes, G. E. Bone, J. Reinertson, E. E. Slaymaker, D. E. Hokanson, and D. E. Strandness, Jr., Noninvasive Ultrasonic Carotid Angiography: Prospective Validation by Contrast Arteriography, Surgery 80:328-335 (1976).

11. R. J. Lusby, J. P. Woodcock, R. Skidmore, W. D. Jeans, D. T. Hope, and R. N. Baird, Carotid Artery Disease: A Prospective Evaluation of Pulsed Doppler Imaging, Ultrasound in Med. and Biology, pp. 365-370 (1981).
12. D. S. Sumner, J. B. Russell, D. E. Ramsey, W. M. Hajjar, and R. D. Miles, Noninvasive Diagnosis of Extracranial Carotid Artery Disease. A Prospective Evaluation of Pulsed-Doppler Imaging and Oculoplethysmography, Arch. Surg. 114:1222-1229 (1979).
13. R. D. Miles, J. B. Russel, J. R. Modi, et al., Computerized Multiplanar Imaging and Lumen Area Plotting for Noninvasive Diagnosis of Carotid Artery Disease, Surgery 93:676-682 (1983).
14. W. Blackshear, D. J. Phillips, B. L. Thiele, et al., Detection of Carotid Occlusive Disease by Ultrasonic Imaging and Pulsed Doppler Spectrum Analysis, Surgery 86:698-706 (1979).
15. G. Fell, D. J. Phillips, P. M. Chikos, J. D. Harley, B. L. Thiele, and D. E. Strandness, Jr., Ultrasonic Duplex Scanning for Disease of the Carotid Artery, Circulation 64: 1191-95 (1981).
16. L. M. Reilly, R. J. Lusby, R. B. Jeffrey, et al., Carotid Plaque Histology Using Real Time Ultrasound. Clinical and Therapeutic Implications, Am. J. Surg., In Press (Aug. 1983).
17. R. J. Lusby, L. D. Ferrell, L. M. Reilly, et al., Stroke: The Significance of Carotid Plaque Haemorrhage with Ulceration, Stroke 14:133 (1983).
18. W. Gee, J. T. Mehigan, and E. J. Wylie, Measurement of Collateral Cerebral Hemisphere Blood Pressure by Ocular Pneumoplethysmography, Am. J. Surg. 130:121-126 (1975).
19. M. M. Kartchner and L. P. McRae, Noninvasive Evaluation and Management of the Asymptomatic Carotid Bruit, Surgery 82: 840-847 (1977).
20. R. N. Busuttil, J. D. Baker, R. K. Davidson, and H. I. Machleder, Carotid Artery Stenosis Haemodynamic Significance and Clinical Course, JAMA 245:1438-1441 (1981).
21. J. S. T. Yao, J. T. Hobbs, and W. T. Irvine, Ankle Systolic Pressure Meaurements in Arterial Disease Affecting the Lower Extremities, Br. J. Surg. 56:676 (1969).
22. J. S. T. Yao, W. R. Flinn, L. A. Queral, and J. J. Bergan, The Use of Doppler Ultrasound in Reconstructive Surgery, in: "Haemodynamics of the Limb I," P. Puel, H. Boccalon, and A. Enjalbert, eds., P563, Societe de la Imprimie Fournie, Toulouse (1979).
23. R. N. Baird, J. P. Woodcock, D. R. Bird, R. J. Lusby, P. W. Davies, and R. Skidmore, Doppler Analysis and the Progression of Arterial Disease, Proceedings of International Symposium on Smoking and Arterial Diseases, R. Greenhalgh, ed., Pitman Medica, pp. 135-141 (1981).
24. R. N. Baird, D. R. Bird, R. Skidmore, P. C. Clifford, and R. J. Lusby, Upstream Stenosis Diagnosed by Doppler Signals from the Common Femoral Artery, Arch. Surg. 115:1316-1322 (1980).

NONINVASIVE ATHEROSCLEROSIS ASSESSMENT FOR CONTROLLED CLINICAL TRIALS

David H. Blankenhorn

Professor of Medicine
University of Southern California School of Medicine
Los Angeles, California 90033

INTRODUCTION

A. Overview

Arterial measurement procedures which have proven useful in controlled clinical trials or show promise for early use in controlled trials will be discussed. Excluded from this discussion are many arterial evaluation procedures used primarily in clinical practice to explore symptoms and select patients for surgery. Procedures now used in clinical trials all provide an image of the vessel or its lumen. The current gold standard for *in vivo* morphometry is selective arterial angiography which is invasive, but is discussed as a basis for comparisonm with other methods. Nuclear magnetic resonance imaging, although not developed to a point where it appears useful in clinical trials, is mentioned because it offers the exciting possibility of both structural imaging and arterial wall metabolic function imaging.

The prime target vessels for controlled clinical trials are coronary arteries, coronary bypass grafts, and the arteries of the neck and lower extremity. All can be imaged with precision by selective arterial angiography, but have varying degrees of accessibility to non-invasive imaging. Table 1 presents the accessibility to imaging with B-mode ultrasound and intravenous (IV) digital subtraction angiography of these vessels.

B. Redundancy in Measurements of Atherosclerosis

In human coronary atherosclerosis, measurements of maximal steno-

TABLE 1

ACCESSIBILITY OF TARGET VESSELS FOR NON-INVASIVE IMAGING

	Vessel	Clinical Use	Controlled Trial
2-Dimensional Reflected Ultrasound:	Common Carotid	Yes	Potentially Possible
	Proximal Superficial Femoral	Yes	Will Need Improvement
	Distal Superficial Femoral	No	Not Currently Possible
Intravenous Digital Subtraction Angiography:	Common Carotid	Yes	Potentially Possible
	Vertebral	Yes	Potentially Possible
	Proximal Superficial Femoral	Yes	Potentially Possible
	Distal Superficial Femoral	Yes	Potentially Possible
	Coronary Bypass Grafts	Occasionally Useful	Will Need Improvement
	Coronary Arteries	No	Not Currently Possible

sis are highly correlated with measurements of percent intimal surface covered by raised lesions. This interesting example of redundant measurements came to light during a recent comparison of autopsy findings with risk factor data in the Framingham Study. Feinleib and associates wished to have microscopic measurements of cross-sectional

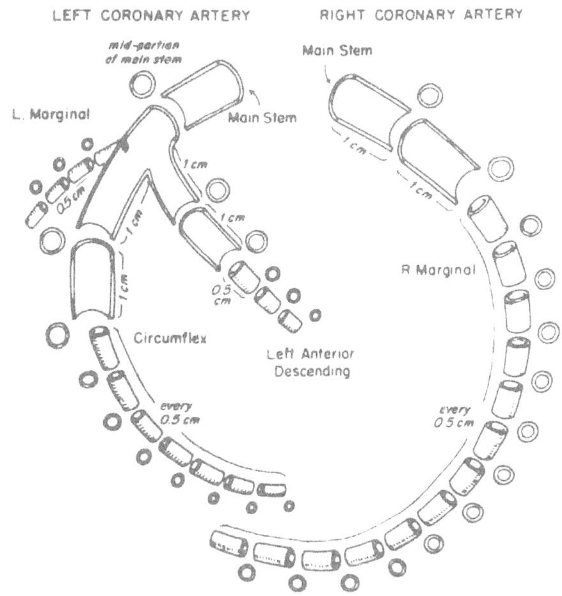

Fig. 1 Sampling procedures used by Feinleib; the coronary artery is cross-cut in areas alternating with segments opened longitudinally.

stenosis, plus simultaneous measurements of percent of inital surface covered by raised lesions in the same subjects.[1] They used the sampling procedure shown in Figure 1, where sections of coronary artery were cross-cut alternated with sections opened longitudinally. In 71 men, percent stenosis was significantly correlated, $r = 0.866$; $p < 0.001$ with percent intimal surface covered by raised lesions; in 54 women the correlation was $r = 0.897$; $p < 0.001$.

Because quantitative arterial imaging is inherently difficult it is important to recognize any aspects of atherosclerosis which offer potential advantage for precise measurements. One potential application of redundant measurements to atherosclerosis assessment in selective coronary angiography is illustrated in Figure 2, where the mid-section of a human right coronary artery is shown during computerized image processing. To estimate stenosis, computer generated edges in a narrowed area are compared with the width of a vessel in a more normal adjacent segment. However, in many coronary angiograms stenotic areas are eccentric and so the apparent degree of narrowing varies according to the angle of view. The currently accepted procedure is to obtain angiograms from a number of angles and take the view showing greatest narrowing as a best estimate. This approach fails when overlapping branches make the stenotic segment visible in only one view, a relatively common occurrence in the

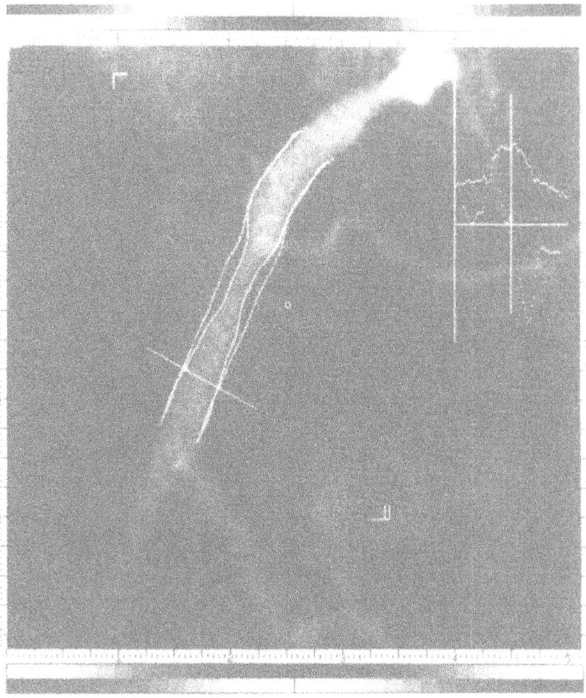

Fig. 2 Human coronary angiogram proximal right coronary artery. Computer generated edge points and "normal" vessel sleeve. At upper right, the vessel density profile and its derivative used for edge finding are shown. The computer generated line perpendicular to the vessel indicates the cross-section at which the vessel density profile is displayed at upper right.

left anterior descending coronary artery. In angiographic segments where stenosis measurements are difficult to obtain, an acceptable alternative may be to measure the length of vessel involved by roughness or narrowing.

The general approach of substituting length of vessel involvement for measures of narrowness may also be useful with ultrasound images. During ultrasound imaging the entire circumference of a vessel can be difficult to obtain in one view because blood within the vessel tends to act as a lens and focuses ultrasound energy away from parts of the vessel wall.[2]

C. Growth of Lesions Toward a Threshold

The essence of a controlled clinical trial based on atherosclerosis assessment is to detect an alteration of lesion growth rate and

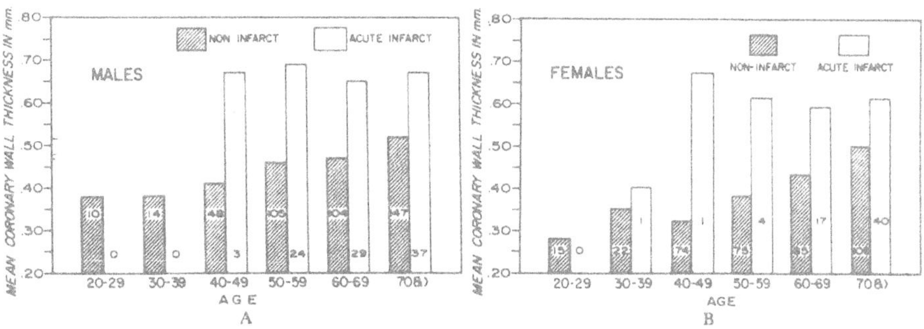

Fig. 3 Coronary arterial wall thickness measured by caliper in coronors' autopsies, as reported by Daoud and co-workers.

the concept that lesions grow toward a symptomatic threshold is helpful in estimating how much lesion growth must be retarded to confer benefit. There is extensive age specific autopsy data which indicates that the limit of coronary atherosclerosis tolerated by the heart of an average individual is reached when approximately 60 percent of the coronary intimal surface is covered by raised plaques. One of the early reports showing a threshold effect for coronary atherosclerosis was based upon coroners' autopsies in Albany, New York,[3] Figure 3. Daoud and coworkers were measuring the thickness of the wall of proximal portions of the coronary arteries. They found a steady increase with age in patients dying from causes other than myocardial infarction, but a constant degree of thickening, which did not change with age when death was due to myocardial infarction.

International Atherosclerosis Project (IAP) data show a similar threshold. The percent of intima covered by raised lesions was measured and a basal group dying of causes other than ischemic heart disease was compared with those dying of ischemic heart disease,[4] Table 2. Persons dying of ischemic heart disease in New Orleans and Oslo have 50-60 percent of the coronary intimal surface covered by raised lesions. Guatemala presents an exception; there is less atherosclerosis in all autopsies, and the threshold for ischemic heart disease appears to be lowered for reasons which are not clear.

The World Health Organization (WHO) Autopsy Study,[5] which included 17,455 autopsies, demonstrated an ischemic heart disease threshold remarkably similar to that reported in Oslo and New Orleans. Five communities (one in Sweden, one in Czechoslovakia, and three in Russia) were included because autopsy rates there were high; 77 percent for all individuals over ten years of age. The average percent of intimal thickening of those dying of ischemic heart disease is compared in Table 3 with a basal group who died of trauma.

Using WHO and IAP autopsy data, it is possible to estimate the

TABLE 2

MEAN PERCENTAGE OF INTIMAL SURFACE INVOLVED WITH RAISED ATHEROSCLEROTIC LESIONS (% RL) IN CORONARY ARTERIES

Location Race Group	Disease Group*	Age Group (% RL) (Years) 35-44	45-54	55-64	65-69
New Orleans	Basal	17	27	31	38
White	CHD	57	60	58	62
Oslo	Basal	16	25	32	38
	CHD	59	60	62	63
New Orleans	Basal	10	18	25	30
Black	CHD	48	58	52	59
Guatemala	Basal	3	5	9	11
	CHD	45	38	30	45

*The basal group contained persons who died of accidental causes or causes not associated with atherosclerosis. The CHD group contained persons whose cause of death was coronary heart disease.

The data are from the International Atherosclerosis Project (J. P. Strong, L. A. Solberg, and C. Restrepo, Atherosclerosis in persons with coronary heart disease, Lab. Invest. 18:527-537, 1968).

difference in average yearly growth rate of atherosclerosis after age 20 in a group of individuals destined to die of ischemic heart disease as opposed to those who will not die of ischemic heart disease. This difference in rate sets a target for the amount of change required if the benefit desired from therapy for atherosclerosis is to delay the onset of ischemic heart disease by retarding lesion growth. Both WHO and IAP data indicates that in developed countries the ischemic heart disease threshold is crossed when approximately 60 percent of the intimal surface is covered by raised lesions. Table 3 indicates that at age 20, the average male has only 1 to 2 percent intimal surface covered by raised lesions. If the average male begins at age 20 to cover 3 percent of intimal surface with new lesions each year, he will reach 60 percent coverage at age 40. If this growth rate is 1.5 percent per year, 60 percent coverage will not occur until age 60. If the growth rate is 1 percent per year, the threshold will not be crossed until age 80. These calculations are simplified by assuming linear growth rates for atherosclerosis, but the results are not

TABLE 3

WHO AUTOPSY DATA PERCENT OF INTIMAL SURFACE COVERED BY RAISED LESIONS

Age	Low Atherosclerosis Group Men	Low Atherosclerosis Group Women	Myocardial Infarction Group Men	Myocardial Infarction Group Women
25	2.6	--	--	--
35	8.8	3.1	43	--
45	17	6.9	53	34
55	30	16	58	55
65	32	27	62	58
75	42	37	64	63
85	45	48	63	65

greatly different if curvelinear functions, such as those published by Solberg and Strong[4] from IAP data are used.

REQUIREMENTS FOR MEASUREMENTS USED IN CLINICAL TRIALS

If some therapy did, indeed, cause 1.5 percent or 2 percent per year difference in atherosclerosis growth rate between a treated and control group, could this be detected in a clinical trial of reasonable size? The answer is yes, if lesions are measured by selective

TABLE 4

THE PROBABILITY OF DETECTING A TRUE DIFFERENCE BETWEEN TEST AND CONTROL GROUPS AT A 5 PERCENT LEVEL OF SIGNIFICANCE

Difference	Years Between Angiograms 1	2	3	4
1.5		0.780	0.822	0.838
2.0	0.815	0.955	0.973	0.977
2.5	0.951	0.995	0.998	0.998
3.0	0.991			
3.5	0.999			

TABLE 5

COMPARATIVE ERROR, ARTERIAL AND VENOUS INJECTION,

CAROTID ANGIOGRAMS IN FOUR DOGS

	1	2	3	4	Avg.
Arterial Injection	1.0	1.0	1.0	1.0	1.0
Venous Injection	2.3	3.2	4.5	2.9	3.2
Venous Injection with Frame to Frame Averaging	1.7	2.6	3.0	1.8	2.2

angiography.[6] Table 4 indicates the chances of detecting (at the 5 percent level of significance) a true difference between test and control groups, each containing 120 subjects with selective angiography. These calculations assume an approximate 4 percent error in stenosis measurement by selective arterial angiography. Table 4 clearly indicates the rationale for testing therapy which is sufficiently aggressive that a reasonably large change in atheroma growth rate can be expected.

NON-INVASIVE IMAGING WITH POTENTIAL FOR CONTROLLED CLINICAL TRIALS

A comparison of IV angiography and selective arterial angiography in the common carotid artery, Table 5, indicates that the error of IV angiography is approximately twice that of selective angiography. This study was performed in our laboratory and employed film to record the angiogram after both IV and selective arterial injection. The images were later digitized and the IV angiograms enhanced by image averaging.[7] In clinical practice IV angiography is carried out somewhat differently, and the images are processed by computer directly from an image intensifier. Data in Table 5 suggest that a controlled clinical trial substituting IV angiography for selective angiography would be feasible, but but would require an increase in the number of subjects required. However, the effective magnitude of difference in atherosclerosis change rate between test and control groups, would remain the predominant factor in determining the power of such a trial.

Ultrasound B-mode imaging is another non-invasive procedure with potential for early use in clinical trials. The instruments in current use employ ultrasound frequencies ranging from 3.5 to 5.0 MHz for cardiac scanning and 5.0 to 11.0 MHz for carotid scanning. The

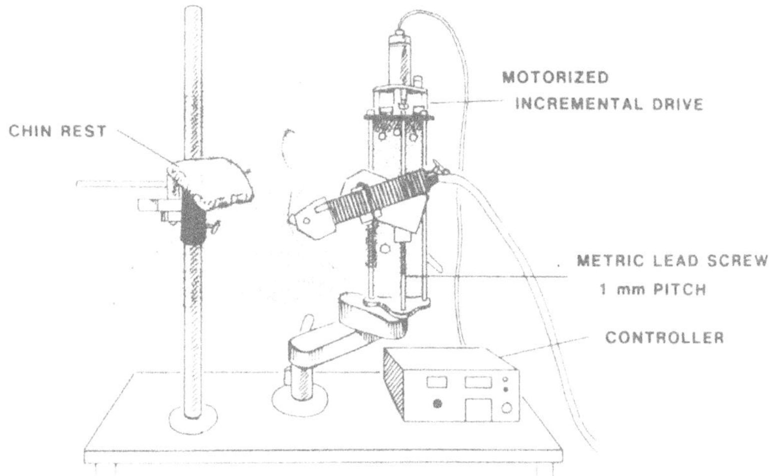

Fig. 4 Mechanical positioner for ultrasound scanning. The head is advanced at 0.2 mm. intervals by a motorized drive as parallel planes are recorded.

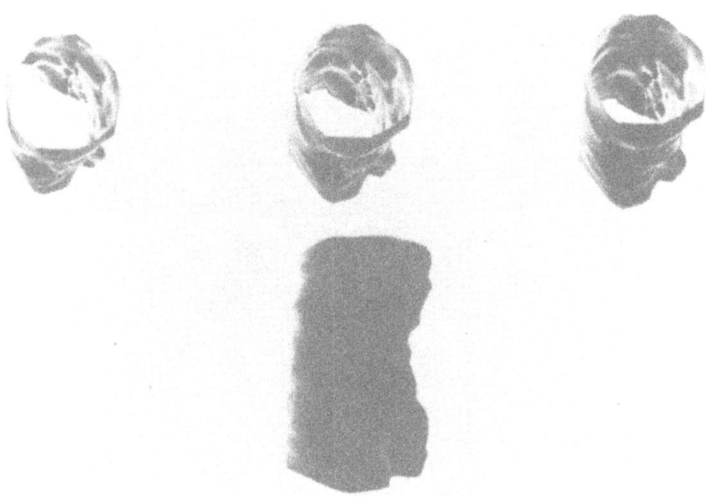

Fig. 5 Three-dimensional reconstruction of ultrasound images obtained with the positioning head. The construction is of a hollow cast covering the intimal surface viewed from the outside or at various angles looking through the cast. The carotid bifurcation is at the bottom of the construction.

production of high resolution images requires the use of high frequency ultrasound which penetrates tissues poorly and can be used only to study vessels lying close to the skin. Highest resolution is obtained when ultrasound travels the shortest axial path between transducer and target vessel and the precision of measurement obtained from this shortest path can be approximately twice that obtained from longer paths. One procedure to optimize the quality of ultrasound measurements is to move the ultrasound head into several stations around the vessel and make measurements only on energy traveling perpendicular to the vessel. A mechanical positioner constructed at the University of Southern California which now is being used for preliminary tests of this approach (Figure 4) produces a series of vessel images in parallel planes. A computer produced three-dimensional reconstruction of one human carotid artery using this positioner is shown in Figure 5.

Computerized axial tomography, nuclear magnetic resonance imaging, and digital subtraction angiography have all been shown to pro-

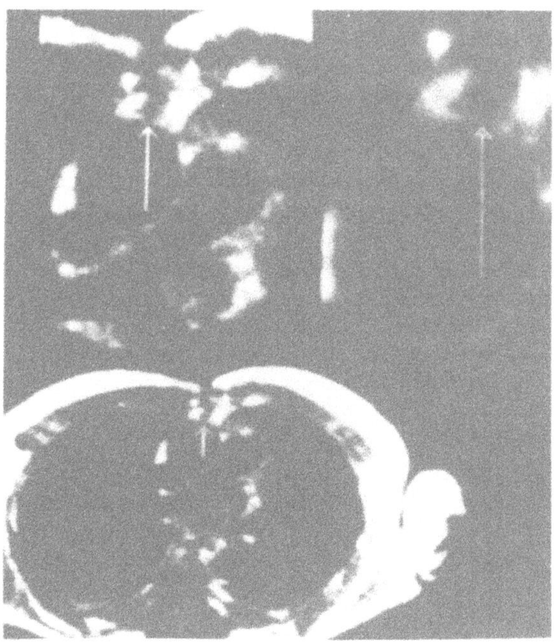

Fig. 6 Nuclear magnetic resonance image transverse section through the thorax of a patient after coronary bypass (arrow). The illustration shows origin from the aorta at three magnifications, as reported by Herfkens and co-workers.

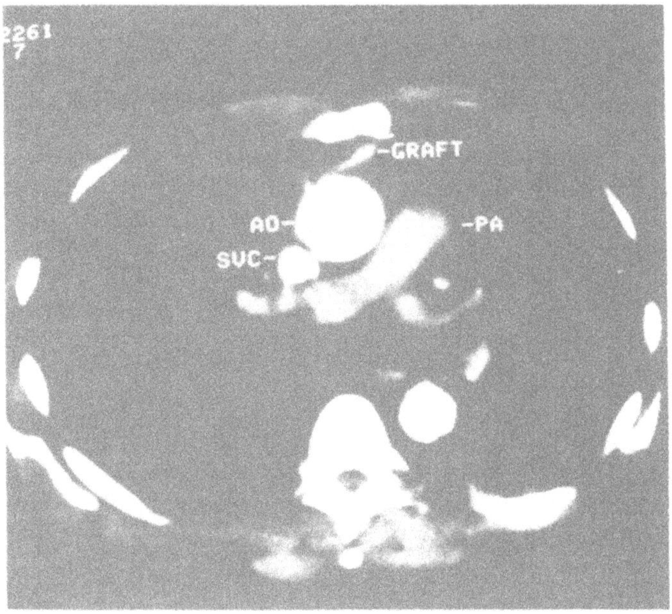

Fig. 7 Contrast enhanced computerized axial tomographic image transverse section through the chest of a patient after coronary bypass surgery, as reported by Herfkens and co-workers.

duce images of coronary artery bypass grafts. These are an attractive target vessel for controlled clinical trials because they can develop advanced atherosclerotic lesions,[8] particularly in patients with elevated plasma lipid levels.[9] The time of onset of exposure of the graft to high levels of atherogenic stimuli is known from the date of operation. Patients who have had coronary artery bypass tend to be compliant to drug and dietary regimens because they wish to maximize the benefits of surgery and delay the possible need for repeat surgery. Nuclear magnetic resonance images (Figure 6), computerized axial tomography enhanced with contrast medium perfusion (Figure 7),[10] and an IV digital subtraction angiogram of coronary artery bypass grafts (Figure 8) are shown. The catheter seen in the digital subtraction angiogram, Figure 8, was used to inject 40 cc of contrast medium into the superior vena cava.

THE NEED TO TEST VIGOROUS THERAPY

A point worth repeating is that a controlled clinical trial using any current imaging procedure is most likely to recognize a true treatment effect if a major difference occurs between treatment and control groups. It follows that lipid active agents most likely to

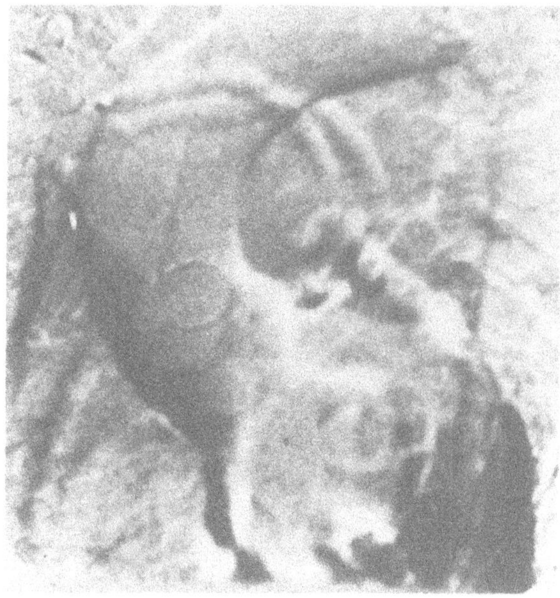

Fig. 8 Digital subtraction angiogram of a patient after coronary bypass surgery. Contrast medium was injected through the catheter shown which is in the superior vena cava. Two grafts are seen originating from the aorta and crossing it to the left coronary system.

show positive results are those which produce large changes in plasma lipids. One potential advantage of small-scale trials which measure atherosclerosis change over large-scale morbidity based trials, such as the WHO trial of clofibrate[11] is that greater degrees of lipid lowering can be achieved. For example, at the University of Southern California, we have a study in progress which will measure femoral, coronary, and carotid atherosclerosis change over two years in 160 men. After a pretrial period to assure an adequate response to drug therapy, angiography is performed and men are randomized to diet plus placebo (16 grams avicell) or diet plus colestipol (30 grams) and niacin (3-12 grams).* Baseline and one year lipid levels in our first 82 subjects are shown in Table 6. If a single parameter, LDL-Cholesterol/HDL-cholesterol, is used as an indicator of coronary risk, the placebo group and test group are separated by 65 percent of the ischemic heart disease risk observed in Framingham.[12]

*The experimental protocol and informed consent forms were approved by the Los Angeles County-University of Southern California Medical Center Human Research Committee.

TABLE 6

EFFECT OF DIET PLUS PLACEBO OR DIET PLUS NIACIN AND COLESTIPOL ON PLASMA LIPIDS

n drug = 41, n placebo = 41

Lipids mg/dl (mean ± sem)	Treatment Group*	Baseline (Visit 3)	One Year on Treatment	Change**	Percent Change
Total	Drug	246 ± 5	185 ± 6	-62 ± 7†	-25
Cholesterol	Control	235 ± 6	236 ± 6	2 ± 5	1
Triglyceride	Drug	165 ± 12	106 ± 8	-58 ± 10†	-35
	Control	169 ± 17	146 ± 14	-23 ± 11††	-14
LDL	Drug	171 ± 5	103 ± 5	-69 ± 7†	-40
Cholesterol	Control	160 ± 5	163 ± 5	3 ± 5	2
HDL	Drug	43 ± 2	61 ± 2	18 ± 2†	42
Cholesterol	Control	43 ± 2	44 ± 2	1 ± 1	2
LDL/HDL	Drug	4.2 ± 0.2	1.8 ± 0.1	-2.4 ± 0.2†	-57
Ratio	Control	4.0 ± 0.2	3.9 ± 0.2	-0.1 ± 0.2	- 3

*Drug represents the combined drug and diet therapy group; and Control, the combined placebo and diet therapy group.

**In each treatment group change is analyzed, using a 2-sided t-test of Ho: expected change is zero. Testing at the .05 level.

†Significant at the .001 level.

††Significant at the .05 level.

SUMMARY

Non-invasive imaging used in controlled clinical trials should be able to detect an average 1.5 to 3 percent change in atherosclerosis growth rate per year. This can now be achieved by selective arterial angiography, an invasive procedure. IV digital subtraction angiography and B-mode ultrasound imaging are the two most promising non-invasive procedures for early application in clinical trials. In carotid artery, the resolution of fine details of lesions by IV angiography is approximately one-half that of selective angiography. The resolving power of ultrasound images depends greatly on frequency of the ultrasound beam and is greatest along the axis of the beam which is perpendicular to the vessel. Nuclear magnetic resonance imaging and computerized axial tomography with enhanced tissue contrast show potentially useful images of coronary artery bypass grafts. Whatever imaging procedure is selected, a major emphasis in trial design should be to produce a large difference in atherosclerosis change rate between test and control groups. A potential advantage of small-scale clinical trials that measure atherosclerosis change is that large reductions in plasma lipid level are possible.

REFERENCES

1. M. Feinleib, W. B. Kannel, C. G. Tedeschi, T. K. Landau, and R. J. Garrison, The relation of antemortem characteristics to cardiovascular findings at necropsy, Athero. 34:145-157 (1979).
2. D. H. Blankenhorn, J. A. Rooney, and P. J. Curry, Non-invasive assessment of atherosclerosis, Prog. Cardiovas. Dis., In Press (1983).
3. A. S. Daoud, R. A. Forentin, and R. Goodale, Diffuse coronary arteriosclerosis versus isolated plaques in the etiology of myocardial infarction, The Am. J. Card. 14:69-74 (1964).
4. L. A. Solberg and J. P. Strong, Risk factors and atherosclerotic lesions. A review of autopsy studies, Arteriosclerosis 3:187-198 (1983).
5. Atherosclerosis of the aorta and coronary arteries in five towns. Bulletin of The World Health Organization 53: No. 5-6, 485-645 (1976).
6. D. H. Blankenhorn and S. H. Brooks, Angiographic trials of lipid-lowering therapy, Arteriosclerosis 1:242-249 (1981).
7. D. H. Blankenhorn, S. H. Brooks, H. P. Chin, D. W. Crawford, J. D. Hestenes, and R. H. Selzer, Atherosclerosis assessment by angiographic image processing and ultrasound, Annual Report, Contract No. N01-HV-2930, Devices and Technology Branch, Division of Heart and Vascular Diseases, N.I.H. 1-105 (1981).
8. A. E. Walts, M. C. Fishbein, H. Sustaita, and J. M. Matloff, Ruptured atheromatous plaques in saphenous vein coronary artery bypass grafts: A mechanism of acute, thrombotic, late graft occlusion, Circ. 65:197-201 (1982).
9. W. M. Shark and R. M. Kass, Repeat myocardial revascularization in coronary disease therapy: Consideration of primary bypass failures and success of second graft surgery, Am. Heart J. 102:303-307 (1982).
10. R. J. Herfkens, C. B. Higgins, H. Hricak, M. J. Lipton, L. E. Crooks, P. Lanzer, E. Botvinick, B. Brundage, P. E. Sheldon,

and L. Kaufman, Nuclear magnetic resonance imaging of the cardiovascular system: Normal and pathologic findings, Radiology 147:749-759 (1983).

11. A cooperative trial in the primary prevention of ischemic heart disease using clofibrate, Report from the Committee of Principal Investigators, Brit. Heart J. 40:1069-1118 (1978).

12. W. P. Castelli, R. D. Abbott, and P. M. McNamara, Summary estimates of cholesterol used to predict coronary heart disease, Circ. 67:730-734 (1983).

STRATEGY, YIELD AND RISKS OF CONTROLLING PLASMA LIPIDS IN THE PRIMARY PREVENTION OF CORONARY HEART DISEASE

M. F. Oliver

Cardiovascular Research Unit
University of Edinburgh
Edinburgh, Scotland

Reduction of plasma cholesterol and cholesterol-containing lipoproteins, or an increase in high density lipoproteins, is widely accepted as the desired goal for the whole population. It is time that a more critical appraisal is made of this aim in terms of the likely yield and practicability of such a policy.

There are several considerations which influence me towards a policy of selective intervention in those at particularly high risk, because of the presence of atherogenic lipoproteins, and against the policy of reducing blood lipids on a mass population and mass intervention basis. These include the actual risk of coronary heart disease (CHD) in relation to blood lipid levels, the current results of mass intervention programmes, the available means for reducing blood lipids and the likely compliance.

RISKS OF CORONARY HEART DISEASE IN RELATION TO PLASMA LIPIDS

We are seriously hampered in reaching any accurate assessment of the relationship of blood lipids to CHD by the pleomorphic nature of the atherosclerotic process and also by the lack of precision of the clinical end-points. I will discuss each briefly.

First, the objective of intervention must be to slow down the occlusive component of coronary atherosclerosis, because it is this which usually determines the onset of clinical features of CHD. Yet the relationship of blood lipids, even hypercholesterolaemia, to occlusive coronary atherosclerosis has not been satisfactorily distinguished from their relationship to widespread distribution of non-occlusive lesions. Were progressively occlusive lesions to be relatively or completely independent of blood lipids levels, then it is not logical to expect an effect on CHD by lowering them. This is not the place to embark on an extensive discussion of the atherosclerotic process, but it is abundantly clear that the platelet-fibrinogen-thrombin interaction has a greater role to play in advanced disease than that of blood lipids. It is not surprising, therefore, to find that serum cholesterol, LDL cholesterol and HDL cholesterol were all only very weakly related to the presence of occlusive coronary atherosclerotic lesions in the Oslo Study.[1]

Second, we are bound to assess any relationship of blood lipids to the risk of CHD by using the generic descriptive term, coronary heart disease, which includes a number of specific syndromes with relatively discrete mechanisms of onset, some of which are most unlikely to have much to do with blood lipid levels. For example, first coronary event, a nonfatal myocardial infarction, fatal coronary attacks, coronary deaths, etc., are among the many terms used to describe the clinical manifestations of previously occult coronary atherosclerosis. An abnormal ECG or sudden cardiac death are others and neither are likely to be closely related to blood lipid levels or to be influenced by their reduction.

Bearing both these reservations in mind, it is not surprising that the actual risk of developing CHD in relation to blood lipid

TABLE 1

PERCENT WITH FIRST CHD EVENT BY INITIAL SERUM CHOLESTEROL IN 8422 MEN

(extracted from Pooling Project[2])

<u>8.6 years follow-up</u>

A. Men aged 40-59 years	
Quintile 1	4
" 2	6
" 3	9
" 4	11
" 5	15
B. Quintile 5	
40-44 years	7
45-49 years	15
50-54 years	16
55-59 years	17
Estimated risk over 25 years (40-64 years)	32

TABLE 2

PERCENT WITH FIRST CHD EVENT OR DEATH BY SERUM CHOLESTEROL

(RATES/1000/YR)

	Pooling Project[2]		Framingham[2]	Israeli Civil Servants[4]	Stockholm Businessmen[5]	Whitehall Civil Servants[3]
Nos.	2140	1922	764	10059	3486	14863
Ages	40-44	50-54	<50	40-65	20-70	40-64
Follow-up	8.6	8.6	20	7	14.5	5
Quintiles of cholesterol						
1	4	11	4	1	12	(1) 8
2	4	9	8	2	13	(2) 8
3	7	9	11	2	12	
4	8	18	13	2	14	(3) 10
5	9	19	15	4	17	(4) 14

There is no statistically significant difference between the underlined figures in each vertical column/

levels is unimpressive. All the major epidemiological surveys indicate, of course, that the chances of developing CHD are increased when serum cholesterol is elevated and, when expressed on the basis of serum cholesterol distribution, those in the top quintile have appreciably more risk than those in the lowest quintiles. But only a minority of those even in the fifth quintile of serum cholesterol distribution will develop CHD in the foreseeable future. For example, the Pooling Project[2] indicates that only about 15% of those with definitely elevated cholesterol concentrations (top quintile) between the ages of 40 and 59 will develop CHD over the next 8.6 years and the estimated risk over a 25-year span is that only one-third of such high risk men, aged 40 to 64, will develop CHD (Table 1). These figures are not altered strikingly when age, raised serum cholesterol and cigarette smoking are also taken into account. Similarly, the five-year risk of developing CHD in the Whitehall Civil Servants Study[3] and in the seven-year Israeli Civil Servants Study[4] was even lower (Table 2).

Another way to emphasize the weak relationship between cholesterol and CHD is to draw attention to the fact that the increment in

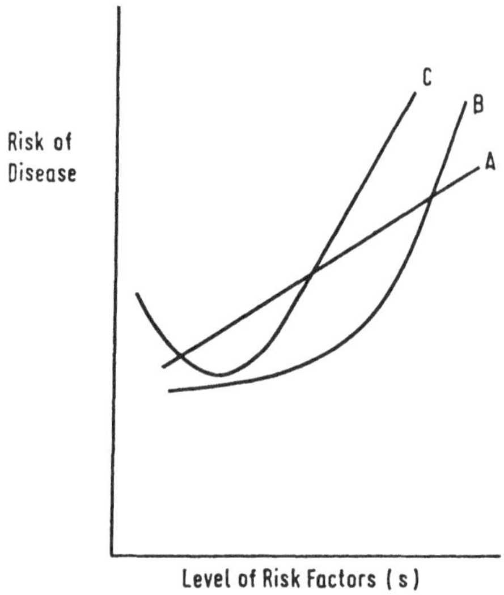

Fig. 1 Shows three hypothetical relationships between risk factors and the risk of disease.
A probably applies for cigarette smoking and CHD.
B probably applies for serum cholesterol and CHD, and also for blood pressure and stroke.
C probably applies for blood pressure and CHD.

(After Epstein, 1980[7]).

the incidence of CHD related to raised serum cholesterol is about 10% over the 8.6 years of the Pooling Project (quintile 5 minus quintile 3). In the Stockholm Businessmen Study[5] where a 14.5-year follow-up was conducted, the increment was only 5%.

The predictability of CHD can be improved by the use of various ratios[6] with total cholesterol/HDL cholesterol being the most sensitive but, even when high, the use of this ratio does little to improve the low specificity. Of course, it might be argued that the fact that the development of CHD can be predicted to occur in 20% of those with raised serum cholesterol means that it is a useful index, but this is not 20% of all those who develop CHD and most do not have any measurable increase in serum lipids.

CONTROL OF PLASMA LIPIDS - FOR EVERYONE OR FOR THOSE AT VERY HIGH RISK?

Epstein[7] has outlined three relevant hypothetical models relating risk to cardiovascular disease (Fig. 1) and I shall use them as a basis for discussing action. If the relationship is direct and linear and with a high correlation coefficient, as in A, then the more the risk is reduced the less the disease. This serves fairly well for the relationship of cigarette smoking to CHD and this is convincing evidence that all should stop smoking. If the relationship is curvilinear, as in B, little more can be expected in terms of reduction of disease when the risk/disease ratio is on to the flat part of the curve. This is the likely model to apply to the relationship of serum cholesterol (or the TC/HDL ratio) to CHD, since there is strong evidence from most studies conducted within a given population that there is no graded relationship between the two, possibly three, lowest quintiles of cholesterol and CHD incidence[8]: the Framingham Study may be an exception but it is much smaller than the others quoted and the results may represent the instability to be expected from a small study. The more linear relationship between cholesterol and CHD when different cultures are contrasted should not be allowed to obscure the weak relationship at low levels within a given population, particularly since the advice to be given should be directed to the population in question. If the relationship is J-shaped, as in C or even U-shaped, there is no argument for lowering the risk factor below the nadir: this is the probable relationship between blood pressure and CHD, particularly when the coronary reserve becomes more fixed as in advancing age, and this is probably a reason why lowering mild hypertension has not reduced CHD mortality.

If it is accepted that model A does not apply to the relationship of serum cholesterol to CHD, the case for reducing serum cholesterol in everyone by, for example, a diet low in saturated fat is weak. It disappears completely if an unnecessary risk such as the life-long use of drugs is to be used.

Therefore, I think that we should develop a selective policy of advice regarding the cholesterol-CHD question.[9] Why is control of raised serum cholesterol or atherogenic lipoproteins regarded differently from that of other causes of vascular disease? Nobody has ever suggested that the diastolic blood pressure of the entire population should be brought down by 10 mmHg in order to reduce the risk of strokes. Nobody has suggested that the entire population should be given anticoagulants to prevent hypercoagulability in the minority. Nobody has suggested that the serum urate of the entire population should be reduced, so as to prevent gout from occurring in a susceptible few.

Let us look at the results of the mass intervention.

RESULTS OF MASS INTERVENTION STUDIES

One of the greatest difficulties in assessing the value of reducing serum cholesterol or cholesterol-containing lipoproteins is that no study has been conducted to determine the effect this has on CHD incidence in the whole population. The Los Angeles Veterans Administration Study,[10] conducted in elderly people, and the Helsinki Mental Hospital Study[11] were both undertaken in institutions and the inmates of these institutions cannot possibly be regarded as representative of the whole population. Furthermore, they were selected on the basis of having raised serum cholesterol concentrations. These are the only two major dietary surveys from which conclusions can be made and, while being critical of them in relationship to population intervention, it should be emphasised that both showed a reduction in the incidence of nonfatal myocardial infarction. Similarly, the WHO clofibrate[12] trial was conducted in a relatively high risk population but also showed that reduction of total cholesterol was associated with a lower incidence of nonfatal myocardial infarction.

In the absence of information concerning the value of lowering serum cholesterol across the board, an alternative approach is to consider the effects of <u>multiple</u> risk factor intervention on a mass scale.

The North Karelia-Kuopio Study showed an aggregated fall of 17% in coronary risk factors over the first five-year period of study[13,14] in North Karelia, the province where intervention was active, compared with Kuopio, the control province, where there was no change in the incidence of CHD. Because these were neighbouring provinces, it was argued that Kuopio had not been a satisfactory control area and also that it would be hard to show a difference between two provinces in a country where the rates were falling overall. The results of the second five years of this study are not much more encouraging.[15] Although between 1969 and 1979 there was an overall decline in the rates by 12% in men and by 26% in women, to what extent this was a result of mass multiple risk factor intervention is unclear. North Karelia has beed singled out for particular comment because of the active intervention programme there and decreases occurred during the eleven-year survey in excess of the mean in men (-24%) and in women (-51%). But in Kuopio and in Vaasa, which were provinces without intensive health education, there were decreases in men of 21% (women 36%) and 22%, respectively. In other words, there was little difference in coronary mortality trends in areas where multiple risk factor intervention was or was not promulgated. Despite this, the authors think the trends reflect an effect of the preventive programme in North Karelia and indicate that long periods of observation are necessary to assess the value of such programmes. An alternative explanation of the differences in the Finnish provinces might be that they reflect the expected degree of random variation from observing 11 samples within a country which is for unknown reasons - not excluding some effect of health education - experiencing a fall in coronary mortality.

The U. S. Multiple Risk Factor Intervention Trial (MRFIT),[16] backed up by a very active programme of advice from physicians, nutritionists, psychologists and the media, showed that it was not possible to reduce coronary mortality by the simultaneous reduction of cigarette smoking, change in diet from saturated to unsaturated fat and improved control of hypertension in 6428 healthy volunteer males compared with initially similar control group of 6438 men. Although there was an impressive reduction in cigarette smoking and a more than expected reduction in blood pressure, there was a surprisingly small reduction in blood cholesterol (-12 mg/dl) in view of the stringent diet of about 30% of fat calories and less than 10% of these from saturated fat. This is the exact diet recommended by the World Health Organisation.[17] The only interpretation of this is that the volunteers, in spite of all the efforts of the nutritionists, psychologists and physicians failed to observe the diet. Alternatively, all the calculations[18] which have proved to be sound for so many years concerning the extent to which dietary cholesterol and dietary fat should be reduced in relationship to the yield of serum cholesterol concentrations are invalid - this seems most unlikely.

The WHO European Coronary Prevention Study[19] has also proved a disappointment. In strict primary prevention terms, there was no significant reduction in CHD in spite of a variable degree of reduction in risk factors. The most promising result was in the Belgian component[20] of 19,409 men: the intervention led to an aggregated reduction of risk factors by nearly 16% with an apparent overall decrease (-24.5%) in coronary incidence but this decrease was made up of a nonsignificant fall in the majority (93%) who were initially healthy and the only significant subgroup where there was a fall in CHD were those who initially had an abnormal ECG. The U.K. section[21] of the study comprised 18,210 men, aged 40-59 years, and they also were given a low saturated fat diet, advice to stop smoking, weight reduction, more exercise and control of hypertension. This led to no more than an overall reduction of risk factors of 4% and no change in coronary incidence.

One problem in interpreting the results of these studies is the use of the multiple logistic function, since when details are given, it often seems that the main power within the product is reduction of cigarette smoking. The influence of reduction of serum cholesterol appears to be of minor importance.

There is still no satisfactory explanation for the remarkable fall in coronary mortality in the United States, which affects both sexes, both major racial groups and all three adult decades equally. While multiple risk factor intervention may have contributed, there is little real evidence to support some of the more extreme views; for example, the notion that these changes were mostly due to reduction of serum cholesterol and this is a consequence of the U. S. dietary changes. Feinleib and Rifkind of the U. S. National Heart, Lung and Blood Institute have recently concluded[22] "it is still unclear whether the reduction in risk factor levels has resulted in a decrease in the number of heart attacks". They prefer the view that the lower case fatality rates may have been partly brought about by

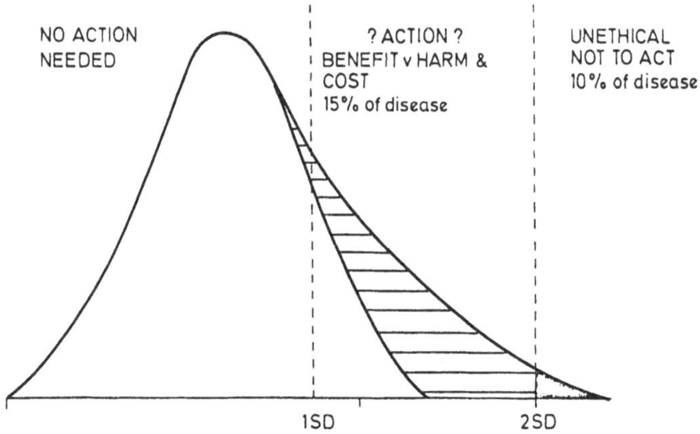

Fig. 2 Shows a diagrammatic distribution curve for plasma atherogenic lipoproteins in the community. While it is probably unethical not to treat the top few percent with grossly elevated concentrations, it may also be unethical to treat those with only moderately elevated values if their risk is not greatly increased and the drugs chosen have not been proved to be safe for indefinite usage.

improvements in specialised medical services. Furthermore, two recent papers from Sweden[23,24] indicated increase in coronary mortality without any commensurate increase in the main risk factors. Indeed, cigarette smoking decreased both in the Gothenburg and Stockholm surveys. This increase in coronary disease has occurred in a country where all the health measures that health educators have put across in the United States and Finland also apply.

IN WHOM AND HOW SHOULD HYPERLIPIDAEMIA BE CONTROLLED?

My answer to this question depends on which policy is to be adopted. The alternatives are illustrated in Fig. 2. Selective action for the top few percent at very high risk would make less impact on CHD incidence in the community than action addressed to a much larger number at only moderate risk. If intervention is to be attempted on a selective basis for those at high risk, then a particularly strong effort should be made to make a fundamental change in the diet along the lines of the World Health Organisation recommendations and also it is wholly justifiable to use drugs. On the other hand, if a policy of mass intervention for the population at large is adopted, then two issues will arise: one is the practicability of making stringent dietary recommendations and the compliance of many not well motivated individuals to these; the other is that the risk of taking drugs may be greater than the uncorrected risk itself, and this is only acceptable in circumstances of very high risk.

DIET

Those who have formed the opinion (and this is all that it is) in favour of a policy of altering the diet of the entire population of developed countries, with the attendant changes necessary in agriculture strategy and economy, advocate action in the absence of any proof that the hypothesis is correct and in the absence of any proof that such a dietary change is safe, particularly when applied to the growing child. They adduce support for their opinion through extrapolation from, for example, the results of short-term feeding studies on serum lipo- and apo-protein concentrations, from the artifical circumstances of regression studies in primates, from an apparent continuous relationship between serum cholesterol or LDL-cholesterol and CHD and from a degree of parallelism which exists with regard to the fall in CHD incidence rates in several countries with a decrease in the consumption of dietary fat. But we should be aware that short-term manipulation of serum lipoprotein concentrations by dietary means has only the remotest relevance to recommendations to be given for life to the public to prevent CHD; the relationship between serum cholesterol and CHD is discontinuous with all major epidemiological studies showing no graded risk for CHD when serum cholesterol is below about 210 mg/dl; and in some countries (Israel[25] and Switzerland[26]) dietary fat consumption has risen as CHD incidence has fallen.

Those who have decided against any dietary action have presumably chosen to disregard the evidence that raised serum cholesterol is a <u>sine qua non</u> for the development of atheroma, that those with genetic failure of LDL receptor formation and those with abnormal apo B/apo A ratio develop CHD prematurely, that reduction of raised serum cholesterol in hypercholesterolaemic heterozygotes[27] by a high P/S diet has led to a significant reduction in CHD incidence, that a diet with a high P/S ratio reduced the CHD incidence in two institutionalised populations and also that the vast amount of epidemiological evidence associating saturated fat and CHD.

Between these extremes of those who are in favour and those who are against dietary changes, there must be a middle course. In view of the lack of acceptability of the WHO recommendations by the volunteers in the MRFIT study and the difficulties in changing a nation's diet to meet the goals, an argument might be made for a moderate change in dietary fat so that 35% of calories are obtained from fat with about 12% from saturated fat. Nevertheless, it has to be emphasised again that even using such a diet on a mass basis has not yet been shown to have any effect on CHD.

Adoption of a much more selective policy of intervention should surely now be the aim. Although directed at fewer numerically, those in whom the risk factor of hyperlipidaemia acts most powerfully are likely to be most benefitted. It would mean screening of a population for severe hypercholesterolaemia and this might be refined in the future by use of apolipoprotein genome probes to identify for example, those with partial failure of low density lipoprotein receptors. Screening should not be insuperable or enormously costly and one result would be to identify individuals who have normal plasma cholesterol levels and permit them to enjoy their food, which is one of the pleasures of life. Identification of the top few percent at really high risk would justify the use of stringent diets and hypolipidaemic drugs. This policy requires all the energy and support possible, since the Oslo Study[27] suggests that it stands a good chance of success.

DRUGS

To date, only one major primary prevention drug trial of the effects of lowering raised plasma lipids has been completed and this is the WHO clofibrate trial.[12] It showed significant reduction in the incidence of non-fatal myocardial infarction and this was commensurate with that to be expected from the degree of reduction of raised plasma cholesterol. It also showed a significant increase (64 more deaths) in non-cardiovascular mortality during clofibrate administration. The increase was not specific for any cause of death. The excess mortality disappeared after completion of the five-year trial[28] (Table 3). The chances of the increase in non-cardiovascular mortality being due to chance are very low indeed. Two alternative explanations have been considered: one is that it results in some way from the mechanisms of action of clofibrate and the other is that it is related to reduction in plasma cholesterol and LDL leading to alteration in the metabolism of membrane and cell cholesterol in aging cells. Both hypotheses remain viable, although the former is the more likely.

The clofibrate trial results represent a major setback for all interested in the use of drugs to modulate atherogenic lipoproteins - pharmacological companies, investigators and clinicians alike - but it has demonstrated the power of a well-designed clinical trial to identify adverse as well as beneficial effects. A related compound, gemfibrozil, is under clinical trial in primary prevention of CHD in Finland and no results can evidently be expected much before 1986.

Meanwhile, several influential pharmaceutical companies have mounted advertising and sales campaigns to promote their particular "fibrate": all of these are structurally related to clofibrate but none have been or are being subjected to the rigour of a controlled long-term clinical trial and it is very difficult - probably impossible - to ascertain whether their usage is also associated with increased non-cardiovascular mortality. The promotion at this time of such drugs seems to be to be irresponsible without formal studies of long-term safety.

Triparanol, or MER-29, had a profound effect on LDL cholesterol but was withdrawn many years ago because it led to accumulation in

TABLE 3

RATIO OF STANDARDISED DEATH RATES* DURING AND AFTER THE WHO CLOFIBRATE TRIAL, BY MAIN CAUSE OF DEATH

CAUSE OF DEATH	During 6 year trial					
	Clofibrate Group (I)	High Cholesterol Control Group (II)	Ratio I/II	Clofibrate Group (I)	High Cholesterol Control Group (II)	Ratio I/II
C.H.D.	1.54	1.57	0.98	4.72	4.33	1.09
Cancer	1.95	1.18	1.65	2.83	2.78	1.02
All causes except CHD	4.15	2.38	1.74	5.24	5.32	0.98
All causes	5.70	3.96	1.44	9.97	9.66	1.03

*Age-standardised death rate per 1000 per annum by the indirect method (age-at-death, aged 40-69).

TABLE 4

DRUGS USED FOR CONTROL OF ATHEROGENIC LIPOPROTEINS IN RELATION TO CORONARY HEART DISEASE

Formal Clinical Trial

Clofibrate	-	reduction of non-fatal myocardial infarction
	-	increased non-cardiovascular mortality
	-	increased gallstone formation
Gemfibrozil	-	on-going trial in Finland reporting in 1986

No Formal Clinical Trial

Bezafibrate	Probucol
Ciprofibrate	Mevinolin
Clinofibrate	Compactin
Beclobrate	Melinamine
Etofibrate	-oryzanol
	Pantethine
	Acipimox

tissue of desmosterol and other oxysterols and, more important, to cataract and blindness.[29]

Nicotinic acid lowers plasma VLDL triglyceride and cholesterol but has not been subjected to a formal clinical trial in primary prevention - nor will it be because of the disagreeable side effects of facial flushing and gastrointestinal effects it causes.

Probucol lowers LDL cholesterol and causes regression of xanthomata but it also lowers HDL cholesterol and possibly increases the Q-T interval in the electrocardiogram. Again, its efficacy and safety remain to be tested by a long-term trial.

For completeness, mention should be made of the anion-exchange resin, colestipol, which was used in a mixed primary and secondary prevention trial[30] with negative results in those initially healthy - and the large continuing trial of cholestyramine conducted by the U. S. Lipid Research Clinics in high risk men.[31] But neither of these resins is absorbed and any adverse effects will be secondary and probably a consequence of altering bile lithogenicity and bile acid reabsorption.

HOW CAN DRUG SAFETY FOR PRIMARY PREVENTION BE IMPROVED?

One way to improve the safety of drugs is to insist on more controlled randomised clinical trials.[32] Only clofibrate and gemfibrozil have been so assessed (Table 4). Physicians must learn to see through the constant claim of drug companies for the benefit of their drug, when they are based on small short-term clinical studies. They argue that, since their drug lowers blood pressure or LDL or raises HDL or whatever, it must be good. First, this does not mean it is harmless. Second, in all probability its "goodness" has never been put to the test. Manipulation of such measurements should not be equated with benefit. The onus of proof of safety and efficacy should lie squarely with the drug house, particularly when the product is to be given to healthy people for years. Third, the pharmokinetics of the drug when given to man are often incompletely studied. They should include, for example, studies of kinetics in terms of plasma concentrations and radioactive labelling, tissue distribution and identification of pharmacologically active metabolites during and after administration of the drug to normal people for periods as long as 12 weeks.

With great care, after years of research and the investment of millions of pounds, responsible pharmaceutical companies produce drugs which seem to be safe. In general, pharmaceutical companies undertake extensive and scrupulous screening tests of a new drug and toxicity is tested at dose concentrations many times in excess of that which will ever be given to humans. Licenses are usually granted by national bodies on the basis that the drug has not been shown to be toxic to animals, that it has not produced any "nasty" effects on orthodox biochemical or haematological tests, that it produces no side effects when given over a few months to man and that it does seem to be valuable in correcting the abnormal measurement at which it is aimed. But post-marketing surveillance is patchy or non-existent. Of course, it is difficult for drug companies to identify what to monitor and for how long, before they can tell the world that their product is perfectly safe and recommend its use for preventing disease in healthy people. What the drug might do to the metabolism of the body when given over years and the extent to which it remains effective in correcting the abnormal measurement can only be identified when it is actually given over many years and to a large number of people. This is a paradox, indeed. A different set of criteria is needed than the orthodox animal toxicity screening and the phase 1 clinical testing. A large and prolonged controlled clinical trial was necessary to demonstrate the increased non-cardiovascular mortality related to use of clofibrate[12] and the male impotence[33] or the increased of arrhythmias[34] induced by thiazide diuretics. Clinical trials are necessary for interpretation of the significance of the "adverse" lipoprotein changes produced by beta-blockers, for example.

It may, however, be an impossible commitment if it is a question of monitoring a change in the prevalence of commonly occurring conditions (as in the clofibrate trial), such as cancer, vascular diseases or premature senility. But, nevertheless, a bigger effort is needed. Another way to improve drug safety, admittedly an expensive one, would be to establish data banks of drug usage.

DATA BANKS OF DRUG USAGE

Never before have drugs been given to so many symptomless, apparently healthy individuals in the hope of preventing diseases. The problem is a unique one for the end of this century. And we have no comprehensive monitoring systems which permit us to look at the repercussions or to provide adequate data to enable responsible decisions to be taken for or against a specific intervention.

I make a plea that a national system for the monitoring of the safety of drugs when given over many years shall be established and established soon.[35] No country has yet established an adequate system of surveillance. An international agency, such as WHO, might help to establish a wider monitoring system which would produce results quicker. Only in this way will it be known when the risk of correcting risk is greater than the uncorrected risk.[31]

REFERENCES

1. I. Holme, S. C. Enger, A. Helgeland, I. Hjermann, Paul Leren, P. G. Lund-Larson, L. A. Solberg, and J. P. Strong, Risk factors and raised atherosclerotic lesions in coronary and cerebral arteries, Statistical analysis from the Oslo Study, Arteriosclerosis 1:250-256 (1981).
2. The Pooling Project Research Group, Relationship of blood pressure serum cholesterol, smoking habit, relative weight and ECG abnormalities to incidence of major coronary events, Final report of the Pooling Project, J. Chron. Dis. 31:201-306 (1978).
3. G. Rose, P. J. S. Hamilton, H. Keen, D. D. Reed, P. McCartney, and R. J. Jarrett, Myocardial ischaemia, risk factors and death from coronary heart disease, Lancet 1:105-109 (1977).
4. U. Goldbourt and J. H. Medalie, Lipoprotein cholesterol and the incidence of coronary heart disease - the Israeli Ischaemic Heart Disease Study, AMA. J. Epidemiol. 109:296-307 (1975).
5. L. E. Bottiger and L. A. Carlson, Risk factors for ischaemic vascular death from men in the Stockholm Prospective Study, Atherosclerosis 36:389-408 (1980).
6. W. P. Castelli, R. D. Abbott, and P. M. McNamara, Summary estimates of cholesterol used to predict coronary heart disease, Circulation 67:730-734 (1983).
7. F. H. Epstein, in: "Prevention and Treatment of Coronary Heart

Disease and its Complications," Excerpta Medica, Amsterdam, pp. 1-11 (1980).

8. M. F. Oliver, The optimum serum cholesterol, Lancet 2:655 (1982).

9. M. F. Oliver, Should we not forget about mass control of coronary risk factors? Lancet 2:37-38 (1983).

10. S. Dayton, M. L. Pearce, S. Hashimoto, W. J. Dixon, and U. Tomiyasu, A controlled clinical trial of a diet high in unsaturated fat in preventing complications in atherosclerosis, Circulation 39,40; Suppl. 2:1-63 (1969).

11. O. Turpeinen, M. J. Karvonen, M. Pekkarinen, M. Miettinen, R. Elosuo, and E. Paavilainen, Dietary prevention of coronary heart disease, The Finnish Mental Hospital Study, Int. J. Epidemiol. 8:99-118 (1979).

12. Report from the Committee of Principal Investigators, A cooperative trial in the primary prevention of ischaemic heart disease using clofibrate, Brit. Heart J. 10:1069-1118 (1978).

13. P. Puska, J. Tuomilehto, J. Salonen, L. Neittaaumaki, J. Maki, J. Virtamo, A. Nissinen, K. Koskela, and T. Takalo, Changes in coronary risk factors during comprehensive five-year community programme to control cardiovascular diseases (North Karelia Project), Brit. Med. J. 4:1173-1178 (1979).

14. J. T. Salonen, P. Puska, and H. Mustaniemi, Changes in morbidity and mortality during comprehensive community programme to control cardiovascular diseases during 1972-77 in North Karelia, Brit. Med. J. 4:1178-1183 (1979).

15. J. T. Salonen, P. Puska, T. E. Kottke, J. Tuomilehto, A. Nissinen, Decline in mortality from coronary heart disease in Finland from 1969-1979, Brit. Med. J. 286:1857-1860 (1983).

16. Multiple Risk Factor Intervention Trial, JAMA 248:1465-1468 (1982).

17. Report of a WHO Expert Committee, Prevention of coronary heart disease, World Health Organisation Technical Report Series 678 (1982).

18. A. Keys, J. T. Anderson, and F. Grande, Serum cholesterol response to changes in the diet. I. Iodine value of dietary fat versus 2S-P, Metabolism 14:747-758; 766-775 (1965).

19. World Health Organisation, European Collaborative Group, Multifactorial Trial in the Prevention of Coronary Heart Disease. 3. Incidence and Mortality Results, Eur. Heart J. 4:141-147 (1983).

20. M. Kornitzer, G. DeBacker, M. Dramaix, F. Kittel, C. Thilly, M. Graffar, and K. Vaylsteek, Belgian Heart Disease Prevention Project: Incidence of mortality results, Lancet 1:1066-1070 (1983).

21. G. Rose, H. D. Tunstall-Pedoe, and R. F. Heller, U. K. Heart Disease Prevention Project: Incidence and mortality results, Lancet 1:1062-1065 (1983).

22. M. Feinleib and B. M. Rifkind, Changing patterns of cardiovascu-

lar disease mortality in the United States, Israel J. Med. Sci. 18:1098-1105 (1982).

23. L. Wellin, B. Larsson, K. Svardsudd, L. Wilhelmsen, and G. Tibblin, Why is the incidence of ischaemic heart disease in Sweden increasing? Study of men born in 1913 and 1923, Lancet 1:1087-1089 (1983).
24. L. Alfredsson and A. Ahlbom, Increasing incidence in mortality from myocardial infarction in Stockholm county, Brit. Med. J. 286:1931-1933 (1983).
25. U. Goldburt and J. D. Kark, Changing patterns of cardiovascular disease mortality in the United States, Israel J. Med. Sci. 18:1077-1097 (1982).
26. E. Guberan, Surprising decline of cardiovascular mortality in Switzerland, 1951-56, J. Epidemiol. Comm. Health 33:114-120 (1979).
27. I. Hjermann, I. Holme, K. V. Byre, and P. Leren, The effect of diet and smoking intervention on the incidence of coronary heart disease, Lancet 2:301-310 (1981).
28. Report of the Committee of Principal Investigators, In preparation.
29. H. O. Perry, R. K. Winkelmann, R. W. P. Achor, and T. J. Kirby, Side effects of triparanol therapy, Am. J. Med. Sci. 244: 556-563 (1962).
30. A. E. Dorr, K. Gunderson, J. C. Schneider, Jr., T. W. Spencer, and W. B. Martin, Colestipol hydrochloride in hypercholesterolaemic patients - effect on serum cholesterol and mortality, J. Chron. Dis. 31:5-14 (1978).
31. Lipid Research Clinics Program, The Coronary Primary Prevention Trial: Design and Implementation, J. Chron. Dis. 32:609-631 (1979).
32. M. F. Oliver, Risk of correcting the risk of coronary disease and stroke with drugs, New Engl. J. Med. 306:297-298 (1982).
33. Medical Research Council Working Party on Mild to Moderate Hypertension, Adverse reactions to bendrofluazide and propranolol for the treatment of mild hypertension, Lancet 2:539-543 (1981).
34. P. K. Whelton, P. Brennan, W. E. Miall, G. Greenberg, B. Subramanian, Thiazide associated cardiac arrhythmias, Circulation 66:Suppl. 2 - 238 (1982).
35. M. F. Oliver, Doctors and the drug industry, Brit. Med. J. 286: 888-889 (1983).

MECHANISMS OF ACTION OF ABSORBABLE HYPOLIPIDEMIC DRUGS

Cesare R. Sirtori

Center E. Grossi Paoletti
University of Milano
20129 Milano, Italy

Absorbable hypolipidemic agents, mostly of the aryloxyacetic acid type, are still used most widely in the general clinical treatment of hyperlipidemia. These compounds will be, therefore, the major object of this presentation. Current hypotheses on the mode of action of these drugs will be analyzed in detail and, moreover, specific problems pertaining to their use will be discussed; among these peroxisomal proliferation, reporting new findings suggestive of specific structural features most and least likely to induce this effect. Finally, aiming to the specific interest of pharmacologists working in this area, the scope and validity of new experimental methodologies, e.g., activation of lipoprotein receptors and changes in high density lipoprotein (HDL) levels, will be examined.

HYPOLIPIDEMIC DRUGS AS "CATABOLIC" ACTIVATORS

Although the mechanism of action of aryloxyacetic acid derivatives (also called "fibrates") is often rated as mysterious, the very potent stimulating activity on lipoprotein lipase (LPL) exerted by all of these agents may provide an adequate explanation for most of their therapeutic and side activities. As already previously indicated,[1] activation of LPL may lead to:

- reduction of plasma triglycerides (TG)
- increased low density lipoprotein (LDL) cholesterol levels in hypertriglyceridemic patients with low baseline LDL[2]
- increased HDL cholesterol
- increased proliferation of peroxisomes in rodent liver

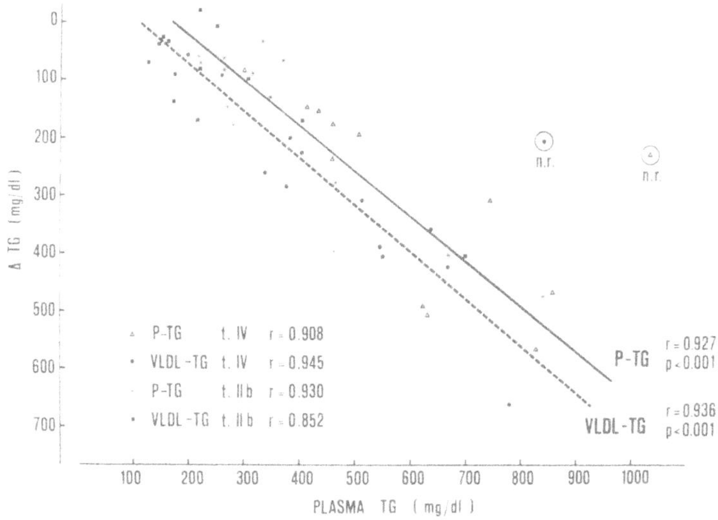

Fig. 1 Correlation between the reduction of plasma triglycerides (Δ TG) and the baseline triglyceridemia after procetofen treatment. Highly significant correlations between Δ TG and both plasma (P-TG) and VLDL-TG are noted for the 13 type IIB and 13 type IV treated patients. Only one type IV patient failed to respond (n.r.).[4]

The catabolic effect on very low density lipoprotein (VLDL) is well exemplified in the case of procetofen, a "fibrate" derivative with a long plasma half-life.[3] Within a study in type IIB and IV patients,[4] a significant correlation between total and VLDL triglycerides and their respective reduction induced by drug therapy could be detected (Fig. 1).

The activation of LPL by "fibrates" may be accompanied by apoprotein changes, the most distinctive of which is the increased apoprotein CII content in VLDL.[5] The apo CII rise, particularly evident in type IV patients, is fully reversible after the end of treatment (Fig. 2). Since apo CII is generally reduced in VLDL from type IV patients, the relative rise of the CII/CIII-1 ratio during drug treatment may be indicative of a specific mode of action. On the other hand, in spite of the well known cofactor activity of apo CII on LPL, there is no clear indication that an increased CII in VLDL may, as a consequence, increase LPL activity.

In addition to the VLDL-TG lowering effect, the increased HDL cholesterol levels following drug treatment may also be related to an activation of LPL.[6] Of less straightforward explanation is the reduction of LDL cholesterolemia, shown repeatedly with clofibrate

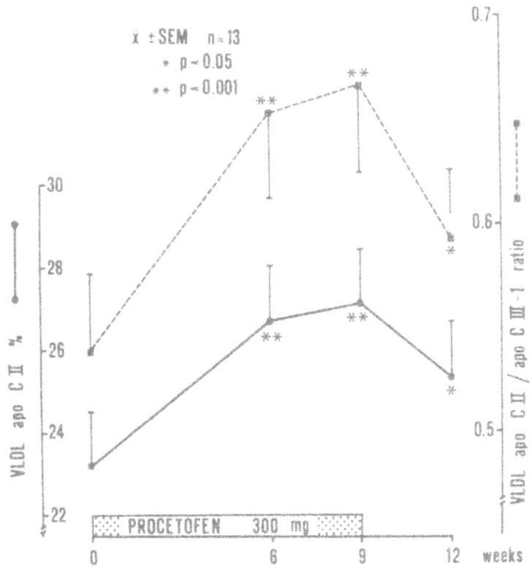

Fig. 2 Progressive increase of the apoprotein C-II content and of the apo C-II/C-III-1 ratio in VLDL during procetofen treatment in patients with type IV hyperlipoproteinemia (same cohort as in Fig. 1). Both apoprotein changes are reversible after the end of treatment.[4]

and, more so, with newer derivatives, i.e., bezafibrate and procetofen.[7,8] A recent comparative evaluation of procetofen and cholestyramine, indicated that the former may induce a more significant LDL cholesterol reduction in type IIA patients.[9] Aside from other postulated mechanisms, with unclear scientific basis, increased LPL may again be linked to reduced LDL cholesterolemia. As reported by Chajek et al.,[10] and also as presented at this Symposium, LPL may activate a receptor-linked mechanism, favoring uptake of cholesterol-rich lipoproteins (chylomicrons or remnants) by different tissues.

Peroxisomal Proliferation

The increased catabolism of VLDL-TG may result in the exposure of the liver to considerable amounts of free fatty acids. Ten years ago, Wolfe et al.[11] indicated that a significant ketosis may be detected in the splanchnic region of clofibrate treated subjects. The phenomenon may become quite dramatic in rodents, a species with an inherent deficiency of oxidative processes.[12]

The peculiar sensitivity of rodents to the toxic effects of compounds requiring extensive oxidative transformations is probably the cause of peroxisomal proliferation. Proliferation of liver peroxisomes in rodents may result simply from the administration of high fat diets.[13] After only a few days of dietary fat enrichment, rodents display a remarkable proliferation of organelles rich in peroxidative enzymes.[13] The phenomenon becomes more extensive in the presence of aryloxyacetic acid derivatives.[14,15] Upon prolonged administration of these agents to selected rodent strains (e.g., the Fisher rat), liver carcinogenicity may ensue.[16]

Proliferation of peroxisomes has been linked recently to an increased liver cell content of enzymes of the fatty acid β-oxidative pathway. In particular, enoyl-L-CoA hydratase (crotonase), is increased by peroxisomal proliferators.[17] The peroxisomal enoyl-CoA hydratase exhibits both enoyl-CoA hydratase and 3-hydroxy acyl-CoA dehydrogenase activities, the heat-labile enoyl-CoA hydratase being particularly detectable in the peroxisomal matrix. The identity between enoyl-CoA hydratase and an 80,000 MW protein, detected in microsomal preparations following treatments with peroxisomal proliferators, has been established.

The apparent species specificity of these findings has tended to downplay similar observations in the clinical setting. Comparative evaluations of liver biopsy specimens before and after treatment with peroxisomal proliferators, failed to show a sizable increase of peroxidative organelles.[18,19] On the other hand, Hanefeld et al.[20] have shown that in individual cases a significant increase of liver peroxisomal content may be detected in the first 4-6 months of clofibrate administration. It would appear that this phenomenon, although on an individual basis, might lead to measurable toxicity when very large numbers of drug users are examined.

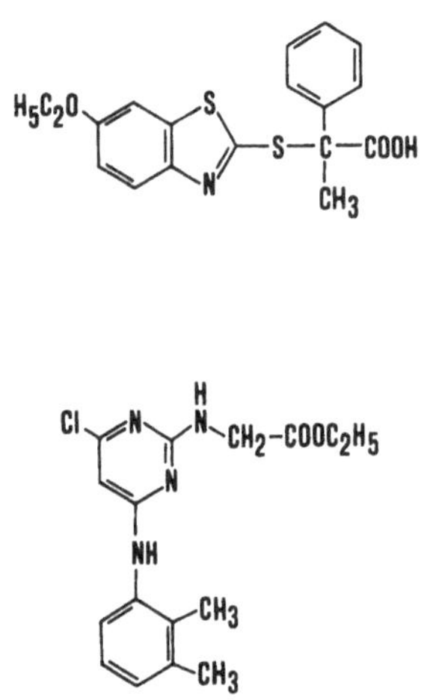

Fig. 3 Structural formulas of EMD 34 853 and of BR-971 (ethylester), two potent hypolipidemic agents not inducing peroxisomal proliferation.

In the search for compounds not exhibiting this disturbing effect, several molecules have been evaluated which apparently do not induce peroxisomal proliferation. Two of these, EMD 34 837 and BR-971 are shown in Fig. 3. Both are powerful lipid lowering agents, but neither increases liver weight to any extent.

The development of BR-971 offers an interesting clue to the understanding of the mechanism of peroxisomal proliferation. BR-971 is a derivative of BR-931, a potent lipid lowering drug, with a similar pyrimidine structure, previously shown to markedly stimulate liver peroxisomal proliferation, and to induce liver hepatomas.[16] In the course of structural studies by X-ray crystallography,[21] it was shown that BR-931 displays a considerable asymmetry in the bond length within the pyrimidine ring, with a consequent loss of aromaticity (Fig. 4). As shown in Fig. 5, the loss of the aromatic structure may lead toward a quinone geometry. This would not be the case of BR-971 which, by X-ray studies, shows a stable aromatic geometry.

The link between loss of aromaticity and proliferation of peroxisomes is not clear. On the other hand, previous findings with clofibrate derivatives, in particular with the p-fluoro analog (Fig. 6), had shown that this latter, probably with a more stable geometry compared to clofibrate, maintains hypolipidemic properties but does not lead to peroxisomal proliferation.[22]

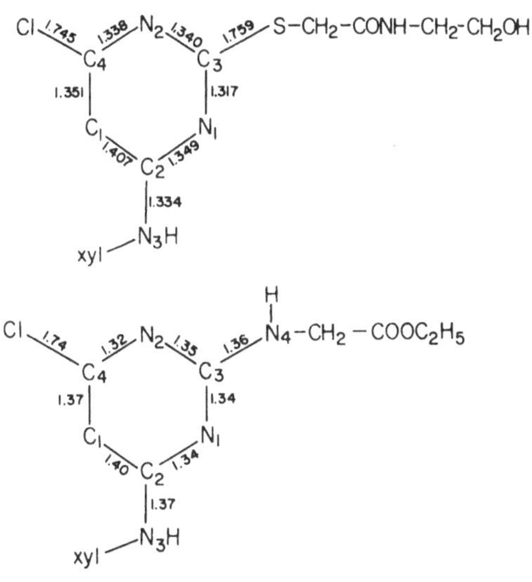

Fig. 4 Bond lengths in the aromatic ring of BR-931 (a powerful peroxisomal proliferation) and of BR-971 (devoid of this activity), as determined by X-ray studies. A considerable asymmetry is noted in the former structure, possibly leading to loss of aromaticity.

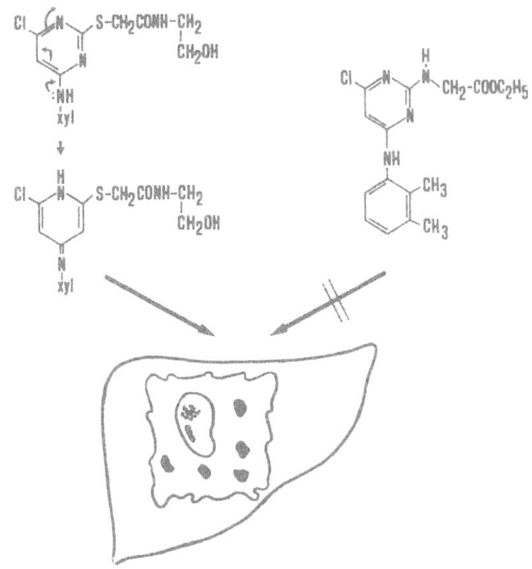

Fig. 5 The unstable molecular geometry of BR-931 (Fig. 4) may possibly lead to loss of aromaticity, and to a quinone geometry. This is not the case for BR-971, which also does not lead to peroxisomal proliferation (see text).

In conclusion, it would appear that peroxisomal proliferation has a dual origin. On the one hand, increased catabolism of TG-rich lipoproteins may expose the liver to a large load of fatty acids, requiring β-oxidation, thus in part inducing increased peroxisomal activity. On the other hand, some structural properties of selected compounds may, by themselves, stimulate the proliferation of the

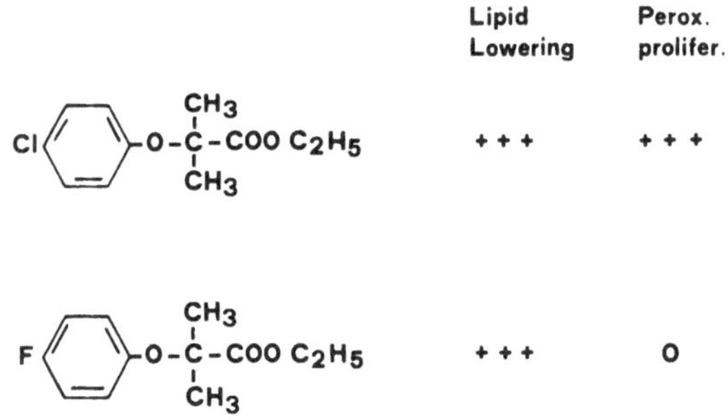

Fig. 6 Different effects of clofibrate and of its p-fluoro analog. Both show powerful lipid lowering activity in rodents, but only clofibrate is a peroxisomal proliferator.[23]

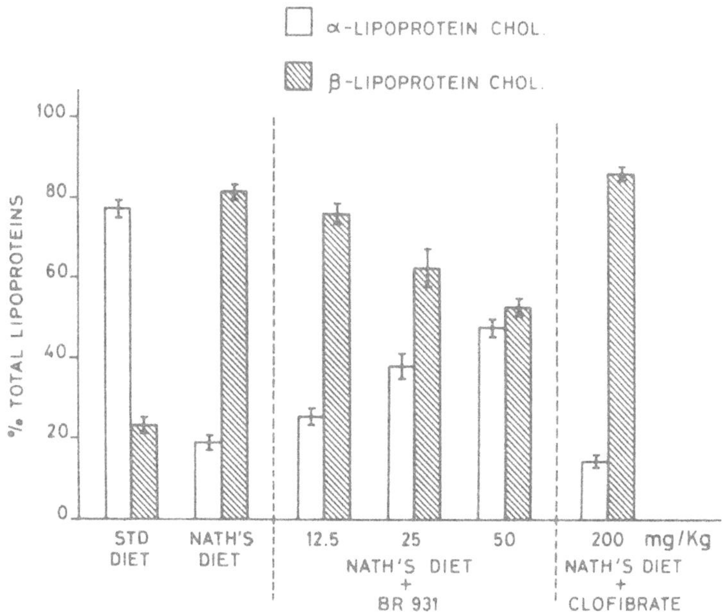

Fig. 7 Example of the evaluation of the effect of two hypolipidemic drugs on high density lipoprotein (α) levels in rats on a high fat diet. The diet _per se_ leads to a dramatic reduction of α-lipoproteins; clofibrate does not appear to influence the ratio between atherogenic (VLDL+LDL, β) and antiatherogenic (HDL, α) lipoproteins; in contrast, progressively higher doses of BR-931 tend to lead this ratio back to normal.[30]

organelles. Interestingly, it appears that in addition to hypolipidemic agents, drugs such as aspirin,[23] food additives, e.g., phthalates,[24] natural compounds such as ursodeoxycholic acid[25] and finally polyunsaturated fatty acids of marine origin[26] may be associated with the proliferation of peroxisomes in rodent liver.

Increased HDL Cholesterol Levels in Rodent Models

The clinical observation of the apparent protection against atherosclerotic processes by elevated HDL cholesterol levels,[27] has led to the wide use of animal models, predictive of this potentially beneficial effect. The rodent model was first tested by Day et al.[28] Administration of several potential hypolipidemic drugs, together with a fat enriched regimen, was followed by the separation of heparin precipitable lipoproteins, allowing a simple mass screening procedure for the identification of compounds with HDL raising properties.

This screening method, with various modifications, has been widely applied. By this technique, it has been generally inferred that clofibrate in rodents does not lead to increased HDL cholesterol levels, in contrast to newer agents.[29] An example of this application, derived from our experience, is reported in Fig. 7.

On the other hand, more recent studies on the function of lipoproteins in different animal species have indicated that in rodents HDL serves a dual purpose. Being the most abundant circulating lipoprotein fraction, HDL have, in fact, both a centripetal and centrifugal role.[30] Separation of fractions serving one or the other role may be achieved by various techniques.[31] The separation of HDL by precipitation and, for that matter, by other techniques, may, therefore, not lead to the measurement of the anti-atherogenic fraction in this animal model.

In a recent comparative evaluation of clofibrate and of EMD 34 853 (see above), we noted discrepant findings between the HDL-cholesterol levels determined by selective precipitation and by ultracentrifuge (d 1.063-1.21). It appears, in fact, that in rodents on a fat regimen, only HDL-cholesterol levels determined after precipitation were increased by EMD 34 853, but not the cholesterol levels of the ultracentrifugally separated lipoproteins. Composition of HDL apoproteins, after ultracentrifugal separation, showed enrichment with apo E of HDL from clofibrate-treated, but not of HDL from EMD 34 853-treated rats.[32] Although recent findings suggest that the apo E poor HDL is probably responsible for the reverse cholesterol transport,[33] further data are necessary to clarify whether the HDL fractions raised by specific drug treatments may indeed exert protective arterial cholesterol deposition.

Induction of High Affinity Receptors for Lipoproteins

An increase in the number of high affinity receptors for lipoproteins, particularly for β-VLDL and LDL, is a typical liver response to cholesterol deprivation, be it a consequence of increased catabolism and elimination (e.g., treatment with anion exchange resins), or to reduced biosynthesius (e.g., HMG-CoA reductase inhibitors).[34,35] In the latter case, particularly in the rodent model, treatment with _mevinolin_ may result in an increase of intracellular HMG CoA reductase activity, as a response to the loss of feedback cholesterol regulation.[36] Even when taking these cautionary considerations into account, several data indicate that absorbable hypolipidemic drugs may increase receptor activity, particularly in the liver. In clinical studies, bezafibrate enhanced the clearance of ^{125}I-labeled LDL in treated type II patients.[37] In the experimental setting, a good animal model may be the rat. With EMD 34 853, we could show a 3-fold increase of the Bmax for β-VLDL from cholesterol-fed rabbits in cell membrane preparations from rats treated

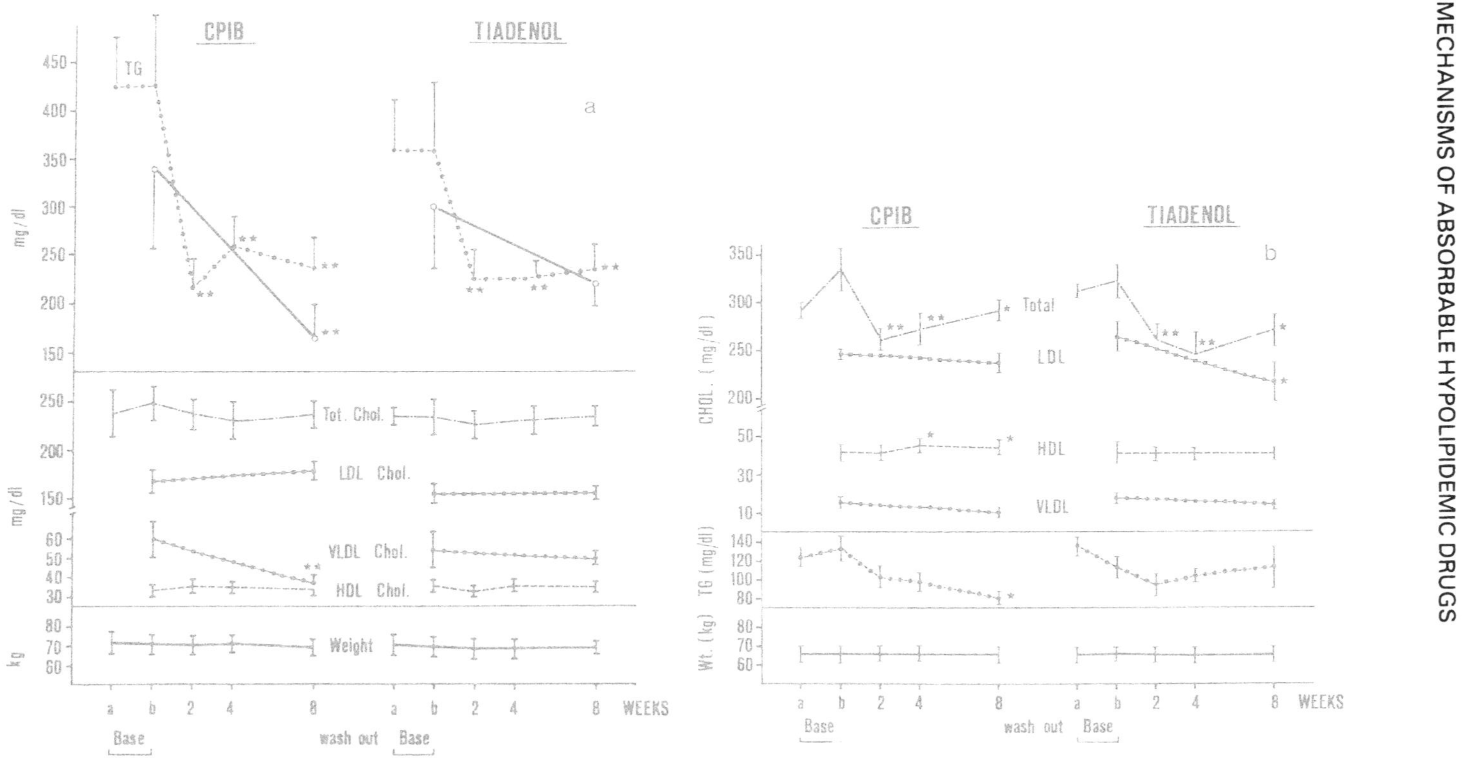

Fig. 8 Plasma lipid and lipoprotein responses to clofibrate (CPIB) and tiadenol in type IV and type IIA patients. In type IV (A), both drugs significantly reduce total triglycerides (TG) (*—*—*), CPIB being more effective than tiadenol; however, only CPIB significantly reduces both VLDL triglyceridemia (o——o) and cholesterolemia (●—●—●). In type IIA patients (B), conversely, both drugs significantly lower total cholesterolemia, but only tiadenol significantly lowers LDL-associated cholesterol (-17.6%).[42]

with a 30 mg/kg dose of the agent.[32] The increased receptor activity is only noted in animals on a normal dietary regimen. Addition of cholesterol to the experimental diet leads to a receptor down-regulation, not amenable to correction by drug treatments.

ABSORBABLE DRUGS NOT AFFECTING LIPOPROTEIN CATABOLISM

Limited attention has been paid to drugs which do not activate LPL activity. The only example, up to now, is that of tiadenol, a bis-thio-decane derivative, shown to possess significant hypolipidemic properties in animal models as well as in human hyperlipoproteinemias.[38,39] In previous studies in type IV patients, we could show that plasma TG reduction was not associated with any significant stimulation of LPL activity.[40]

In a comparative study of clofibrate and tiadenol, given in random order to patients with different forms of hyperlipoproteinemia, clofibrate constantly reduced VLDL cholesterol and TG levels, whereas this effect was generally not significant with tiadenol[41] (Fig. 8). In contrast, the latter exerted a specific cholesterol lowering activity in the LDL fraction of type II patients. This last finding is in line with the demonstration of a marked cholesterol lowering activity of the agent in familial type II patients.[42] It may be concluded tentatively that tiadenol, and possibly other agents with similar mechanism, while not affecting lipoprotein breakdown, may reduce the secretion of lipoprotein particles by the liver, with a major effect on LDL levels.

CONCLUSION

Studies with absorbable hypolipidemic drugs, in the past 15 years, have provided significant contributions to the understanding of the physiology and pathology of lipid transport. The mechanism of most of these agents appears to be related to a stimulation of the breakdown of TG-rich lipoproteins, i.e., a "catabolic" effect. This mechanism may explain most if not all of the experimental and clinical observations. It may also help to understand the peroxisomal proliferation, consequent to treatment with many of these drugs. Proliferation of peroxisomes may also be related to specific structural features of the agents, i.e., unstable aromatic arrangement.

Newer technologies in the developmental studies of newer agents have evaluated lipoprotein modifications, particularly the increased HDL levels. The significance of this last finding should be rated in terms of the lipoprotein metabolism in the animal. An increase of liver receptor activity for lipoproteins is generally a consequence of a marked reduction of cholesterol transport. On the other hand, detection of an increased receptor activity confirms the potential for a drug under study, to markedly affect cholesterol synthesis and distribution.

In conclusion, studies on lipid lowering drugs may benefit significantly from a collaborative effort between basic, clinical and biochemical investigators. Newer drugs, designed with the knowledge collected in the past two decades, may offer significant advantages in terms of safety and efficacy for patients selected for treatment.

REFERENCES

1. C. R. Sirtori, Lancet i:1362 (1981).
2. L. A. Carlson, A. G. Olsson, and D. Ballantyne, Atherosclerosis 26:603 (1977).
3. J. P. Desager and C. Harvengt, Int. J. Clin. Pharmacol. Biopharm. 16:570 (1978).
4. G. Franceschini, M. Sirtori, G. Gianfranceschi, T. Frosi, G. Montanari, and C. R. Sirtori, Artery, submitted for publication.
5. P. Schwandt, P. Weisweiler, M. Drosner, and P. Janetschek, Atherosclerosis 42:245 (1982).
6. J. R. Patsch, A. M. Gotto, Jr., T. Olivecrona, and S. Eisenberg, Proc. Natl. Acad. Sci., U.S.A., 75:4519 (1978).
7. A. G. Olsson and P. D. Lang, Atherosclerosis 31:429 (1978).
8. S. Roessner and L. Oroe, Atherosclerosis 38:273 (1981).
9. A. Lehtonen and J. Viikari, Artery 10:353 (1982).
10. G. Friedman, T. Chajek-Shaul, O. Stein, T. Olivecrona, and Y. Stein, Biochim. Biophys. Acta 666:156 (1981).
11. B. M. Wolfe, J. P. Kane, R. J. Havel, and H. P. Brewster, J. Clin. Invest. 52:2146 (1973.
12. J. M. Tolmasoff, T. Ono, and R. G. Cutler, Proc. Natl. Acad. Sci., U.S.A., 77:2777 (1980).
13. H. Ishii, N. Fukumori, S. Horie, and T. Suga, Biochim. Biophys. Acta 617:1 (1980).
14. J. K. Reddy, D. L.Azarnoff, and C. R. Sirtori, Arch. Int. Pharmacodyn. Ther. 234:4 (1978).
15. N. D. Lalwani, M. K. Reddy, S. A. Qureshi, C. R. Sirtori, Y. Abiko, and J. K. Reddy, Human Toxicol. 2:27 (1983).
16. J. K. Reddy, D. L. Azarnoff, and C. Hignite, Nature 283:397 (1980).
17. M. Bendayan, M. K. Reddy, T. Hashimoto, and J. K. Reddy, J. Histochem. Cytochem. 31:509 (1983).
18. M. Hanefeld, C. Kemmer, W. Loenhardt, K. D. Kjuze, W. Joross, and H. Haller, Atherosclerosis 37:157 (1980).
19. F. A. De La Iglesia, J. E. Lewis, R. A. Buchanan, E. L. Marcus, G. McMahon, Atherosclerosis 43:19 (1982).
20. M. Hanefeld, C. Kemmer, and E. Kadner, Atherosclerosis 46:239 (1983).

21. R. Destro, C. Scolastico, and C. R. Sirtori, Manuscript in preparation.
22. D. L. Azarnoff, J. K. Reddy, C. Hignite, and T. Fitzgerald, in: "Proceedings VI Int. Congress of Pharmacology," Vol. 4. H. Vapaatalo, ed., IUPHAR, Helsinki, p. 137 (1975).
23. H. Ishii and T. Suga, Biochem. Pharmacol. 28:2829 (1979).
24. J. K. Reddy, D. E. Moody, D. L. Azarnoff, and M. S. Ras, Life Sci. 18:941 (1976).
25. S. F. Salen, G. Zaki, and G. Salen, Hepatology 3:201 (1983).
26. E. N. Christiansen, T. Flatmark, and H. Kryvi, Eur. J. Cell Biol. 26:11 (1981).
27. G. J. Miller and N. E. Miller, Lancet i:16 (1975).
28. C. E. Day, P. E. Schurr, D. E. Emmert, R. E. Ten Brink, and D. Lednicer, J. Med. Chem. 18:1075 (1975).
29. C. R. Sirtori, P. Gomarasca, G. D'Atri, S. Cerutti, G. Tronconi, and C. Scolastico, Atherosclerosis 30:45 (1978).
30. Y. Stein, M. C. Glangeaud, M. Fainaru, and O. Stein, Biochim. Biophys. Acta 431:347 (1976).
31. T. L. Innerarity and R. W. Mahley, Biochemistry 17:1440 (1980).
32. H. Nowak, E. Bosisio, M. Galbussera, and C. R. Sirtori, Manuscript in preparation.
33. V. Gordon, T. L. Innerarity, and R. W. Mahley, J. Biol. Chem. 258:6202 (1983).
34. J. Shepherd, C. J. Packer, S. Bicker, T. D. V. Lowrie, and H. G. Morgan, N. Engl. J. Med. 302:1219 (1980).
35. P. T. Kovanen, D. W. Bilheimer, J. L. Goldstein, J. J. Jaramillo, and M. S. Brown, Proc. Natl. Acad. Sci., U.S.A., 78:1194 (1984).
36. M. S. Brown, J. Faust, J. L. Goldstein, I. Kaneko, and A. Endo, J. Biol. Chem. 253:1121 (1978).
37. J. M. Stewart, C. J. Packard, A. R. Lorimer, D. E. Boag, and J. Shepard, Atherosclerosis 44:355 (1982).
38. D. Kritchevsky, S. A. Tepper, S. A. Czarnecki, and J. A. Story, Pharmacol. Res. Comm. 11:475 (1979).
39. J. Rouffy and J. Loeper, Therapie 27:433 (1972).
40. G. Franceschini, A. Poli, A. L. Catapano, E. Gatti, M. Sirtori, G. Gianfranceschi, and C. R. Sirtori, Atherosclerosis 40:245 (1981).
41. M. Sirtori, G. Montanari, G. Gianfranceschi, M. G. Malacrida, P. Battistin, G. Morazzoni, E. Tremoli, S. Colli, P. Maderna, and C. R. Sirtori, Atherosclerosis 49:149 (1983).
42. G. Baggio, G. Briani, R. Fellin, S. Martini, M. R. Baiocchi, and G. Crepaldi, Artery 5:486 (1979).

DIETARY FACTORS AFFECTING LIPOPROTEIN METABOLISM

Paul J. Nestel

Baker Medical Research Institute
Commerical Road
Prahran, Victoria, 3181, Australia

This paper will discuss several facets of dietary influence on plasma lipids and lipoproteins. Recent developments that will be considered include, 1) the effect of fish oils on lipid metabolism; 2) the stimulation by dietary cholesterol of lipoprotein transport; 3) the interactions of dietary fats and dietary cholesterol; 4) the modification of triglyceride production by inhibiting glucoside hydrolysis; 5) the effect of dietary casein on lipoprotein and cholesterol clearance.

FISH OILS AND LIPOPROTEIN METABOLISM

The fatty acids of fish oils differ from those of land animals and vegetable oils. Marine fatty acids, especially from cold waters, are rich in polyunsaturated fatty acids (PUFA) of the omega-3 (ω-3) series and contain up to six double bonds. Vegetable oils tend to be rich in linoleic acid (ω-6, two double bonds). Thus cod liver oil contains >50% of fatty acid as ω-3, while safflower oil contains >50% as ω-6.

Recent dietary studies with marine PUFA have shown a striking reduction in plasma lipids, especially in triglyceride within very low density lipoproteins (VLDL).[1,2] Patients with severe hypertriglyceridemia respond most satisfactorily.

The mechanism for this profound lipid-lowering effect is unknown. We have studied the effect of a diet rich in fish oil on the rate of production of the triglyceride-transporting very low density lipoprotein (VLDL) in normal and in hypertriglyceridemic subjects who received up to 30% of daily energy needs from a fish oil preparation.

The oil was rich in eicosapentaenoic acid and docosahexaenoic acid, omega-3 fatty acids with 5 and 6 double-bonds respectively.

Compared to a diet enriched with safflower oil, the fish oil diet lowered VLDL lipids and B apoprotein concentrations profoundly as early as 1 week later. HDL lipids and A_1 apoprotein were also lowered but the effect on LDL concentration was inconsistent. Triglyceride levels became normal in hypertriglyceridemic subjects. The reductions in the lipids and in apoprotein B in VLDL and in IDL have been observed previously with linoleate-rich (ω-6) diets[3-5] but the effects with ω-3 PUFA are far greater. The cholesterol in HDL and

TABLE 1

TRANSPORT OF VLDL APOPROTEIN B AT END OF EACH OF THE SAFFLOWER OIL AND FISH OIL DIETS IN 4 NORMAL AND 2 HYPERTRIGLYCERIDEMIC SUBJECTS

SUBJECTS	Diet	Pool*	Irreversible Fractional Removal	Flux
		mg	day^{-1}	mg/d
1	S	148	3.15	468
	F	49	5.82	285
2	S	300	5.30	1588
	F	40	6.37	254
3	S	133	6.24	829
	F	18	9.60	173
4	S	202	7.08	1430
	F	54	11.28	609
5†	S	2160	2.08	4492
	F	762	1.95	1486
6†	S	774	4.38	3390
	F	515	2.87	1478

S = safflower oil; F = fish oil;

*Data for kinetics in pool A, the rapidly equilibrating pool.

†Hypertriglyceridemic subjects.

TABLE 2

EFFECTS OF FISH OIL ON TRIGLYCERIDE SECRETION FROM PERFUSED RAT LIVER

Addition to Diet	n	VLDL TG Secretion µmol/g/hr
None	4	1.84 ± 0.12
Safflower	5	2.10 ± 0.18
Fish Oil	4	0.87 ± 0.10 **

Wong, Nestel, Topping 1983

apoprotein A_1 reductions have also been reported with ω-6 PUFA[6] which again were exceeded by ω-3 PUFA.

The production of VLDL apoprotein B, calculated from reinjected ^{125}I labeled VLDL was significantly lower in all subjects after 1-3 weeks of fish oil compared with safflower oil (Table 1).

Reduced formation has also been put forward to explain the triglyceride lowering effect of ω-6 PUFA. We have previously demonstrated a lesser utilization of linoleic acid than of palmitic acid for triglyceride formation.[7] Recently Lewis and co-workers have reported a reduced flux of VLDL apoprotein B with ω-6 PUFA diets.[8] In preliminary studies we have observed significantly reduced VLDL triglyceride flux following injections of radioglycerol in subjects fed MaxEPA oil (Reardon, Nestel and Boston, unpublished).

Further studies have been carried out with perfused rat livers. Livers from rats fed either a standard commercial chow (controls) or diets supplemented with 15% (w/w) fish or safflower oils were perfused with undiluted rat blood. The hepatic release of very low density lipoprotein triglyceride mass was significantly depressed in animals fed the fish oil-supplemented diet but not in those fed safflower oil (Table 2). Rates of hepatic lipogenesis were measured from the incorporation of ^3H_2O into fatty acids, and showed the lowest rates for fish oil fed rats (Table 3).

By contrast, ketogenesis was increased by fish oil feeding (Table 3). The results in the rat livers indicate that the lowering of plasma triglyceride by fish oil reflects: (a) diminished secretion of triglyceride by the liver; (b) dimished lipogenesis; (c) increased fatty acid oxidation possibly in peroxisomes. The diversion of highly

TABLE 3

EFFECTS OF FISH OIL ON LIPID METABOLISM IN PERFUSED RAT LIVERS

Addition to Diet	n	Lipogenesis μmol fatty acid/g/hr	Ketogenesis μmol/g/hr
None	4	3.10 ± 0.22	2.46 ± 0.01
Safflower	5	2.43 ± 0.19*	2.68 ± 0.19
Fish Oil	4	1.34 ± 0.13**	3.45 ± 0.21**

Wong, Nestel, Topping 1983

polyunsaturated fatty acids to pathways of oxidation from those of esterification, contribute to the fall in VLDL.

EFFECTS OF DIETARY CHOLESTEROL ON LIPOPROTEIN TRANSPORT

The rise in plasma cholesterol through increased cholesterol consumption reflects changes in cholesterol within several lipoproteins. Although this occurs mostly in low density lipoprotein (LDL) in man, both intermediate density lipoprotein (IDL) and high density lipoprotein (HDL) may also show an increase in cholesterol content. We[9] have recently reported additional changes in VLDL composition that include enrichment with cholesteryl ester and apoprotein E and an increased affinity for heparin by a proportion of VLDL particles. In subjects eating 1700 mg cholesterol daily, these cholesteryl ester, apoprotein E-rich particles accumulated in plasma within two weeks. This subpopulation of VLDL, smaller than normal triglyceride rich VLDL resemble the more evident particles in cholesterol-fed animals, termed -VLDL.[10] The question arises whether these are remnants of VLDL, or even of chylomicrons, or independently secreted smaller lipoproteins approximating IDL. Direct secretion of IDL with cholesterol feeding has been demonstrated in rats.[11]

From our studies of VLDL apoprotein B kinetics in subjects eating 1700 mg daily cholesterol, that revealed no rise in production,[9] we reasoned that the cholesteryl ester-rich VLDL were therefore secreted directly from the liver, representing retransport of dietary cholesterol. We therefore measured the transport of IDL apoprotein B in 8 men during two dietary periods containing either 200 mg or 1700 mg cholesterol per day.[12] Radioiodinated IDL were reinjected and trans-

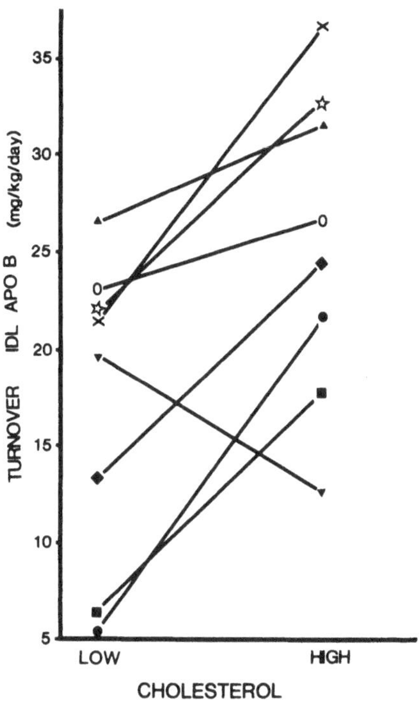

Fig. 1 Production of Apoprotein B in Intermediate Density Lipoprotein (IDL) with low and high cholesterol intakes. (P. Nestel and T. Billington, Metabolism 32:320 (1983).

port calculated from specific radioactivity-time curves of apoprotein B in reisolated IDL. With cholesterol loading, the IDL cholesterol and apoprotein B concentrations rose in 7 of 8 subjects. IDL transport was stimulated consistently and significantly ($p < 0.01$), rising by at least 50% in 5 subjects (Figure 1). Furthermore, the change in plasma total cholesterol concentration was significantly correlated with the change in IDL transport ($r = +0.70$, $p < 0.05$). Since LDL are derived from IDL, the cholesterol-induced rise in IDL formation may explain the increase in LDL concentration with dietary cholesterol. We tested this indirectly, by estimating the fractional rate of appearance of IDL radioactivity within LDL and observed this to be greater with the higher intake of cholesterol (Figure 2).

INTERACTIONS OF DIETARY FATS AND DIETARY CHOLESTEROL

Recently published studies by Schonfeld et al.[4] have confirmed the important interaction between the amounts of dietary cholesterol and the degree of unsaturation of the dietary fat on the plasma LDL concentration. The rise in the serum cholesterol at a given choles-

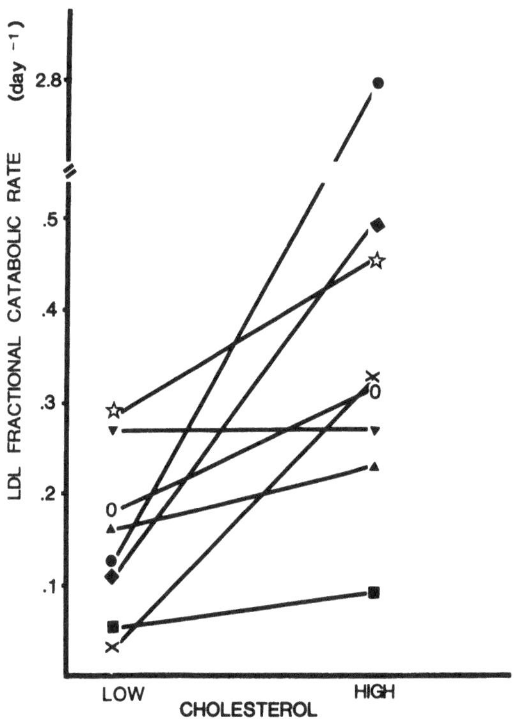

Fig. 2 Fractional rate of transfer of IDL Apo-B radioactivity to low density lipoprotein (LDL), with low and high cholesterol intakes.

sterol intake is less with increasing unsaturation of dietary fatty acids.[13] The total amount of dietary fat also affects the cholesterolemic response to dietary cholesterol, being less at low than at high intakes of fat.[14] These critical interactions are often overlooked in studies on free living subjects which claim that dietary cholesterol exerts little if any influence on the serum cholesterol concentration.

REDUCTION IN TRIGLYCERIDE PRODUCTION WITH GLUCOSIDE HYDROLASE INHIBITION

This class of drugs, that includes acarbose, an inhibitor of alpha-glucoside hydrolase, may offer a new approach to the treatment of diabetic hypertriglyceridemia, since, when given with a carbohydrate meal it reduces the glycemia and insulinemia.[15] Because hypertriglyceridemia is influenced by dietary carbohydrate and related to the degree of insulinemia we have tested the usefulness of acarbose in modifying the severity of carbohydrate-induced hypertriglyceridemia (Nestel, Bazelmans, Reardon and Boston, unpublished).

Eight men were given diets comprising 65-67% of energy as carbohydrate (mainly starch and sucrose) for 3-4 weeks. Triglyceride production was measured over the final two days of each period, using radioglycerol as label and analyzing the VLDL triglyceride specific radioactivity curves by compartmental kinetics.

The carbohydrate diet led to a significant mean increase in triglyceride level for the group. While the diet led to greater expansion in the VLDL triglyceride pool with placebo (3496 $\pm$ 1198 mg, mean $\pm$ SEM) than with acarbose (2963 $\pm$ 1028 mg), the difference was not signficant. The fractional catabolic rates were on average similar with placebo (0.42 $\pm$ 0.05 hr^{-1}) and acarbose (0.41 $\pm$ 0.09 hr^{-1}) but the production or flux of VLDL triglyceride was significantly lower with acarbose:placebo (13.4 $\pm$ 2.6 $mg.kg^{-1}.hr^{-1}$) versus acarbose (9.7 $\pm$ 1.7 $mg.kg^{-1}.hr^{-1}$).

DIETARY CASEIN AND SOY PROTEIN ON CHOLESTEROL AND LIPOPROTEIN METABOLISM

The substitution of vegetable protein for animal protein leads to a small but significant reduction in serum cholesterol level in healthy subjects[16] but appears to be more effective in hypercholesterolemia.[17] The most responsive animal model is the rabbit which becomes markedly hypercholesterolemic with dietary casein. Cholesterol catabolism is reduced in such rabbits[18] but the recent finding by Chao et al.[19] that casein also suppresses the activity of the specific receptor for LDL in rabbit liver represents a major advance in this area. They have also shown that the initial lipoprotein abnormality with casein feeding is accumulation of LDL.

We have studied the effects of casein feeding in a less susceptible animal model, the cholesterol-fed rat (Cohn and Nestel, unpublished). Younger, more responsive rats showed an initial accumulation of VLDL cholesterol when casein was substituted for soy protein. Cholesterol absorption was similar with both sources of protein as was total exchangeable cholesterol transport (calculated by compartmental analysis). However, the irreversible removal rate of cholesterol was significantly less in the casein-fed rats, indicating that clearance of lipoprotein cholesterol, rather than overproduction, was responsible for casein-induced hypercholesterolemia in rats (Table 4).

DIETARY FIBER LOWERS SERUM CHOLESTEROL

Several reports have shown that viscous gums and leguminous fibers

TABLE 4

CHOLESTEROL KINETICS (COMPARTMENTAL ANALYSIS) IN CASEIN-FED AND SOY-FED RATS SUPPLEMENTED WITH DIETARY CHOLESTEROL AND COCONUT-OIL

	Plasma cholesterol $mg.dl^{-1}$	Absorption %	Mass Pool A mg	Production $mg.d^{-1}$	Fractional clearance, d^{-1}
Casein-fed	201 ± 11	40 ± 5	71.9 ± 7.3	21.8 ± 1.1	0.32 ± 0.03
Soy-fed	51 ± 7	41 ± 4	43.9 ± 7.2	23.1 ± 1.8	0.49 ± 0.04

Cohn & Nestel, 1983

Cholesterol kinetics measured after injection of ^{14}C-cholesterol.

Cholesterol absorption measured from plasma ratios of orally administered ^{3}H-cholesterol and intravenously administered ^{14}C-cholesterol.

TABLE 5

EFFECTS OF DIETARY FIBER ON PLASMA LIPIDS, GLUCOSE AND INSULIN AND ON INSULIN SENSITIVITY

	High Fiber	Low-Fiber
Fasting FFA (μM/l)	453 ± 33*	432 ± 50
Fasting Glucose (mM)	4.6 ± 0.1	4.6 ± 0.1
Fasting Insulin (μU/ml)	6 ± 1	5 ± 1
Fasting Cholesterol (mg/dl)	133 ± 10#	156 ± 13
Fasting Triglyceride (mg/dl)	100 ± 16	131 ± 35
Insulin Sensitivity	11 ± 1.5	12 ± 1.9
(mg glucose/kg.min/μU insulin/ml)		

*Mean ± SEM

#Significantly lower on high-fiber ($p < 0.05$)

lower plasma cholesterol levels in man.[14,20] It is unlikely that this is importantly related in man to increased steroid excretion because the two effects can be dissociated.[21] We have examined the possibility that the lipid lowering effect may be related to improved carbohydrate tolerance and insulin sensitivity. We have compared these parameters in healthy, normolipidemic men on two diets rich in starch, one containing 16 g and the other 100 g fiber (Nestel, Nolan and Bazelmans, unpublished).

Whereas the serum cholesterol was significantly lower with the fiber-rich diet (Table 5), glucose tolerance (4 hr 75 g glucose tolerance test) and insulin sensitivity (insulin infusion, euglycemic clamp technique) were similar with both diets.

REFERENCES

1. T. O. von Lossonczy, A. Ruiter, H. C. Bronsgeest-Schoute, C. M. Van Gent and R. J. J. Hermus, The effect of a fish diet on serum lipids in healthy human subjects, Am. J. Clin. Nutr. 31:1340-1346 (1978).
2. W. S. Harris, W. E. Connor, and S. H. Goodnight, Jr., in: "Progress in Lipid Research," Ralph Holman, ed., Pergamon Press, Oxford, England, 20:75-79 (1982).
3. E. H. Ahrens, J. Hirsch, W. Insull, T. T. Tsaltas, R. Blomstrand, and M. L. Peterson, The influence of dietary fats on serum-lipid in man, Lancet 1:943-953 (1957).
4. G. Schonfeld, W. Patsch, L. L. Rudel, C. Nelson, M. Epstein, and R. E. Olson, Effects of dietary cholesterol and fatty acids on plasma lipoproteins, J. Clin. Invest. 69:1072-1080 (1982).
5. G. L. Vega, E. Groszek, R. Wolk, and S. M. Grundy, Influence of polyunsaturated fats on composition of plasma lipoproteins and apolipoproteins, J. Lipid Res. 23:811-822 (1982).
6. J. Shepherd, C. J. Packard, J. R. Patsch, A. M. Gotto, Jr., and O. D. Taunton, Effects of dietary polyunsaturated and saturated fat on the properties of high density lipoprotein and the metabolism of apolipoprotein A-I, J. Clin. Invest. 60: 1582-1592 (1978).
7. P. J. Nestel and P. Barter, Metabolism of palmitic and linoleic acids in man: differences in turnover and conversion to glycerides, Clin. Sci. 40:345-350 (1971).
8. Y. Levy, S. Rao, C. Whiting, E. Janus, N. Miller, and B. Lewis, Dietary effects on very low density (VLDL) and low density (LDL) lipoprotein apoprotein B (APO B) metabolism in man, Eur. J. Clin. Invest. Suppl. p.19 (1981).
9. P. Nestel, N. Tada, T. Billington, M. Huff, and N. Fidge, Changes in very low density lipoproteins with cholesterol loading in man, Metabolism 31:398-405 (1982).
10. R. W. Mahley, Alterations in plasma lipoproteins induced by cholesterol feeding in animals including man, in: "Disturbances in Lipid and Lipoprotein Metabolism," J. M. Dietschy, A. M. Gotto, and J. A. Ontko, eds., Williams & Wilkins Co., Baltimore, 181-197 (1978).
11. L. L. Swift, N. R. Manowitz, G. D. Dunn, and V. S. LeQuire, Isolation and characterization of hepatic Golgi lipoproteins from hypercholesterolemic rats, J. Clin. Invest. 66:415-425 (1980).
12. P. J. Nestel and T. Billington, Increased transport of intermediate density lipoprotein with cholesterol loading, Metabolism 32:320-322 (1983).
13. P. J. Nestel, in: "'Atherosclerosis IV' Proceedings of Fourth International Symposium," G. Schettler, Y. Goto, Y. Hata, and G. Klose, eds., Springer-Verlag, Berlin, pp. 442-444 (1977).
14. B. Lewis, F. Hammett, M. Katan, R. M. Kay, I. Merkx, A. Nobels, N. E. Miller, and A. V. Swan, Towards an improved lipid-

lowering diet: additive effects of changes in nutrient intake, Lancet 2:1310-1313 (1981).

15. D. J. A. Jenkins, R. H. Taylor, D. V. Goff, H. Fielden, J. J. Misiewicv, D. L. Sarson, S. R. Bloom, and K. G. Alberti, Scope and specificity of acarbose in slowing carbohydrate absorption in man, Diabetes 30:951-954 (1981).
16. K. K. Carroll, P. M. Giovannetti, M. W. Huff, O. Moase, D. C. K. Roberts, and B. M. Wolfe, Hypercholesterolemic effect of substituting soybean protein for animal protein in the diet of healthy young women, Amer. J. Clin. Nutr. 31:1312-1321 (1978).
17. C. R. Sirtori, E. Gatti, O. Mantero, F. Conti, E. Agradi, E. Tremoli, M. Sirtori, L. Fraterrigo, L. Tavazzi, and D. Kritchevsky, Clinical experience with the soybean protein diet in the treatment of hypercholesterolemia, Amer. J. Clin. Nutr. 32:1645-1658 (1979).
18. M. W. Huff and K. K. Carroll, Effects of dietary protein on turnover, oxidation, and absorption of cholesterol, and on steroid excretion in rabbits, J. Lipid Res. 21:546-558 (1980).
19. Y. S. Chao, T. T. Yamin, and A. W. Alberts, Effects of cholestyramine on low density lipoprotein binding sites on liver membranes from rabbits and endogenous hypercholesterolemia induced by a wheat starch-casein diet, J. Biol. Chem. 25:3623-3627 (1982).
20. D. Kritchevsky and J. A. Story, Fibre, hypercholesterolaemia, and atherosclerosis, Lipida 13:366-369 (1978).
21. T. L. Raymond, W. E. Connor, D. S. Lin et al., The interaction of dietary fibers and cholesterol upon the plasma lipids and lipoproteins, sterol balance, and bowel function in human subjects, J. Clin. Invest. 60:1429-1437 (1977).

INHIBITION OF CHOLESTEROL ABSORPTION BY NATURAL PRODUCTS

George V. Vahouny

Department of Biochemistry
The George Washington University
School of Medicine and Health Sciences
Washington, D.C. 20037

There have been numerous reports on the hypocholesteremic properties of a variety of materials derived from biological sources and foods. These include vegetable oils (e.g. 1) and in particular, the plant sterols,[1,2] fish and shellfish oils,[3,4] and the sterols contained in these oils,[5,6] plant fibers and specific fiber components, such as the pectins (e.g. 7) and more recently, some of the acetylated aminopolysaccharides derived from the exoskeleton of certain shellfish.[8,9] These communications reflect on the continuing interest in describing the importance of components of natural foods in maintaining circulating lipid levels and reducing diet - induced hypercholesteremias.

In the case of unabsorbable materials such as plant sterols and dietary fibers, the hypocholesteremic properties are largely ascribed to interference with one or more aspects of the solubilization and/or absorption of intestinal cholesterol, whether dietary or endogenous.[2,10] Although plant and marine oils may also influence cholesterol absorption, their hypocholesteremic properties have also been ascribed to other aspects of the metabolism of circulating lipoproteins.[3]

The present communication is concerned only with evaluation of the direct effects of a variety of "natural" products and derivatives on intestinal absorption of cholesterol into the lymphatic circulation of the rat. The test materials include specific plant sterols, shellfish sterols, plant fibers and acetylated aminopolysaccharides, and specific vegetable and marine oils. In some cases, only acute responses have been evaluated, while in others, the chronic "adaptive" responses to longer term feeding of the test materials have also been studied. Portions of these studies are elaborated in greater detail in specific publications.[10-15]

EXPERIMENTAL PROCEDURES

For acute studies, adult male albino rats (200-300 g) were allowed food and water ad libitum, and maintained at 25°C with a 12-h light-dark cycle. Animals were subjected to cannulation of the left thoracic lymphatic channel under sodium pentobarbital anesthesia as described previously.[11,12] In addition, an indwelling catheter was placed in the stomach for continuous infusion of saline-5% glucose (3 ml/h) and introduction of the test emulsions. At 9:00 a.m. the next day, each animal was administered 3 ml of the aqueous test emulsion via the stomach catheter, the saline-glucose infusion was reestablished, and lymph was collected on ice for specified periods up to 24 h.

The aqueous test emulsions[11,12] contained the following components: 50 mg [1,2-^{3}H] cholesterol (5μ Ci); 50 mg bovine serum albumin; 288 mg sodium taurocholate; 291 mg [1-^{14}C] oleic acid. For specific studies, additions to this basic emulsion included: 50 mg of either cholestyramine or chitosan; 50 mg of β-sitosterol, stigmasterol or fucosterol; 50 mg oyster sterols. Where indicated, the cholesterol was replaced by the plant sterol or shellfish sterols, and the oleic acid was substituted for by either corn oil, salmon oil, arachidonic acid or 5,8,11,14-eicosapentaenoic acid.

For chronic feeding effects, animals (150-200 g) were provided, ad libitum for 4-6 weeks, a defined diet which was prepared and pelleted by Bio-Serv (Frenchtown, N.J.) and consisted of the following components in g/100 g: dextrose, 55; casein, 25; corn oil, 14; modified USP XIV salt mix, 5; and vitamin mix, 1. Where indicated, the diets also included: 1% or 5% cholestyramine or chitosan; 10% white wheat bran; 10% alfalfa meal; 5% highly metoxylated pectin; 5% guar gum. After the feeding periods, animals were subjected to cannula- of the left thoracic lymph duct and handled as described above.

Lymph samples were extracted in cholorform-methanol (2:1 v/v) according to Folch, et al.[16] Where indicated, aliquots of the lipid extract were analyzed directly for radioactivity by liquid scintillation spectrometry,[12] for distribution of isotope in major lipid classes,[11,12] for fatty acid composition of major lipid classes by derivatization and gas liquid chromatography,[17] and/or for individual sterols by gas-liquid chromatography.[13,14]

All data represent means ± SEM, and differences between groups were analyzed for significance by Student's t-test. p values of <0.05 were considered significant.

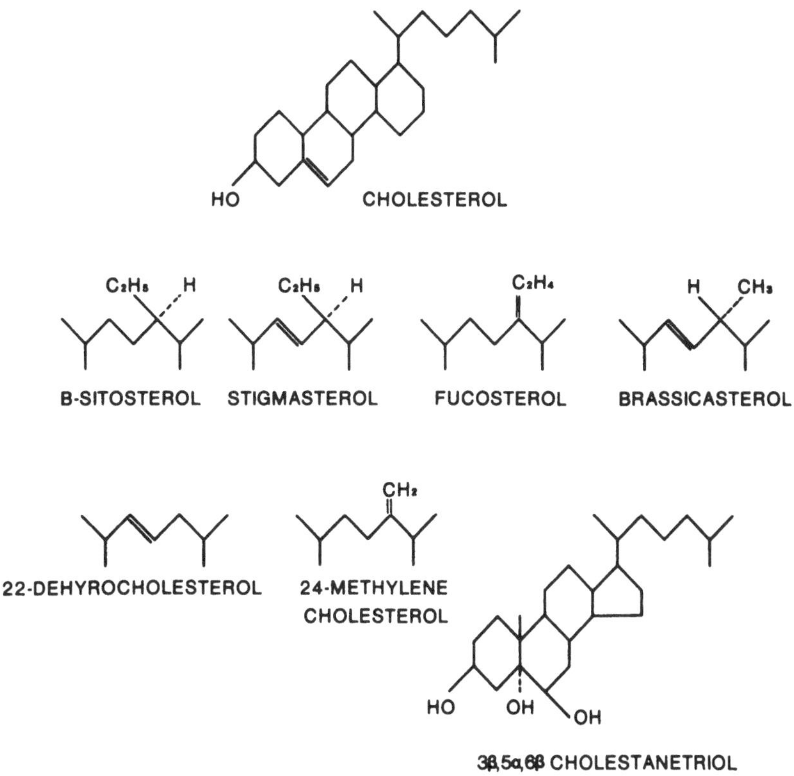

Fig. 1 Structural differences between cholesterol, plant sterols and major sterols of shellfish.

RESULTS

Effects of Plant and Marine Sterols

The structural analogues employed in the present studies are shown in Fig. 1. These included a sterol with ring modifications (3β, 5α, 6β- cholestanetriol) and several sterols with side chain modifications. Derivatives of cholesterol included β-sitosterol (24α-ethyl), fucosterol (24-ethylidine) and 24-methylene cholesterol, while derivatives of 22-dehydrocholesterol included stigmasterol (24α-ethyl) and brassicasterol (24β-methyl).

The purity of the individual sterols, composition of the shellfish sterols, and absorbability of the fed sterols are summarized in Table 1. Methods for purification and identification by gas-liquid chromatography-mass spectrometry are described elsewhere.[13,14]

With the side-chain modified analogues, 22-dehydrocholesterol and 26-carbon sterols were absorbed almost as efficiently as cholesterol.

TABLE 1

ABSORPTION OF STEROL ANALOGUES AND EFFECTS ON CHOLESTEROL ABSORPTION

STEROL ANALOGUE	COMPOSITION	RELATIVE ABSORBABILITY (CHOLESTEROL = 100)	DEPRESSION OF CHOLESTEROL ABSORPTION
	%		%
β-Sitosterol	95.6	7.0	54
Stigmasterol	96.3	10.3	54
Fucosterol	94.4	8.4	0
Cholestane triol	100	4.5	58
Oyster Sterols			
cholesterol	34.9	--	
24-methylene cholesterol	20.7	61	
Brassicosterol	18.7	36	
Plant sterols	9.8	< 10 (54, 24-methylene cholesterol to 26 carbon sterols)	39 (24-methylene cholesterol to 26 carbon sterols)
22-dehydrocholesterol	8.2	83	
26 carbon sterols	7.7	92	

Absorption of individual sterols were determined by lymphatic recovery after a 50 mg intragastric dose of each sterol or mixture in an aqueous emulsion (12). Effects on cholesterol absorption were determined by employing mixture of 25-70 mg of cholesterol and each test sterol. Data are modified from Vahouny et. al. (11,13,14).

Substitutions at the carbon 24 position of cholesterol resulted in varying degrees of unabsorbability. This progressed from 24-methylene cholesterol (61% of cholesterol) to brassicasterol (24β-methyl-22-dehydrocholesterol; 36% of cholesterol). Despite the increased water-solubility characteristics of cholestanetriol,[11] this derivative was also poorly absorbed, based on lymphatic recovery of the fed sterols.

In general administration of equal levels of test sterols with cholesterol, the test sterols resulted in a significant depression of cholesterol absorption (Table 1, column 3). Thus, β-sitosterol, stigmasterol and cholestanetriol, all of which are poorly absorbed, caused a 50-60% depression of cholesterol absorption. The oyster sterols, of which 35% were cholesterol, and only 28.5% were poorly absorbed sterols (brassicasterol and plant sterol), caused a 39% depression in cholesterol absorption.

The interesting exception was fucosterol (24-ethylidine cholesterol), which despite its similar solubility characteristics to other plant sterols and equivalently poor absorbability, had no effect on cholesterol absorption.

Effects of Cholestyramine, Chitosan and Plant Fibers

Cholestyramine is a synthetic anion-exchange resin which sequesters bile acids and other micellar components[18,19] and can acutely depress cholesterol absorption in the rat.[20] Because of this direct intralumenal effect, cholestyramine has been employed as positive control for comparing acute and chronic effects of polysaccharides on cholesterol absorption in the present studies.

As shown in Table 2, when 50 mg cholestyramine was included in the aqueous emulsion used for intragastric administration, choles-

TABLE 2

EFFECTS OF CHOLESTYRAMINE, CHITOSAN AND DIETARY FIBER DERIVATIVES ON CHOLESTEROL ABSORPTION IN THE RAT

AGENTS TESTED	DEPRESSION OF CHOLESTEROL ABSORPTION
	%
ACUTE STUDIES	
Cholestyramine	47 ± 9
Chitosan	51 ± 16
CHRONIC FEEDING STUDIES	
Cholestyramine, 1%	28 ± 3
Cholestyramine, 5%	69 ± 3
Chitosan, 1%	18 ± 10
Chitosan, 5%	63 ± 4
White Wheat Bran, 15%	21 ± 7
Alfalfa, 15%	49 ± 6
Pectin, 15%	31 ± 7
Cellulose, 15%	62 ± 6

terol absorption over the 24-h lymph collection period was depressed by 47%. Under the same conditions, administration of 50 mg chitosan, a partially deacetylated derivative of the aminopolysaccharide, chitin,[15] caused a similar (51%) depression of cholesterol absorption.

In addition to these acute responses to direct inclusion of the agents in the test emulsions, the adaptive effects of chronic feeding of the agents in defined diets was investigated. Cholestyramine or chitosan was included as 1% and 5% of the diet and provided ad libitum for four weeks. Controls received the same diets without these agents. Animals were subjected to cannulation of the thoracic lymphatic duct and fasted overnight. The animals were then given the test emulsion containing cholesterol but without the agents under study.

After feeding 1% of cholestyramine or chitosan four weeks, cholesterol absorption in the fasted animals was depressed by 28 and 18%, respectively (Table 2). In animals fed 5% levels of the agents, cholesterol absorption was reduced by 69% and 63%, respectively.

Dietary fiber derivatives were only investigated for their long-term adaptive effects because of the difficulty of adding sufficient

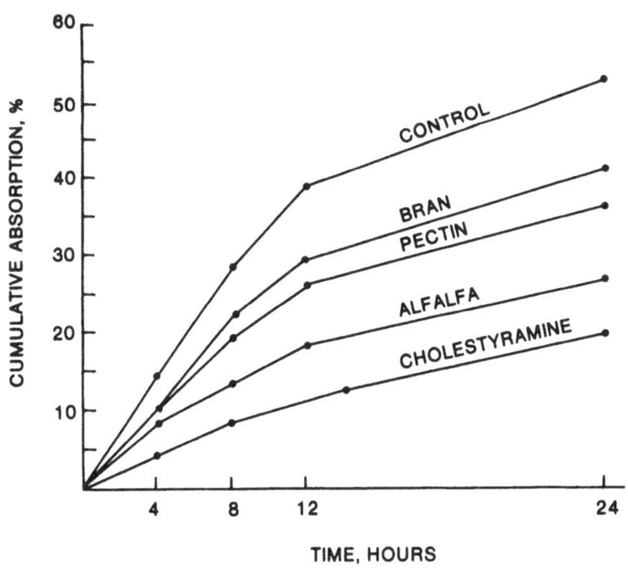

Fig. 2 Cumulative absorption of cholesterol in animals fed semi-synthetic diets containing no dietary fiber (control) or containing 15% levels of white wheat bran, methoxylated pectin, alfalfa meal, or cellulose.

quantities of these materials to the intragastric test emulsion. Animals were fed ad libitum for 5-6 weeks on either the defined diet with no additions (controls), or the diet containing 15% levels of white wheat bran, alfalfa meal, cellulose, or methoxylated pectins. Cholesterol absorption was then determined in surgically prepared and fasted animals.

As shown in Table 2, cholesterol absorption was depressed by 21% in animals fed wheat bran, by 31% in animals given pectin, by 49% in animals fed alfalfa meal and by 76% in rats given cellulose. As shown in Figure 2, the effect of prior feeding of these agents on subsequent cholesterol absorption was expressed throughout the 24-h lymph collection period, suggesting an adaptive response of the intestine to the diet. Furthermore, these responses to diets containing individual fiber components were reproducible.[12]

Since the intragastric emulsions employed in these studies also contained oleic acid, the recovery of [1-^{14}C] oleic acid in lymph lipids was also determined. As shown in Figure 3, there was a direct correlation between effects of various agents on cholesterol absorption and fatty acid recovery in thoracic duct lymph. Thus, the effects of all agents tested in these studies appeared to be on lipid absorption or lipoprotein transport in general, rather than on cholesterol absorption per se.

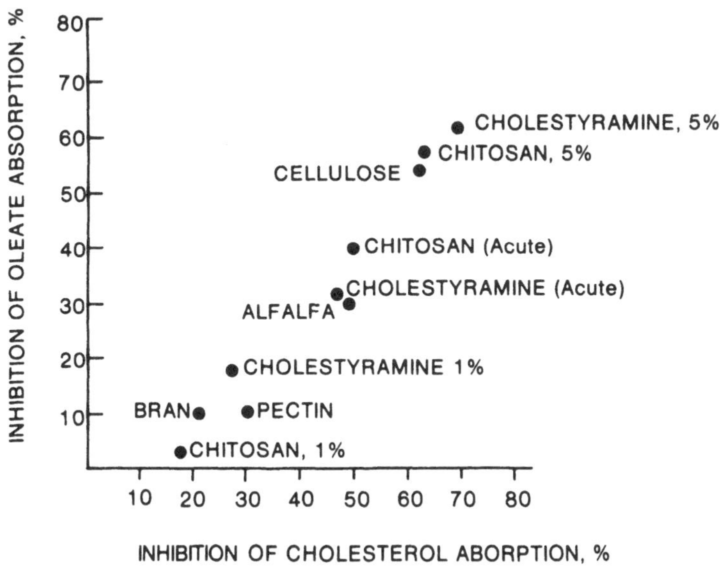

Fig. 3 Correlation of effects of various agents on cholesterol absorption and fatty acid absorption into thoracic duct lymph in rats. Specific conditions for studies on each agent is given under "Experimental Procedures".

Effects of Oleic Acid, Polyunsaturated Acids and Polyunsaturdated Oils on Cholesterol Absorption

Because of the increased interest in biological responses to marine oils containing ω-3 eicosapentaenoic acid (e.g. 3), comparative studies have been conducted on the relative absorbability of polyunsaturated acids and their effects on cholesterol absorption.

In studies with the free fatty acids, oleic, arachidonic (5,8,11,14-eicosatetraenoic acid), or 5,8,11,14,17-eicosapentaenoic acids were included in the test emulsions at levels of 0.3 m mol, and were administered intraduodenally.[21] Lymphatic recovery of the [1-^{14}C] labeled fatty acid and of [1,2-^{3}H] cholesterol (25 mg) was determined over a 24-h collection period.

The data in Table 3 indicated that the two polyunsaturated acids are absorbed as efficiently as oleic acid, and demonstrate a lymph lipoprotein distribution identical to that of the monounsaturated acid. The extent of cholesterol absorption with oleic acid (59.1 ± 3.2) is typical of that obtained in earlier studies using similar experimental conditions. Absorption of cholesterol from emulsions containing either arachidonic or eicosapentaenoic acids was not significantly different from that obtained with oleic acid.

TABLE 3

ABSORBABILITY OF POLYUNSATURATED FATTY ACIDS AND EFFECTS ON CHOLESTEROL ABSORPTION

MEASUREMENT	OLEIC ACID	ARACHIDONIC ACID	EICOSAPENTAENOIC ACID
Fatty Acid Recovery In Thoracic Duct Lymph, %	76.2 ± 1.7	81.6 ± 4.0	85.6 ± 3.0
Lipoprotein Distribution, %			
Chylomicrons + VLDL (d < 1.006 g/ml)	94.4 ± 1.1	93.7 ± 0.7	94.6 ± 0.5
LDL (1.006>d < 1.063 g/ml)	4.2 ± 1.0	4.8 ± 0.3	4.2 ± 0.7
HDL (1.063>d < 1.21 g/ml)	1.4 ± 0.2	1.8 ± 0.2	1.2 ± 0.2
Cholesterol Absorption,%	59.1 ± 3.2	45.8 ± 3.8	58.1 ± 59

TABLE 4

COMPARATIVE ABSORPTION OF CORN AND SALMON OIL FATTY ACIDS AND EFFECTS ON CHOLESTEROL ABSORPTION

MEASUREMENT	LIPID ADMINISTERED		
	OLEIC ACID	CORN OIL	SALMON OIL
COMPOSITION (MAJOR FATTY ACIDS) %			
16:0		10	20
18:1 ω 9	99.8	25	26
18:2 ω 6		57	3
18:3 ω 6		5	
22:1			10
20:5 ω 3			10
22:6 ω 3			12
FATTY ACID RECOVERY IN LYMPH, % of dose	71.1 ± 9.0	32.7 ± 5.4	14.0 ± 1.3
CHOLESTEROL ABSORPTION OF Dose	53.0 ± 5.3	20.6 ± 3.2	10.1 ± 2.0

Rats with thoracic lymphatic drainage were intragastrically administered an aqueous emulsion (12) containing 50 mg cholesterol and 282 mg of either oleic acid, corn oil or salmon oil. Recovery of fatty acids and cholesterol was determined by gas-liquid chromatographic analysis of 6-h fasting lymph samples and 24 h collections after administration of the lipid dose.

For comparing the absorbability of corn oil and salmon triglycerides and their effects on cholesterol absorption, oleic acid (1 m mol) was used as control and was administered intragastrically in an emulsion containing 50 mg cholesterol. Analysis of emulsion indicated that 99.8% of the added fatty acid was oleic acid, and recovery through derivatization and gas-liquid chromatography was 98.6%. With this intragastric feeding, 71.1 ± 9.0% of the fed oleic acid was recovered in the 24-h lymph collection, and 53.0 ± 5.3% of the administered cholesterol was absorbed (Table 4).

Using the same analytical approach with emulsions containing 282 mg corn oil, 95.9% of the corn oil fatty acids were recovered and of this, 91.9% was as triglyceride. The fatty acid composition of the corn oil indicated that almost 92% of the fatty acids were composed of linoleic (57%), oleic (25%) and palmitic (10%) acids. Intragastric administration of an emulsion containing 282 mg corn oil and 50 mg cholesterol resulted in recovery of only 32.7 $\pm$ 5.4% of the corn oil fatty acids (Table 4), indicating limited digestibility and absorbability of the corn oil glycerides under these conditions. Also, absorption of cholesterol was only 20.6 $\pm$ 3.2%, or less than half that observed with oleic acid emulsions.

Analysis of salmon oil-containing emulsions showed that 81.6% of the fatty acids were contained in triglycerides, with lesser amounts in unesterified fatty acids (9%), sterol esters (5.6%), and phospholipid (3.7%). Of the total salmon oil fatty acids, 19.5% was as palmitic, 26.3% was oleic, 10.2% was 22:1, and 23.6% was ω-3 fatty acids. Of the latter, 42% was eicosapentaneoic acid and 45% was docosahexaenoic acid.

Intragastric administration of 282 mg of salmon oil (259 mg fatty acid equivalents) resulted in only 14.0 $\pm$ 1.3% recovery of the potentially available fatty acids in lymph, and under these conditions, cholesterol absorption was only 10.1 $\pm$ 2.0% of the administered dose.

DISCUSSION

The present approach for assessing potential influences of a variety of biologically-derived materials on cholesterol absorption has been extensively exploited for defining pathways and mechanisms of sterol transfer from intestinal lumen to lymph.[2,22] Acute effects of the agent can be investigated by addition to a standardized aqueous emulsion containing oleic acid, cholesterol and bile salt, and quantitative administration via indwelling catheters into either the stomach or duodenum. The chronic "adaptive" effects of prolonged feeding of the materials under study is investigated by intragastric administration of the standardized aqueous emulsion to surgically-prepared animals, which have been fasted overnight in order to avoid direct intragastric effects of the agent. Within the limitations of this approach, a variety of natural materials or their derivatives have been tested with respect to their acute and/or chronic effects on direct lymphatic absorption of administrered exogenous cholesterol.

Acute studies with highly purified plant sterols[14] clearly demonstrate that sitosterol and stigmasterol exhibit limited absorbability, and will markedly depress absorption of administered cholesterol. Similar effects are exhibited by 3β, 5α, 6β-cholestanetriol, which is also poorly absorbed. The studies with shellfish sterols was based on earlier reports of the hypocholesteremic properties of clam and oyster sterols.[13] The mixture of purified oyster sterols used in the present studies contained about one-third cholesterol, one-third of efficiently absorbed sterols, and the remainder of poorly absorbed sterols (brassicasterol and plant sterols). Administration of this complex mixture with cholesterol still resulted in about 40% depression of the absorption of cholesterol.

To date, studies with a variety of sterols, both absorbable and unabsorbable, suggest that poorly-absorbed sterols uniformly depress absorption of cholesterol by mechanisms as yet undescribed.[1,2] These potentially include competition for micellar solubilization, for membrane translocation or for sterol esterification.[1,2] The present data with fucosterol, however, suggests a more complex explanation, since this sterol is also poorly absorbed, but has no discernable effect on cholesterol absorption. The importance of this general area of study is emphasized by the human hereditary defect referred to as β-sitosterolemia and xanthomatosis, in which there is an apparent loss in intestinal selectivity of absorbable and non-absorbable sterols.[23]

With respect to undigestible polysaccharides, such as those contained in dietary fibers, data on the hypocholesteremic and antiatherogenic properties of these materials are not complete.[7,24] In general, insoluble fiber sources, such as wheat bran and cellulose given in reasonable doses, have subtle or negligible effects on hyperlipidemias, while viscous derivatives, such as pectins, routinely exhibit hypolipidemic properties.[7,24] The varied effects of different fibers on gastric emptying, intestinal transit, and a variety of hormonal and enzymatic reponses of the intestine do not allow a simple and uniform explanation of the action of these plant cell wall derivatives.[25] This is further exemplified in the present studies, in which long-term administration of various dietary fiber derivatives, prior to studies on cholesterol absorption in fasted animals, all displayed from sublte to dramatic effects on both sterol and oleic acid absorption. These data together with those obtained in acute and chronic studies with model compounds, such as cholestyramine and chitosan, suggest that there adaptive changes in the intestine to administration of unabsorbable polysaccharides. These changes result in modified absorption of lipids in general as well as delayed absorption of certain water-soluble nutrients, such as glucose.[25]

The dramatic acute and chronic effects of chitosan on absorption of both cholesterol and oleic acid require additional attention. This aminopolysaccharide behaves as a weak anion exchanger, in contrast to cholestyramine, but also has viscosity properties similar to the pectins and guar gum. These combined physical and chemical properties suggest a potentially important therapeutic application of this and comparable derivatives of chitin.

Recent interest in the fats of certain cold water marine animals is derived from the finding that the unusual diet of certain Eskimo populations may be protective against thrombosis and coronary heart disease.[3] These oils are characterized by an unusual content of ω-3 fatty acids, such as 5,8,11,14,17-eicosapentaenoic acid. Both vegetable oils and marine oils have comparable hypocholesteremic effects on humans[26] despite major differences in their fatty acid composition. The discovery that platelet thromboxanes derived from eicosapentaenoic acid have different aggregability properties than those derived from arachidonic acid[27] has generated broad interest in the properties of marine oils.[3]

Little is known regarding the absorbability and mechanisms of hypocholesteremia of the marine oils. Early studies on marine oils from various sources[28,29] suggest that these oils are inefficiently digested by pancreatic lipase,[28] and that somewhat drastic conditions are required in vitro hydrolysis of triglycerides containing ω-3 fatty acids.[29] It has been suggested that this resistance to lipolysis is due to steric hindrance by the terminal methyl group of eicosapentaenic acid, which is located largely in the 1 and 3 positions of glycerides.[28] The reltive indigestibility of these oils might interfere with normal oil-micellar partitioning of lipid in the intestinal lumen, and could result in reductions in cholesterol absorption.

The data presented in this report clearly indicate that eicosapentaenoic acid, presented in low doses as the unesterified acid, is absorbed as efficiently as is oleic acid or arachidonic acid. Furthermore, the lipoprotein distributions of all three free fatty acids are identical, and all three are largely (86-90%) incorporated into triglyceride fraction of the d <1.006 g/ml lymph lipoproteins. Cholesterol absorption is also comparable in the presence of the polyunsaturated acids.

Similar studies with higher doses of oleic acid results in fatty acid and cholesterol absorption data comparable to those obtained with the low doses of free fatty acid. With high doses of corn oil, however, there is a marked reduction in corn oil fatty acid recovery in lymph suggesting that conditions for efficient lipolysis in vivo are limiting. Under these conditions, cholesterol absorption is also reduced, most likely as a result of altered oil-micellar partitioning of the sterol. Using an equivalent dose of salmon oil, the lymphatic recovery of fatty acids, including eicosapentaenoic acid was less than half that of corn oil, and only 20% of that with oleic acid. The absorption of cholesterol under these conditions was only half that with corn oil and 20% that with the free fatty acid. This limited digestibility of certain marine oils is also reflected by the relatively low "fat tolerance" curves observed in human studies.[30] Further studies are required to elucidate other aspects of the availability, transport and metabolic characteristics of the ω-3 fatty acids of these oils.

ACKNOWLEDGMENTS

Portions of these studies were supported by grants from United States Department of Agriculture (82 CRCR 1001) and the United States Public Health Services (HL-02033). Colleagues participating in individual studies included: Drs. William Connor and Don Lin (University of Oregon Health Sciences Center, Portland); Drs. David Kritchevsky and Jon Story (The Wistar Institute, Philadelphia); Dr. Ivan Furda (General Mills, Minneapolis) and Drs. Marie M. Cassidy and F. Lightfoot (George Washington University).

The author also wishes to acknowledge the excellent technical assistance of Messrs. Timothy Roy and S. Satchithanandam and Mrs. I. Chen in portions of these studies.

REFERENCES

1. O. J. Pollak and D. Kritchevsky, Sitosterol, in: "Monographs on Atherosclerosis," T. B. Clarkson, D. Kritchevsky and O. J. Pollak, eds., Karger, Basel, pp. 1-215 (1980).
2. G. V. Vahouny and D. Kritchevsky, Plant and marine sterols and and cholesterol metabolism, in: "Nutritional Pharmacology," G. Spiller, ed., Alan R. Liss, New York, pp. 32-72 (1981).
3. S. H. Goodnight, W. S. Harris, W. E. Conner, and D. R. Illingworth, Polyunsaturated fatty acids, hyperlipidemia and thrombosis, Arteriosclerosis 2:87-113 (1982).
4. N. Iritani, E. Fukuda, and K. Inoguchi, Influences of oyster and clam feeding on lipid metabolism in the rat, J. Nutr. Sci. Vitaminol. 25:205-211 (1979).
5. E. Reiner, R. D. Idler, and J. D. Wood, A hypocholesteremic factor in marine sterols, Can. J. Biochem. 38:1499-1500 (1960).
6. D. R. Idler, L. M. Safe, and G. A. Mackinnon, Scallop sterols are hypocholesterolemic relative to cholesterol for the chick, J. Fish. Res. Bd. Cab. 27:601-603 (1970).
7. G. V. Vahouny, Dietary fiber, lipid metabolism and atherosclerosis, Fed. Proc. 41:233-240 (1982).
8. J. J. Nagyvary, J. D. Falk, M. L. Hill, M. L. Schmidt, A. K. Wilkins, and E. L. Bradbury, The hypolipidemic activity of chitosan and other polysaccharides in rats, Nutr. Repts. Intern. 20:677-684 (1979).
9. M. Sugano, T. Fujikawa, Y. Hiratsuji, K. Nakashima, N. Fukuda, and Y. Hasegawa, A novel use of chitosan as a hypocholesteremic agent in rats, Am. J. Clin. Nut. 33:787-793 (1980).
10. G. V. Vahouny, Dietary fiber and intestinal absorption of lipids, in: "Dietary Fiber in Health and Disease," G. V. Vahouny and D. Kritchevsky, eds., Plenum Press, New York, pp. 203-227 (1982).
11. M. Ito, E. W. Connor, E. J. Blanchette, C. R. Treadwell, and G. V. Vahouny, Inhibition of lymphatic absorption of choles-

terol by cholestane-3β, 5α, 6β-triol., J. Lipid Res. 10:694-702 (1969).

12. G. V. Vahouny, T. Roy, L. L. Gallo, J. A. Story, D. Kritchevsky, and M. M. Cassidy, Dietary fibers III. effects of chronic intake on cholesterol absorption and metabolism in the rat, Am. J. Clin. Nut. 33:2182-2191 (1980).
13. G. V. Vahouny, W. E. Connor, T. Roy, D. S. Lin, and L. L. Gallo, Lymphatic absorption of shellfish sterols and their effects on cholesterol absorption, Am. J. Clin. Nut. 34:507-513 (1981).
14. G. V. Vahouny, W. E. Connor, S. Subramaniam, D. S. Lin, and L. L. Gallo, Comparative lymphatic absorption of sitosterol, stigmasterol and fucosterol and differential inhibition of cholesterol absorption, Am. J. Clin. Nut. 37:805-809 (1983).
15. G. V. Vahouny, S. Satchithanandam, M. M. Cassidy, F. B. Lightfoot, and I. Furda, Comparative effects of chitosan and cholestyramine on lymphatic absorption of lipids in the rat, Am. J. Clin. Nut., In Press (1983).
16. J. Folch, M. Lees, and G. H. S. Sloane-Stanley, Simple method for the isolation and purification of total lipides from animal tissues, J. Biol. Chem. 226:497-509 (1957).
17. S. L. Gartner and G. V. Vahouny, Endogenous triglyceride and glycogen in perfused rat hearts, Proc. Soc. Exp. Biol. Med. 143:556-560 (1973).
18. G. V. Vahouny, R. Tombes, M. M. Cassidy, D. Kritchevsky, and L. L. Gallo, Dietary fibers V. binding of bile salts, phospholipids and cholesterol from mixed micelles by bile acid sequestrants and dietary fibers, Lipids, 15:1012-1018 (1980).
19. G. V. Vahouny, R. Tombes, M. M. Cassidy, D. Kritchevsky, and L. L. Gallo, Dietary fiber VI. binding of fatty acids and monolein from mixed micelles containing bile salts and lecithin, Proc. Soc. Exp. Biol. Med. 166:12-16 (1981).
20. S. A. Hyun, G. V. Vahouny, and C. R. Treadwell, Effect of hypocholesteremic agents on intestinal cholesterol absorption, Pro. Soc. Exp. Biol. Med. 112:496-501 (1963).
21. G. V. Vahouny, E. M. Blendermann, L. L. Gallo, and C. R. Treadwell, Differential transport of cholesterol and oleic acid in lymph lipoproteins, J. Lipid Res. 21:415-424 (1980).
22. C. R. Treadwell and G. V. Vahouny, Cholesterol absorption, in: "Handbook of Physiology, The Alimentary Canal," American Physiological Society, Bethesda, Volume III; pp. 140-1438 (1968).
23. A. K. Bhattacharyya and W. E. Connor, β-sitosterolemia and xanthomastosis, A newly described lipid storage disease in two sisters, J. Clin. Invest. 53:1033-1043 (1974).
24. R. M. Kay, Dietary fiber, J. Lipid Res. 23:221-242 (1982).
25. G. V. Vahouny and D. Kritchevsky, eds., "Dietary Fibers in Health and Disease," Plenum Press, New York (1982).
26. W. S. Harris, W. E. Connor, and M. P. McMurry, The comparative reductions of plasma lipids and lipoproteins by dietary

polyunsaturated fats: salmon oil versus vegetable oils, Metabolism 32:179-184 (1983).
27. P. Needleman, A. Raz, M. S. Minkes, J. A. Ferrendelli, and H. Sprecher, Triene prostaglandins: prostacyclin and thromboxane biosynthesis and unique biological properties, Proc. Nat. Acad. Sci., U.S.A., 76:944-948 (1979).
28. N. R. Bottino, G. A. Vandenburg, and R. Reiser, Resistance of certain long-chain fatty acids of marine oils to pancreatic lipase hydrolysis, Lipids 2:689-693 (1967).
29. A. Brockerhoff, R. J. Hoyle, and P. C. Hwang, Incorporation of fatty acids of marine origin into triglycerides and phospholipids of mammals, Biochim. Biophys. Acta. 144:541-548 (1967).
30. W. S. Harris, W. E. Connor, and S. H. Goodnight, Jr., Dietary fish oils, plasma lipids and platelets in men, in: "Progress in Lipid Research. Essential Fatty Acids and Prostaglandins," R. T. Holman, ed., Pergamon Press, New York, pp. 75-79 (1982).

EFFECTS OF NICOTINIC ACID AND ITS DERIVATIVES ON LIPID METABOLISM AND OTHER METABOLIC FACTORS RELATED TO ATHEROSCLEROSIS

Goeran Walldius and Gustaf Wahlberg

King Gustaf V Research Institute
and Department of Medicine, Karolinska Hospital
Stockholm, Sweden

INTRODUCTION

In the late 1930's nicotinic acid (NAc) was first used in milligram doses in the treatment of pelagra. Not until the mid-50's gram doses of NAc were used. Altschul was the first to describe that gram doses of NAc had a profound hypocholesterolemic effect in man.[1] Carlson and Oroe, 1962, found that NAc had antilipolytic properties which might contribute to the hypolipidemic mode of action of the drug.[2] Since then there has been a great interest in the effects of this drug on lipid and lipoprotein metabolism also expanding over the years to include studies on various other metabolic and hemodynamic factors related to atherosclerosis. Several excellent reviews have been published.[3-8] A major summary of pharmacological and physiological results were presented already (1971).[9] In our review some of these findings and several recent results on various metabolic and hemodynamic risk factors for atherosclerosis are summarized.

PHARMACOLOGY OF NICOTINIC ACID

Nicotinic acid (pyridin-3-carboxylic-acid) was studied in detail already in the early 60's and 70's as summarized by Fumagelli.[10] The drug is readily absorbed and reaches in plasma a peak within approximately 15-30 minutes in the form of free NAc. Several metabolites are recognized. The drug is rapidly distributed in the various tissues including kidney and adipose tissue with a slower metabolism of liver and brown fat. It also penetrates through the blood brain barrier.

The antilipolytic effect of the drug has often been taken as a measure of the physiological effects of the compound. The peak of the drug reached in plasma coincides with the free fatty acid (FFA) lowering in blood. Thus plain NAc has a very rapid and profound FFA lowering effect as compared to slow release preparations of NAc which have somewhat lower FFA lowering and also lesser rebound effect than plain NAc. Several of these slow release preparations reach a peak in plasma many hours after the drug is taken and furthermore the peak lowering of FFA is later and not as impressive as with plain NAc.

ADMINISTRATION OF THE DRUG - SIDE EFFECTS

The drug causes flush and gastrointestinal upset as the major side effects. In order to avoid these problems, also being discussed later, the drug has to be given in slowly increasing doses from 0.25 g x 3-4 up to 1 g x 3-4 daily within one week. In patients with extreme hyperlipidemia 8-12 grams daily can be given with a good dose response effect. We often do this on a metabolic ward to motivate and to inform the patient. The slower the doses of the drug are increased the better. The initial problems are flush and itching in the face and scalp which usually recedes in a couple of days. It is wise to avoid coffee together with the intake of the drug. A simultaneous administration of antacids may reduce some of the side effects. Patients with gastritis or pathological liver tests should be treated carefully. Also, subjects with uncontrolled (mainly insulin treated) diabetes may respond adversely to the drug.

Approximately 80-90% of the patients manage to reach the average treatment dose of 3-4 grams daily. In our hands and from other reports as well, the drop-out rate is about 20% including early and late drop-outs. There are more drop-outs early in the treatment if plain NAc derivatives are given. On the contrary, more patients finish their treatment after a couple of months when being on slow release preparations. In fact slow release preparations often cause unexpected flush and nausea which to many subjects is more disturbing than the well known early flush in the morning which is the rationale for having subjects taking plain NAc.

In some patients abnormal liver tests (GOT and GPT) occur. More frequently we find uric acid elevations most often of a moderate degree but sometimes, nevertheless, necessitating alpurinol. In few cases disturbed vision may call for ophthalmological check-ups.

This drug can be combined by other lipid lowering drugs as clofibrate and bile acid sequestering agents.

EFFECTS ON TOTAL SERUM LIPIDS

The cholesterol lowering effects of NAc were first described by Altschul.[1] Since then numerous reports have confirmed the cholesterol lowering potency of the drug.[3-8,11-13] The drug is effective in all serum lipoprotein abnormalities including type IIA, IIB, III, IV and V. The drug is often preferred in severe hypertriglyceridemia because of its dose response lipid lowering affects. Also in normolipidemic patients the drug reduces both cholesterol and triglycerides between 10 and 20%. The percentage reduction in the other types of hyperlipoproteinemia average 10-70% for cholesterol and up to 90% for triglycerides.[14] The relative lipid lowering effects are obviously higher, the higher the initial lipid values are. Also, slow release preparations have about similar lipid lowering effects as plain NAc at least in moderate types of hyperlipidemia.

EFFECTS ON SERUM LIPOPROTEINS

As discussed above NAc has lipid lowering effects in all types of hyperlipoproteinemias. Thus VLDL-triglycerides and VLDL-cholesterol fall as does LDL-cholesterol in subjects with elevated LDL-cholesterol. However, in subjects with initially low LDL-cholesterol (that is, values below 2.7 mmol/l), LDL-cholesterol is moderately increased, especially so in type IV patients.[13] The elevation is, however, not excessive and rarely gives rise to any kind of hypercholesterolemia. This LDL-cholesterol elevating effect has been taken to indicate that the drug affects the lipolytic process of VLDL particles resulting in an increased formation of LDL-cholesterol. It is not known if this moderate LDL-cholesterol increase is negative concerning the development of atherosclerosis since there is a simultaneous increase also in the anti-atherogenic HDL-cholesterol.

The effects on HDL-cholesterol and its subfractions have been less studied than the effects of NAc on other lipoproteins. In 1974 Olsson and co-workers reported that HDL-cholesterol increased both in type IIA and type IIB patients and in equal degree on plain NAc and slow release preparations.[15] The HDL increases were especially marked in patients with type IV and type V since in these patients the initial HDL-cholesterol is often very low.

We have recently studied 38 patients with various types of hyperlipoproteinemia treated with 3-4 grams of NAc for 6 weeks (Wahlberg et al., In preparation). They were weight stable during the treatment. In these patients there were significant triglyceride and cholesterol reductions in VLDL- and VLDL-cholesterol. Total HDL increased in all types of hyperlipoproteinemia. This increase was explained by an increase in what is thought to be the most anti-atherogenic particle that is HDL_2, see Table 1. There was an inverse relation between changes in HDL_2 and HDL_3 cholesterol, $r = -0.62$, $p<0.01$. The increase in HDL_2-cholesterol was positively correlated with the initial HDL_3-cholesterol concentration, $r = 0.57$, $p<0.01$. In a similar study previously presented on fewer patients HDL_3-cholesterol was found to increase on NAc.[16] Various results on HDL_2

TABLE 1

EFFECTS OF NICOTINIC ACID 3 GRAMS DAILY FOR 6 WEEKS ON SERUM LIPOPROTEIN CONCENTRATIONS IN PATIENTS WITH TYPE IIA (n=7), IIB (n=2) AND TYPE IV (n=20)

	T¹⁾TG²⁾	TC³⁾	VLDL-TG	VLDL-C	LDL-C	THDL-C	HDL_2-C	HDL_3-C
Δ %	-46***	-19***	-63***	-60***	-17***	+48***	+113***	-5

1) T = total
2) TG = triglycerides
3) TC = cholesterol

*** = $p<0.001$

(Wahlberg, Walldius, Kirstein, and Olsson, In preparation)

and HDL_3 metabolism might depend on the selection of patient material, the treatment time as well as initial values and lipoprotein types. Kostner recently reported that NAc does not effect LP(a).[17]

EFFECTS ON LIPOPROTEIN TURNOVER

The mode of action of NAc on lipoprotein turnover has recently been summarized.[14,18] Grundy presented evidence that NAc in type IIA does not affect the frational catabolic rate of lipoproteins as studied by I^{125}-labelled LDL disappearance.[18] However, since the concentration of LDL-cholesterol decreased, these results taken together with the previous findings suggest that the synthesis of LDL-cholesterol decreases on NAc. This may be a consequence of the reduced synthesis of VLDL induced by NAc since VLDL is the precursor for LDL.[3,14,18]

Grundy also reported that in familiar combined hyperlipidemia the synthesis of VLDL-triglycerides was decreased by NAc.[18] These findings are in line with previous suggestions by Carlson.[3,6] Since NAc is antilipolytic, the reduced inflow of FFA to the liver will result in a decreased VLDL synthesis from FFA. In Grundy's studies not only triglyceride synthesis decreased but also VLDL-triglyceride fractional catabolic increased on NAc.[18] Such results have also previously been presented.[19] This could be explained by increased peripheral removal among other things in adipose tissue,[11,20-22] as discussed below.

EFFECTS ON APOLIPOPROTEINS

Yovos et al. recently presented evidence in type IIB and type IV patients that 6 months of NAc treatment increased apo-CII and decreased apo-CIII in VLDL.[23] Carlson and Wahlberg have shown that NAc in type V increased the relative proportion of apo-CII to CIII in the VLDL molecules.[24]

As yet there is little information on apo-B during NAc treatment. However, it seems reasonable to believe that apo-B is decreasing during treatment, at least in patients with initially high LDL-cholesterol values.

Packard has presented results in type IV patients that there is an increase in apo-AI due to a fall in its fractional catabolic rate. However, apo-AII was unaffected.[16]

The apo-E subspecies and apo-E-III to apo-E-II area ratio did not change significantly in Yovos studies on patients with type IIB or type IV hyperlipidemia.[23]

EFFECTS ON BILE ACID METABOLISM

Miettinen[25] reported that in 22 patients with familiar hypercholesterolemia that the NAc induced fall of serum cholesterol was associated during a transition period with a significant increase in the fecal elimination of cholesterol in the form of neutral but not acid steroids. In liver biopsy specimens they found that NAc reduced the cholesterol content but not the triglycerides. Angelin recently reported that there was no consistent influence of bile acid production in hypercholesterolemia.[26] However, NAc reduced the enhanced bile acid synthesis in type IV and also increased the molar concentration of cholesterol in the bile.

ANTILIPOLYTIC EFFECTS OF NICOTINIC ACID

In the early 60's the first studies on the antilipolytic effects were described by Carlson and co-workers.[22] Carlson and Oroe found that NAc lowered the concentration of FFA of fasting humans and of dogs and furthermore suggested that the hypolipidemic effect of NAc might be the result of its FFA lowering activity.[2,3,6] Since then the inhibition of lipid mobilization has been observed in several species under various conditions.[7] With plain NAc per os or after intravenous injections there is a rapid fall of FFA which stays low for several hours. Thereafter, there is an overshoot or rebound of increased FFA. The fall of FFA as well as the rebound afterwards seems to be less profound with slow release preparations.[7,27] The cause for the rebound is unknown but has been suggested to be due to an alphareceptor effect.[28] This suggestion has been put forward since one has found that phentolamin completely abolished the rebound and also partially inhibited the initial depression of FFA.[28] During long-term treatment with NAc the drug still seems to have antilipolytic effects. Whether this is caused by decreased lipid mobilization from adipose or works by other mechanisms is currently not known. We have previously reported that during long-term treatment the rate of fatty acid mobilizing lipolysis, if anything, seems to increase.[29] These findings fit with the results presented by Froeberg et al. of an increased FFA 24-hour profile during long-term treatment with NAc.[30]

The mode of action of NAc in reducing rate of basal and stimulated lipolysis *in vitro* and in the early phase of the treatment *in vivo* has been discussed at length.[7,31] There are reports suggesting that NAc stimulates cyclic AMP phosphodiesterase thereby decreasing the amount of cyclic AMP needed for activating the hormone sensitive lipase. Other studies favor the idea of an increased inhibition of the formation of cyclic AMP due to decreased adenylate cyclase activity.[32,33] Aktories and Jakobs recently presented evidence to suggest that at least in rat and hamster adipocytes there is a common membrane receptor for NAc and heterocyclic carboxylic acids related to adenylate cyclase.[33] In their studies they also found that adenylate cyclase inhibition being dependent on the presence of a GTP binding protein (see Aktories et al. in this meeting) can desensitize following both *in vivo* and *in vitro* administration of an inhibitory agent.

EFFECTS ON PLASMA TRIGLYCERIDE BOUND FATTY ACID REMOVAL

Lipoprotein lipase is a major regulator of the removal process of the triglyceride bound fatty acids from plasma to peripheral tissues, mainly muscles and adipose tissue. If the activity of lipoprotein lipase is low, there will be a diminished removal of triglycerides and hence serum triglyceride levels may rise. Lipoprotein lipase can be measured by different methods either after injection of heparin *in vivo* which releases not only lipoprotein lipase but also hepatic lipase or by direct measurements of lipoprotein lipase in adipose tissue by different methods. Some but not all of these studies have come to the conclusion that in hypertriglyceridemia lipoprotein lipase activity of adipose tissue is low. Nicotinic acid seems to increase in the lipoprotein lipase activity at least in animal specimens as studied by Nikkilae.[34] The effects on human adipose tissue is less well known.

Although lipoprotein lipase is a major regulator of the removal process, the released fatty acids have to be taken up and incorporated into a peripheral tissue before the fatty acids are effectively removed from plasma. We have studied this fatty acid removal and esterification process in human adipose tissue for years. A method was developed in which we can measure the fatty acid incorporated into adipose tissue (FIAT) on needle biopsy specimens.[20] This pro-

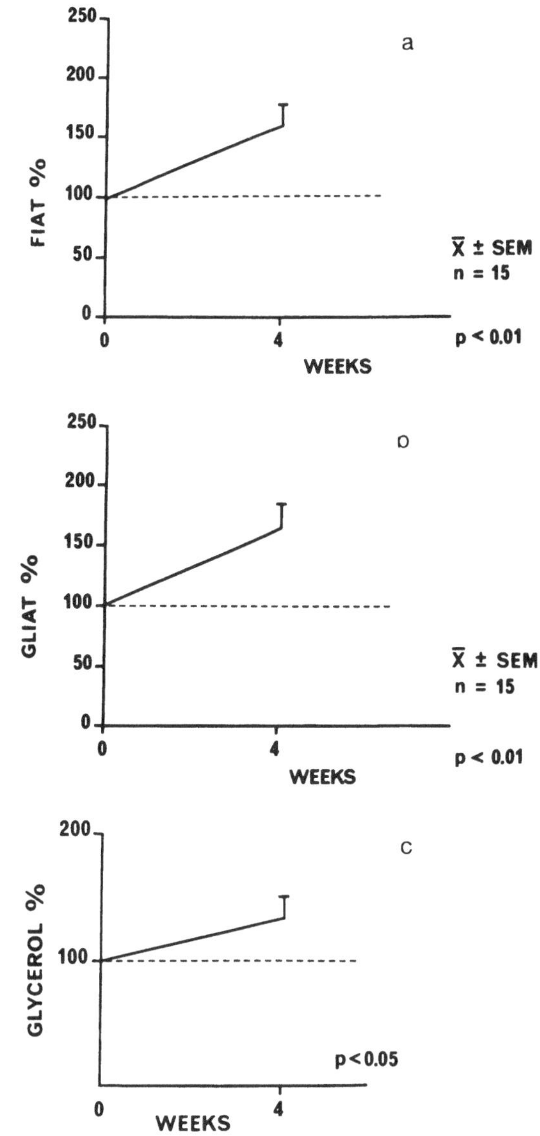

Fig. 1 Effects of nicotinic acid 3-4 grams daily on a) fatty acid (FIAT) and b) glucose (GLIAT) incorporation into and c) lipolysis (glycerol release) from human adipose tissue.[36,22]

cess describes how the fatty acids are removed (esterified) into the storage pool in adipose tissue which is di- and triglycerides. In this method we simultaneously measure the glucose incorporation into adipose (GLIAT) since alpha-glycerophosphate generated in glycolysis is needed for a fatty acid incorporation into adipose tissue. In several studies we have found that both FIAT and GLIAT are low both in severe hypertriglyceridemia[29,35] and in more moderate forms of triglyceride disorders.[11,21,22] There seems to be a negative correlation between the FIAT/GLIAT processes and serum triglycerides levels.[11,21,22] A low fatty acid incorporation (esterification) may therefore contribute to the existence (development?) of hypertriglyceridemia.

From both in vitro studies where NAc has been added as well as in short- and long-term studies of patients being treated with 3-4 grams daily of NAc, we have found that both FIAT and GLIAT increase significantly.[11,22,36] These studies may be taken to indicate that NAc increases the removal of fatty acids that is the step after lipoprotein lipase. However, to our surprise during long-term treatment for 4-6 weeks, we did not only find an increased uptake of fatty acids and glucose during NAc treatment, but also an unexpected increase of fatty acid mobilizing lipolysis[36] (See Fig. 1).

These effects were seen either with NAc alone[36] or when combined with fenofibrate.[22] All of these results taken together thus suggest that the fatty acid turnover rate of adipose tissue is increased by NAc. It is currently not known, however, if the removal process exceeds the fatty acid mobilizing lipolysis. Taken together with the earlier mentioned findings by Froeberg et al.,[30] it is thus possible that our adipose tissue data indicating an increased lipolytic rate goes well along with their findings of an increased 24-hour profile of FFA in plasma. Obviously it is not certain that NAc works by the same mode of action in short-term studies as during the long-term treatment. During such states, other metabolic regulations seem to occur simultaneously.

EFFECTS ON CARBOHYDRATE METABOLISM

It has long been known that NAc induces a decreased glucose tolerance measured after per oral glucose[37] or intravenous glucose loads.[36] Also insulin during a glucose load is increased in healthy subjects.[37] These effects regress upon withdrawal of the drug. This may depend upon increased glucose output from the liver or it may be related to interactions in the peripheral metabolism of FFA and glucose. If there is an increased FFA profile after NAc, as mentioned above, this substrate may be the preferred substrate in muscles (Randle effect), also explaining the increase of glucose in plasma. These results are supported by earlier findings of an increased oxidation of longchain fatty acids by NAc.[38] Since NAc increased glucose incorporation into adipose tissue, it seems less likely that the decreased glucose tolerance is due to an increased resistance of adipose tissue towards glucose and insulin.[36] Furthermore, patients treated with NAc do not generally become obese; for this reason, there will be no increase in cell size and thus indirectly probably no increase in receptor numbers.

EFFECTS ON MUSCLES

Nicotinic acid treatment decreases the amount of stored triglycerides in heart muscle and in red but not white fibers of skeletal muscles.[39] One possible explanation for this decrease is that if adipose tissue lipolysis is reduced, the triglyceride stores in muscle tissue may be used as substrates in the oxidative metabolism. This may be made possible by the simultaneous effect of NAc stimulating muscle circulation (see below). It seems extremely important to further analyze how the drug effects adipose and muscle metabolism during long-term treatment in order to understand how the important triglyceride stores in these tissues are metabolized and distributed during long-term treatment. Teleologically it would be attractive to believe that fatty acids previously stored as triglycerides are oxidized in excess of glucose during long-term treatment since then the body gets rid of lipids and hence is less susceptible to "lipid accumulation" in other tissues.

EFFECTS ON PROSTAGLANDIN METABOLISM

Nicotinic acid causes vasodilation. Kaijser et al. have found that this effect is mediated by prostaglandin derivatives since pretreatment of the patients with prostaglandin inhibitors such as indometazin reduces the flush.[40] From _in vitro_ studies on rat epididymal fat, Puglisi et al. have found that NAc release prostacyclin.[41] Recently Olsson and co-workers have measured the production of 6-keto-PGF_1-alpha as well as PGF_2-alpha in patients with type IV hypertriglyceridemia after 2 and 28 days of treatment. They found that NAc increased the release of prostacyclin metobolites after 2 days of treatment, probably explaining the increased tendency for flush. These effects were however lost during one month's treatment which goes well along with the low tendency for flush after prolonged treatment. The authors conclude that this early effect of NAc is prostacyclin mediated but not involved in FFA inhibition neither in serum lipid lowering.[42]

EFFECTS ON PLATELET AGGREGATION

Nagakava last year reported that in 16 patients with atherosclerosis 750 mg/day of an NAc derivative resulted in a lowered ADP, collagen, and adrenalin induced platelet aggregation.[43] Similar results with a new derivative which is a combination of clofibrate analogue and NAc (Etofibrate, this meeting) suggest that this drug also reduces platelet aggregation.

CLINICAL STUDIES WITH NIOTINIC ACID

The heart uses both FFA and glucose in its oxidative metabolism.

The heart cannot actively chose its substrate but is under the passive influence of the concentration gradient of FFA. If the FFA concentration increases, FFA are used for oxidation in excess of glucose. In stressed states the FFA concentration is increased; therefore exposing the heart for its possibly deleterious metabolic effects.[44] In decreased states where the muscle bloodflow is reduced, for example, in angina pectoris, the heart is probably even more sensitive to excess of FFA in relation to glucose. Studies performed by Lassers et al. have shown that by reducing the FFA concentration with NAc in acute studies it is possible to have more efficient glucose extraction.[45] These studies have given valuable information of how to use the drug in acute coronary care. Thus Rowe et al. have found that by reducing lipolysis with a NAc analogue it is possible to reduce also ventricular arrhythmias during myocardial infarction.[46] Similar results have been obtained by Kjekshus et al. in experimental animals where NAc has been shown to decrease ST-segment elevations as a measure of ischemia.[47] Obviously both metabolic effects of NAc such as FFA reduction as well as vasodilating effects may explain the obvious beneficial effects of NAc in acute studies.

NICOTINIC ACID IN REGRESSION STUDIES

Jakobsson et al. reported their findings on 18 months treatment of minipigs consuming different diets with clofibrate and/or NAc.[48] They found that the right coronary artery reduced its cholesterol ester content when NAc was given. They also noted a reduced frequency of sudden death indicating a favorable effect of long-term treatment. In men there is now an interesting ongoing study on the development of early atherosclerosis as measured by a combined X-ray and computer technique. In this study Olsson et al. follow the effect of combined NAc and fenofibrate treatment given to symptom-free subjects with different types of hyperlipoproteinemia.[49]

NICOTINIC ACID IN SECONDARY PREVENTION TRIALS

In the coronary drug project studying male survivors after myocardial infarction, NAc reduced serum cholesterol by 10 and serum triglycerides by 26%.[50] Although there were no significant differences in the rate of ischemic heart deaths, there was a highly significant reduction of non-fatal myocardial infarctions in the NAc treated group. This effect was significant, contrary to that for clofibrate which only reduced serum lipids by 6%. The goal seems obvious: with lipid lowering therapy, one has to reduce serum atherogenic lipoproteins effectively if this shall influence the life expectancy in relation to atherosclerotic diseases. Recently Rosenhamer and Carlson have published their results on a combined NAc and clofibrate trial after myocardial infarction. There is a significant reduction both of non-fatal as well as fatal infarctions.[51]

SUMMARY

Nicotinic acid treatment thus induces several beneficial effects on serum lipoproteins and on hemodynamic factors related to the risk for development of atherosclerosis. It effectively reduces the atherogenic lipoproteins VLDL and LDL and also increases the anti-atherogenic HDL, mainly the HDL_2 fraction. The drug seems to be active not only in decreasing the synthesis of various lipoproteins but also to enhance the removal into peripheral tissues, thereby speeding up the catabolic events of serum lipoproteins. The mode of action of NAc in adipose and muscle tissue needs further evaluation to better understand the complex interplay between free fatty acid and glucose and insulin metabolism. The recent findings of a stimulation of prostacyclin formation as well as a reduction in platelet aggregation are newly discovered favorable effects of the drug that needs to be further examined. Although the drug seems to induce some undesirable side effects (reversible), its several favorable anti-atherosclerotic properties should stimulate both experimental and clinical research with this drug. Hopefully newer derivatives with even better toler-may be developed.

REFERENCES

1. R. Altschul, A. Hoffer, and J. D. Stephen, Arch. Biochem. 54:558 (1955).
2. L. A. Carlson and L. Oroe, Acta Med. Scand. 172:641 (1962).
3. L. A. Carlson, J. Boberg, and B. Hoegstedt, in: "Handbook of Physiology," Chapter 63, A. E. Renold and C. F. Cahill, eds., p. 625-644 (1965).
4. L. A. Carlson and G. Walldius, in: "Pharmacological Control of Lipid Metabolism," W. L. Holmes, R. Paoletti, and D. Kritchevsky, eds., Plenum Publishing Corp., New York (1972).
5. L. A. Carlson and A. G. Olsson, in: "Progress in Biochemical Pharmacology," Vol. 15, S. Eisenberg, ed., Karger, Basel, p. 238-257 (1979).
6. L. A. Carlson, in: "Drugs, Lipid Metabolism, and Atherosclerosis," D. Kritchevsky, R. Paoletti, and W. L. Holmes, eds., Plenum Publishing Corp., New York, p. 225-238 (1978).
7. F. P. Kupiecki, Progr. Biochem. Pharmacol. 6:274 (1971).
8. L. A. Carlson, Progr. Biochem. Pharmacol. 3:151 (1967).
9. Metabolic Effects of Nicotinic Acid and its Derivatives, K. F. Gey and L. A. Carlson, eds., Hans Huber Publishers, Bern-Stuttgart-Vienna (1971).
10. R. Fumagalli, in: "Metabolic Effects of Nicotinic Acid and its Derivatives," K. F. Gey and L. A. Carlson, eds., Hans Huber Publishers, Bern-Stuttgart-Vienna, p. 33-49 (1971).
11. L. A. Carlson and G. Walldius, Europ. J. Clin. Invest. 6:195 (1976).
12. L. A. Carlson, A. G. Olsson, L. Oroe, S. Roessner, and G.

Walldius, in: "Atherosclerosis III, G. Schetter and A. Weizel, eds., p. 768-781 (1974).

13. L. A. Carlson, A. G. Olsson, and D. Ballantyne, Atherosclerosis 26:603 (1977).

14. L. A. Carlson, in: "Treatment of Hyperlipoproteinemia," L. A. Carlson and A. G. Olsson, eds., Raven Press, In Press (1983).

15. A. G. Olsson, L. Oroe, and S. Roessner, Atherosclerosis 19:61 (1974).

16. J. Packard, J. M. Stewart, J. L. H. C. Third, H. G. Morgan, T. D. V. Lawrie, and J. Shepard, Biochim. Biophys. Acta 618:53 (1980).

17. G. Kostner, C. Klein, and F. Krempler, in: "Treatment of Hyperlipoproteinemia," L. A. Carlson and A. G. Olsson, eds., Raven Press, In Press (1983).

18. S. M. Grundy, in: "Treatment of Hyperlipoproteinemia," L. A. Carlson and A. G. Olsson, eds., Raven Press, In Press (1983).

19. J. Boberg, L. A. Carlson, S. Froeberg, A. Olsson, L. Oroe, and S. Roessner, in: "Metabolic Effects of Nicotinic Acid and Its Derivatives," K. F. Gey and L. A. Carlson, eds., Hans Huber Publishers, Bern-Stuttgart-Vienna, p. 465-470 (1971).

20. G. Walldius and P. Rubba, Scand. J. Clin. Lab. Invest. 36:357 (1976).

21. G. Walldius, Acta Med. Scand. Suppl. 591:1-47 (1976).

22. G. Walldius, H.-E. Norbeck, and G. Wahlberg, in: "Metabolic Risk Factors for Ischemic Vascular Disease, L. A. Carlson and B. Pernow, eds., Raven Press, New York, p. 225-238 (1982).

23. J. G. Yovos, S. T. Patel, J. M. Falko, H. A. I. Newman, and D. S. Hill, J. Clin. Endocrinol. Metab. 54:1210 (1982).

24. L. A. Carlson and G. Wahlberg, Atherosclerosis 31:77 (1978).

25. T. A. Miettinen, in: "Metabolic Effects of Nicotinic Acid and its Derivatives, K. F. Gey and L. A. Carlson, eds., Hans Huber Publishers, Bern-Stuttgart-Vienna, p. 677-686 (1971).

26. B. Angelin, in: "Treatment of Hyperlipoproteinemia," L. A. Carlson and A. G. Olsson, eds., Raven Press, In Press (1983).

27. J. N. Pereira, J. Lipid Res. 8:239 (1967).

28. W. G. Blackard and S. A. Heldingsfelder, Metabolism 18:226 (1969).

29. G. Walldius, in: "Treatment of Hyperlipoproteinemia," L. A. Carlson and A. G. Olsson, eds., Raven Press, In Press (1983).

30. S. O. Froeberg, J. Boberg, L. A. Carlson, and M. Ericsson, in: "Metabolic Effects of Nicotinic Acid and its Derivatives," K. F. Gey and L. A. Carlson, eds., Hans Huber Publishers, Bern-Stuttgart-Vienna, p. 167-181 (1971).

31. T. W. Butcher, in: "Metabolic Effects of Nicotinic Acid and its Derivatives," K. F. Gey and L. A. Carlson, Hans Huber Publishers, Bern-Stuttgart-Vienna, p. 347-355 (1971).

32. I. F. Skidmore, D. Kritchevsky, and P. Schoenhoefer, in: "Metabolic Effects of Nicotinic Acid and its Derivatives," K. F. Gey and L. A. Carlson, Hans Huber Publishers, Bern-Stuttgart-Vienna, p. 371-377 (1971).

33. K. Aktories and K. H. Jakobs, Naunyn-Schmiedeberg's Arch. Pharmacol. 318:241 (1982).
34. E. A. Nikkilae, in: "Metabolic Effects of Nicotinic Acid and its Derivatives," K. F. Gey and L. A. Carlson, eds., Hans Huber Publishers, Bern-Stuttgart-Vienna, p. 487 (1971).
35. L. A. Carlson, I, Eriksson, and G. Walldius, Acta Med. Scand. 194:363 (1973).
36. G. Wahlberg and G. Walldius, in: "Nicotinic Acid and its Derivatives in the Prevention of Atherosclerosis," M. Mancini, ed., Farmaci, Suppl. 3, p. 41-46 (1981).
37. Z. N. Gaut, H. M. Solomon, and O. N. Miller, in: "Metabolic Effects of Nicotinic Acid and its Derivatives," K. F. Gey and L. A. Carlson, eds., Hans Huber Publishers, Bern-Stuttgart-Vienna, p. 923-927 (1971).
38. M. A. Mishkel and W. F. Webb, J. Biochem. Pharmacol. 16:897 (1967).
39. S. O. Froeberg, in: "Metabolic Effects of Nicotinic Acid and its Derivatives," K. F. Gey and L. A. Carlson, eds., Hans Huber Publishers, Bern-Stuttgart-Vienna, p. 449-456 (1971).
40. L. Kaijser, B. Eklund, A. G. Olsson, and L. A. Carlson, Medical Biology 57:114 (1979).
41. L. Puglisi, G. F. Caselli, F. Maggi, M. G. Ciapponi, and M. R. Accomago, Abstract, Sixth International Symposium on Atherosclerosis (1982).
42. A. G. Olsson, L. A. Carlson, E. Aenggard, and G. Ciabattoni, Lancet 2:265 (1983).
43. Y. Nagakava, H. Orimo, and M. Harasawa, Abstract, Sixth International Symposium on Atherosclerosis (1982).
44. M. F. Oliver, in: "Modern Trends in Cardiology - 3," M. F. Oliver, ed., Butterworths, London, p. 89 (1975).
45. B. W. Lassers, M. L. Wahlqvist, L. Kaijser, and L. A. Carlson, J. Appl. Physiol. 33:72 (1972).
46. M. J. Rowe, J. M. M. Neilson, and M. F. Oliver, Lancet 1:295 (1975).
47. J. K. Kjekshus and O. D. Mjos, J. Clin. Invest. 52:1770 (1973).
48. L. Jakobsson and L. Lundholm, Abstract, Sixth International Symposium on Atherosclerosis (1982).
49. A. G. Olsson, in: "Treatment of Hyperlipoproteinemia," L. A. Carlson and A. G. Olsson, eds., Raven Press, In Press (1983).
50. The Coronary Drug Project Research Group, JAMA 231:350 (1971).
51. G. Rosenhammer and L. A. Carlson, Atherosclerosis 37:129 (1980).

HMG-CoA REDUCTASE INHIBITORS

Akira Endo

Department of Agricultural and Biological Chemistry
Tokyo Noko University
Fuchu-shi, Tokyo, Japan

INTRODUCTION

Since in humans the greater part of the cholesterol in the body is synthesized *de novo* in the liver and intestine, the search for drugs to inhibit cholesterol biosynthesis has long been pursued as a means to lower the level of plasma cholesterol and so help to prevent and treat atherosclerosis. The major rate-limiting step in the biosynthesis of cholesterol is the reduction of 3-hydroxy-3-methylglutaryl (HMG)-CoA to mevalonate which is catalyzed by the enzyme HMG-CoA reductase. This enzyme, therefore, is a prime target for pharmacological intervention.

Endo and his associates first discovered an inhibitor of sterol synthesis in the culture broth of the fungus *Penicillium citrinum* (Endo et al., 1976b). This compound, designated ML-236B (compactin), was shown to be a specific potent inhibitor of HMG-CoA reductase. Compactin has been shown to be highly effective in the treatment of hypercholesterolemia. Further, it has been useful as a research tool for studying the regulation of cholesterol and other isoprennoid biosynthesis.

ISOLATION OF COMPACTIN (ML-236B) RELATED COMPOUNDS

Endo (1979) isolated another active compound (named monacolin K) from the fungus *Monascus ruber*. Later, the same compound (named mevinolin) was also isolated by Alberts et al. (1980) from *Aspergillus terreus*. Along with these two main products, several metabolites were isolated from cultures of these fungi: ML-236A and ML-236C (Endo et al., 1976b) and dihydrocompactin (Lam et al., 1981)

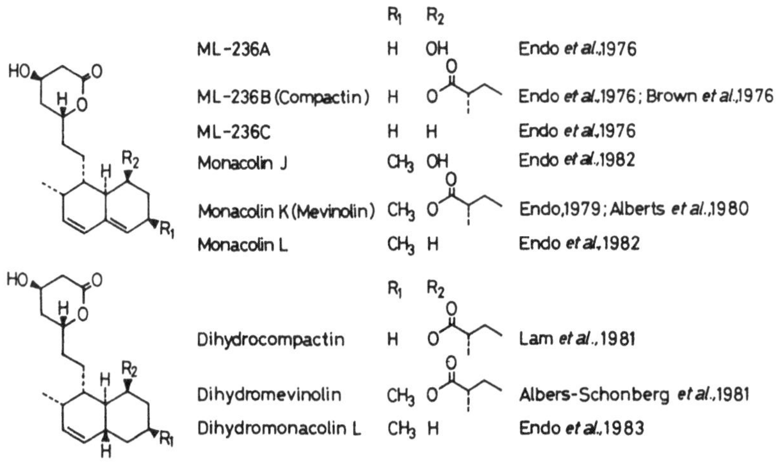

Fig. 1 Compactin (ML-236B)-related compounds isolated from fungi.

from P. citrinum; dihydromevinolin from A. terreus (Albers-Schonberg et al., 1981); monacolin J and L (Endo, 1983) and dihydromonacolin L (Endo, unpublished data) from M. ruber. All these metabolites are structurally related to each other (Fig. 1) and are specific inhibitors of HMG-CoA reductase.

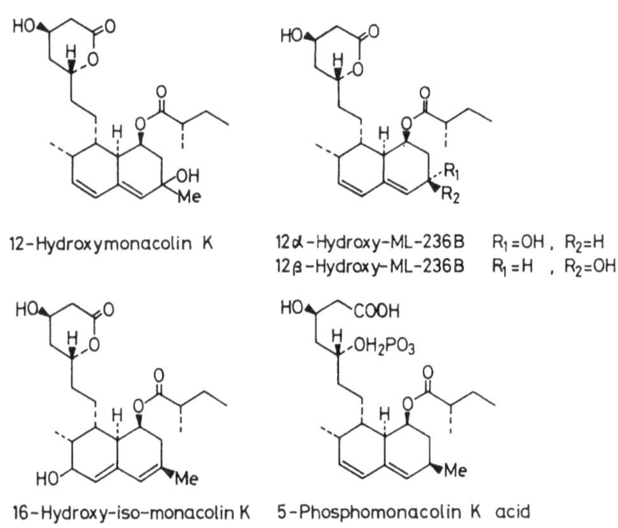

Fig. 2 Compactin-related compounds produced by microbial conversion.

Shown in Fig. 2 are compounds which are derived from either compactin or monacolin K by microbial conversion. 12α-hydroxy-ML-236B and 16β-hydroxy-iso- and 12-hydroxy-monacolin K are produced by growing the fungus Mucor hiemalis in a culture medium that contains, in addition to other nutrients, ML-236B and monacolin K, respectively (Serizawa et al., 1983a). ML-236B is also converted to 12β-hydroxy-ML-236B by Syncephalastrum nigricans (Serizawa et al., 1983b) and monacolin K to 5-phosphomonacolin K acid (Endo and Yamashita, 1983).

Of the compactin-related compounds described above, compactin and monacolin K are major metabolites produced in the fermentation broth. These two compounds, as well as dihydrocompactin, dihydromevinolin, 12α- and 12β-hydroxy-ML-236B and 12-hydroxymonacilin K, inhibit sterol synthesis in a cell-free system 50% at a concentration of 4 - 10 ng/ml and are more potent in inhibitory activity than the rest of the derivatives. All these seven compounds have an α-methylbutyrate residue in the structure, which appears to play a significant role in the inhibition of HMG-CoA reductase activity. The structures of the acid from compactin-related compounds include a portion that resembles the structure of the HMG portion of HMG-CoA, the substrate in the HMG-CoA reductase reaction (Fig. 3).

Recently, new producing microorganisms of compactin have been isolated by Endo et al. (1983), which include Paecilomyces sp. and Hypomyces chrysospermus. These two fungal strains are particularly suited for use in the production of compactin, since no mycotoxin has been isolated from culture broth of these fungi. Other producers, Penicillium citrinum and P. brevicompactum (Brown et al., 1976), are known to produce mycotoxins (Ciegler et al., 1971).

In addition to compactin-related compounds, several compounds, which include citrinin (Endo and Kuroda, 1976; Tanzawa et al., 1977) and adenosin 2'-monophospho-5'-diphosphoribose (Tanzawa and Endo, 1979), inhibit HMG-CoA reductase.

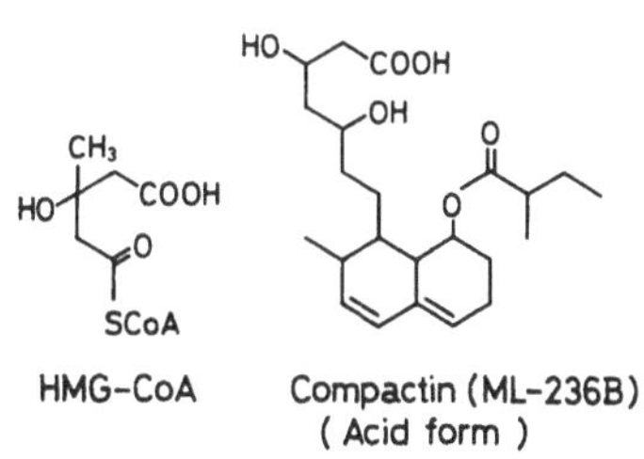

Fig. 3 Structures of compactin and HMG-CoA.

MECHANISM FOR HMG-CoA REDUCTASE INHIBITION

HMG-CoA reductase catalyzes the two-step reduction of HMG-CoA to mevalonate in the presence of NADPH.

$$\text{HMG-CoA} + 2\text{NADPH} \rightarrow \text{Mevalonate} + \text{CoA} + 2\text{NADPH}$$

The inhibition of HMG-CoA reductase by compactin-related compounds is competitive with respect to HMG-CoA and noncompetitive with respect to NADPH (Endo et al., 1976a; Endo, 1980). The Ki value for compactin is 1.2 nM. Under the same conditions, the Km value for HMG-CoA was 9.1 μM. Thus the affinity of the enzyme for the inhibitors is 8,000-fold, or more, higher than its affinity for the natural substrate HMG-CoA.

Using compactin and adenosine 2'-monophospho-5'-diphosphoribose, it is indicated that the two substrates bind to the enzyme (rat liver) in an ordered manner (Tanzawa and Endo, 1979): reductase first interacts with HMG-CoA to make a binary complex, which, in turn, forms a ternary complex with one molecule of NADPH. A bi-uni-uni-ter-ping-pong mechanism is proposed as a model of the overall reaction. Rodgers and Rudney (1982) suggested that the binding of compactin (or mevinolin) to HMG-CoA reductase induced a conformational change in the enzyme and a related alteration in antigenicity.

Of the enzymatic reactions in which HMG-CoA is involved as a substrate, both HMG-CoA cleavage enzyme (EC 4.1.3.4) and HMG-CoA synthase (EC 4.1.3.5) are not inhibited by compactin at higher concentrations up to 10 μM (Endo, unpublished observation).

USES AS A RESEARCH TOOL

Compactin has been shown to inhibit sterol synthesis in a variety of cultured cells which include human skin fibroblasts and L cells (Kaneko et al., 1978; Brown et al., 1978; Haba et al., 1981), human T lymphocytes (Cuthbert and Lipsky, 1980), human intestinal mucosa cells (Betteridge et al., 1978), Chinese hamster ovary (CHO) cells (Goldstein et al., 1979), Leidig tumor cells (Freeman and Ascoli, 1982), bovine granulosa cells (Savion et al., 1982), rat hepatocytes (Kempen et al., 1983; Pullinger and Gibbons, 1982) and bovine aortic endothelial cells (Cohen et al., 1982a and 1982b). In most cells studied, sterol synthesis from ^{14}C-acetate is significantly inhibited by compactin at a concentration of 0.005 - 0.02 μg/ml.

Compactin has revealed a hitherto unsuspected aspect of mevalonate metabolism in cultured cells. It blocks the production of mevalonate so that the cells now depend on exogenous mevalonate and are phenotypic auxotrophs. Analysis of this adaptive response has disclosed that not only cell growth, but also regulation of HMG-CoA

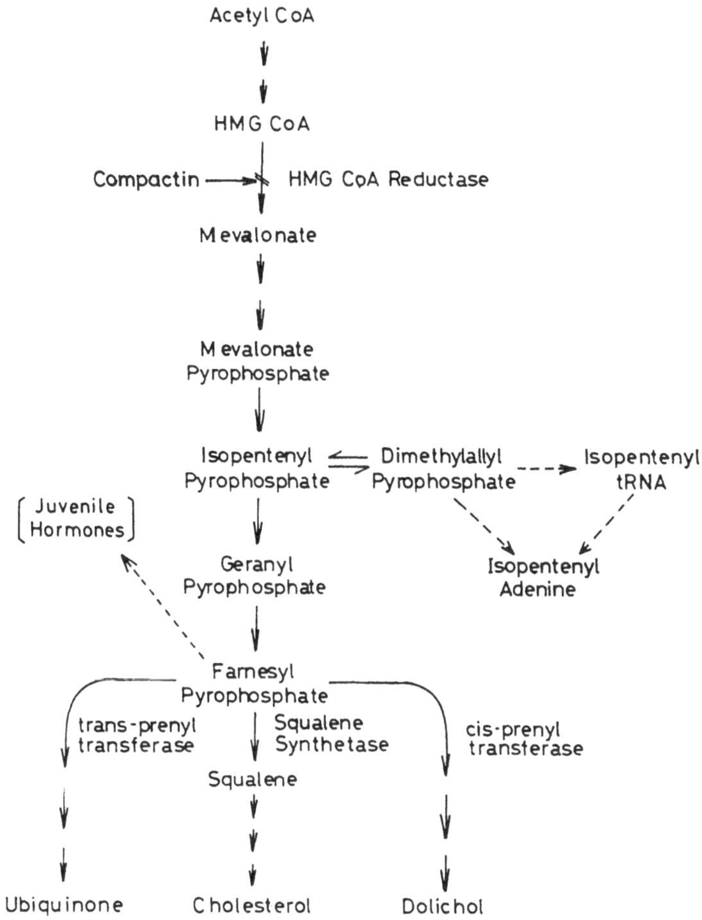

Fig. 4 Synthetic pathway for cholesterol and other isoprenoids derived from mevalonate.

reductase in cultured cells requires, in addition to cholesterol, one or more non-cholesterol products normally synthesized endogenously from mevalonate.

As shown in Fig. 4, mevalonate is a precursor of ubiquinone and dolichol as well as cholesterol. Further, according to current evidence, isopentenyl adenosine (and ispentenyl adenine) is synthesized from mevalonate <u>via</u> dimethylallyl pyrophosphate (Brown and Goldstein, 1980).

A. Growth Inhibition

Kaneko et al. (1978) first reported that high levels of compactin inhibited the growth of L cells and human fibroblasts. Growth could be restored by the addition of mevalonate in the presence of lipoprotein cholesterol. These authors posturated that the cells might require a small amount of active HMG-CoA reductase in order to synthesize a mevalonate-derived substance other than a sterol that is required for growth.

Quesney-Huneeus et al. (1979) extended these observations by studying baby hamster kidney (BHK) cells. When the cells were incubated in the presence of compactin, they failed to enter the S-phase of growth as evidenced by an inhibition of the incorporation of ^{3}H-thymidine into DNA. The addition of cholesterol in the form of lipoproteins failed to overcome this compactin-mediated inhibition of DNA synthesis. On the other hand, when the cells were given mevalonate, along with lipoproteins, DNA synthesis was restored within minutes. Of known mevalonate metabolites examined as possible mediators by which mevalonate controls DNA replication, only isopentenyladenine and its 4'-hydroxylated analogue, zeatin, could substitute for mevalonate in restoring DNA replication in compactin-blocked cells (Quesney-Huneeus et al., 1980). In addition, isopentenyladenine, like mevalonate, stimulated DNA synthesis specifically during the S-phase of the cell cycle. These findings indicate that isopentenyladenine or a closely related derivative may mediate the regulatory role of mevalonate in DNA replication. Requirement for a mevalonate-derived product in compactin-inhibited cells were also shown with cultured monkey arterial smooth muscle cells and Swiss 3T3 cells (Habenicht et al., 1980) and cultured mouse spleen lymphocytes (Perkins et al., 1982).

In the case of human T lymphocytes, inhibition of mevalonate production by compactin had little effect on the initial cell activation and blast transformation, while the subsequent enlargement and cell division were suppressed (Cuthbert and Lipsky, 1980). These inhibitions could be prevented by mevalonate. Compactin also caused inhibition of DNA synthesis that could be abolished by mevalonate. Effects of isopentenyladenine and other metabolites derived from mevalonate in these systems have not yet been reported (Cuthbert and Lipsky, 1981).

Carson and Lennarz (1979) investigated the effect of compactin on the embryonic development of the sea urchin (Strongylocentrotus purpuratus). In the presence of compactin, the embryo underwent abnormal gastrulation. However, when exogenous dolichol was added to the culture medium along with compactin, the embryos gastrulated normally. Supplementation of cholesterol or ubiquinone or both did not prevent the compactin-mediated developmental lesion. The data indicate that dolichol, which is known to be involved in the synthesis of N-glycosidically linked glycoproteins, is an essential factor in the embryonic development of the sea urchin.

Growth of CHO cells in the presence of LDL is totally inhibited by compactin at a concentration of 40 μM (Brown and Goldstein, 1980). The addition to the culture medium of mevalonate restored full growth of the cells, but squalene failed to prevent this growth inhibition. Thus, it is unlikely that the putative factor derived from mevalonate is any distal intermediate in the sterol synthetic pathway. In this connection, Ryan et al. (1981) studied the inhibitory effect of compactin on the growth of CHO-K1 cells. At 8 μg/ml of compactin, the growth inhibition was prevented by the addition of mevalonate or free cholesterol to the culture medium. Addition of dolichol and ubiquinone had no effect when added in the presence or absence of cholesterol. When compactin was added to the culture medium at 50 μg/ml, only mevalonate was capable of preventing the cytotoxic effect of the drug. Neither cholesterol alone or cholesterol with added dolichol, ubiquinone, and isopentenyladenine was effective in preventing cell death. Thus, it is unlikely that these three products are growth-limiting in CHO-K1 cells.

From the studies described above, it is unlikely that the mevalonate-derived substance, which acts cumultatively with cholesterol to cell growth, is common to most animal cells. Rather, it may vary in different cells with their specific requirement for different metabolites derived from mevalonate.

B. Induction of HMG-CoA Reductase

When HMG-CoA reductase activity of human fibroblasts was inhibited by compactin, where mevalonate production was completely inhibited, the striking increase in the cellular levels of HMG-CoA reductase occurred (Brown et al., 1978). The induced HMG-CoA reductase could not be fully suppressed even when the cells were given LDL; the suppression was about 85% (Brown and Goldstein, 1980). The added LDL was effective in delivering cholesterol to the compactin-treated cells. However, despite an abundance of intracellular cholesterol, the amount of HMG-CoA reductase remained relatively high. In the presence of compactin the enzyme could be fully suppressed only when the cells were given mevalonate in addition to the LDL-cholesterol. These results suggest that the increased amount of HMG-CoA reductase enzyme in compactin-grown cells appears to be produced as a result of the cellular deprivation of one or more of the non-cholesterol products that are normally synthesized from mevalonate.

The induction of high levels of HMG-CoA reductase activity by compactin required protein synthesis. Thus, the increase in the reductase activity was completely blocked by cycloheximide (Brown et al., 1978). At the present time, however, it is not known whether mevalonate inhibits _de novo_ synthesis of HMG-CoA reductase protein or not. Further, no evidence is presently available to indicate that the reversible inactivation through phosphorylation (Gibson and Ingebritsen, 1978; Nordstrom et al., 1977) is involved in this mechanism.

The regulator that acts cumultatively with cholesterol to suppress HMG-CoA reductase could be mevalonate or any one of the products derived from its metabolism. Some of the likely candidates for this feedback regulation include ubiquinone (Brown and Goldstein, 1980), dolichol (James and Kandutsch, 1979) and lanosterol (Kaneko and Endo, unpublished observation).

C. Compactin-Resistant Cells

Using stepwise selection procedure, Ryan et al. (1981) have obtained several variant cell lines of CHO-K1 cells which are resistant to 8 μg/ml of compactin, a value that is nearly 100 times higher than that sufficient to cause growth inhibition of the parent cell line. The variant cell lines are able to overcome the cytotoxic effects of compactin by a mechanism which leads to overaccumulation of HMG-CoA reductase which, in turn, permits normal mevalonate metabolism and cholesterol synthesis to take place. In the process of characterizing one of the related-cell lines, designated C100, Hardeman et al. (1983b) succeeded in identifying an Mr 92,000 protomer of HMG-CoA reductase. In addition, the authors suggested that the previously reported Mr values of the enzyme { 62,000 (Ness et al., 1981) and 53,000 (Sinensky et al., 1981)} were artifacts of sample preparation for $NaDoSO_4$ gel electrophoresis and proteolysis during enzyme isolation. Recently another variant cell line of CHO-K1 cells resistant to 40 μM (16 μg/ml) compactin was developed by Chin et al. (1982a). In this line, designated UT-1, HMG-CoA reductase increased by 500-fold as compared to that of the parent cells and accounted for approximately 2% of total cell protein in the cell. To accommodate the increased amounts of reductase, UT-1 cells developed marked proliferation of tubular smooth endoplasmic reticulum membranes, as revealed by immunofluorescence and electron microscopy. The tubular membranes were packed in crystalloid hexagonal arrays. Despite this marked increase, enzyme activity was rapidly suppressed by LDL and the crystalloid membranes disappeared.

This decrease in reductase activity in UT-1 cells is due to a profound suppression of synthesis of the enzyme (Faust et al., 1982). By using UT-1 cells as an enriched source of mRNA for molecular cloning of the cDNA for the reductase, Chin et al. (1982b) showed that the primary translational product of reductase mRNA was an Mr 90,000 protein and that LDL suppressed the reductase in the cells by drastically reducing the level of its mRNA. These findings are consistent with the data that the overproduction of HMG-CoA reductase in C100 cells is the result of increased enzyme synthesis due to elevated levels of translatable mRNA (Hardeman et al, 1983a). A similar translational regulation of the elevated levels of HMG-CoA reductase by compactin was also suggested with rat hepatocytes by Koizumi et al. (1982).

Masuda et al. (1982) isolated 3 mutants of Chinese hamster cell line V79 which showed a 4- to 5-fold higher resistance to compactin than the parent cell line. These mutuants showed a defect in internalization of ^{125}I-LDL into the cells, although their binding activity for ^{125}I-LDL was comparable to that of the parental cells.

UT-1 cells also have a markedly increased amount of another protein with an Mr of 53,000 that may represent cytosolic HMG-CoA synthase, the enzyme preceding the reductase in the cholesterol biosynthetic pathway. Synthesis of this protein is also suppressed by LDL and sterols, and its level is much higher in UT-1 cells than in parental CHO cells (Luskey et al., 1982).

D. Other Uses

Compactin has been used to estimate the contribution of *de novo* synthesis of cholesterol as the source for progesterone biosynthesis in cultured Leyding tumor cells (Freeman and Ascoli, 1982). It also has been used in cultured bovine granulosa cells (Savion et al., 1982) and for bile acid formation in cultured rat hepatocytes (Kempen et al., 1983). In these studies, it was shown that cholesterol derived from *de novo* synthesis was used for steroid biosynthesis when intracellular stores of cholesterol were depleted or lipoproteins were absent in the culture medium. Oram et al. (1981) used compactin to block supply of cholesterol in their study of the effects of high density lipoprotein on cholesterol efflux from cultured fibroblasts. Pullinger and Gibbons (1982) reported the compactin's effect on the rate of VLDL secretion in rat hepatocytes.

HYPOCHOLESTEROLEMIC ACTIVITY

A. In Animals

The efficacy of compactin as a hypocholesterolemic drug was first evaluated in the rat. It turned out, however, that with one exception the drug failed to reduce plasma cholesterol levels even at high doses up to 500 mg/kg (Endo et al., 1979). The only exception was when rats were treated with Triton WR-1339, a detergent that is known to cause hyperlipidemia in these animals (Kuroda et al., 1977; Endo et al., 1979). The administration of compactin caused a significant decrease in fecal excretion of bile acids and in the hepatic levels of cholesterol 7α-hydroxylase, the rate-limiting enzyme in bile acid synthesis. In addition, as observed with cultured cells treated with compactin, a marked increase (7- to 10-fold) in the activity of hepatic HMG-CoA reductase was produced by compactin, so that net synthesis of sterols in the liver was unimpaired. The lack of hypocholesterolemic activity of compactin in the rat could be attributed, at least partly, to these unexpected changes in the activity of the two hepatic microsomal enzymes (Endo et al., 1979). Increases in hepatic HMG-CoA reductase activity was also shown in rats fed a rat chow diet containing mevinolin (monacolin K) and cholestyramine (Tanaka et al., 1982). Compactin also showed no hypocholesterolemic effects in other rodents, including the mouse and hamster (Endo et al., 1979; Endo et al., unpublished observation.

However, compactin is effective in other animal species. In dogs, this drug produced a rapid reduction of both plasma cholesterol and phospholipid levels when administered at a dose of 10 mg/kg (Tsujita et al., 1979). Triglyceride was not consistently lowered. Fecal excretion of bile acids was, unlike in the rat, significantly elevated. Of the lipoprotein classes, β- and pre-β-lipoproteins were preferentially lowered. Kovanen et al. (1981) reported that treatment of the dogs with monacolin K (mevinolin) produced a 1.5 to 2-fold increase in LDL receptor activity of the liver. This increase correlated with an increase in the fractional rate for intravenously administered ^{125}I-LDL, suggesting that the increased hepatic receptors were responsible for the enhanced clearance of LDL from plasma. In addition, treatment of dogs with the drug reduced the synthetic rate for the lipoprotein. The data suggest that the inhibition of cholesterol synthesis by compactin can trigger an increase in LDL receptors, thereby reducing LDL levels in plasma.

In cynomolgus monkeys, compactin was also effective in lowering plasma cholesterol levels at a dose of 20 mg/kg (Kuroda et al., 1979). Levels of triglycerides and phospholipids were not significantly affected. Of the lipoprotein classes, a β-lipoprotein corresponding to LDL was preferentially reduced. The drug also produced a slight increase in fecal excretion of bile acids in the monkeys. In laying hens, compactin was effective in reducing plasma cholesterol when the animals were fed with a diet supplemented with compactin (0.06%). A 20% reduction of cholesterol content of eggs produced was obtained after 4 weeks (Endo, unpublished observation).

Of the animal species other than man tested so far, the rabbit is the most sensitive to compactin. At a dose of 5 mg/kg, a significant decrease in plasma cholesterol concentrations was obtained in normal healthy rabbits after 2 weeks of drug treatment (Watanabe et al., 1981). In normal rabbits fed a cholesterol free, low-fat semisynthetic diet, mevinolin (monacolin K) produced a 37% decrease in serum cholesterol levels at a dose of 2 mg/kg (Kroon et al, 1982).

Watanabe and co-workers have developed a strain of rabbit (called WHHL rabbit) with inborn hyperlipidemia (Watanabe, 1980). The mode of inheritance of the trait was shown to be autosomal recessive. At the age of one month, plasma cholesterol and triglyceride levels of the homozygous animals were as high as 518 and 511 mg/dl, respectively; this is 8- and 9-fold higher than those for normal animals. Cultured fibroblasts (Tanzawa et al., 1981) and membranes from the liver and adrenal glands (Kita et al., 1981) of WHHL rabbits lacked high-affinity LDL receptors. When compactin was administered to these animals at 5 mg/kg, plasma cholesterol concentrations were reduced by 21% (Watanabe et al., 1981).

B. In Man

In healthy man, compactin is well tolerated and exerts a rapid and profound cholesterol-lowering effect (Shigematsu et al., 1979). Similar effects are obtained with mevinolin (monakolin K) (Tobert et al., 1981; Tobert et al., 1982).

Of the various types of hypercholesterolemia, familial hypercholesterolemia (FH), characterized by a marked increase in LDL, is notoriously resistant to drug therapy. Hyperlipidemia is present at birth in such persons and cardiovascular disease often, but not always, occurs prematurely. Yamamoto et al. (1980) first studied the efficacy of compactin in patients with FH. In patients with heterozygous FH, a 27% decrease (on the average) in plasma cholesterol was obtained after 4 to 8 weeks of treatment at a daily dose of 1 to 2 mg/kg. The cholesterol levels started to decrease within 2 weeks of treatment. Mabuchi et al. (1981) reported a detailed study of compactin's effects in FH. At a daily dose of 0.5 to 1 mg/kg, they observed a 29% decrease in plasma LDL levels (Fig. 5). Plasma HDL levels did not change. Serum ubiquinone-10 concentrations did not change, but LDL levels of ubiquinone-10 decreased by 50%.

The combination of a bile acid-binding resin (cholestyramine or colestipole) and an HMG-CoA reductase inhibitor (compactin or mevinolin) produces a much greater decrease of LDL levels than can be obtained by either agent alone (Mabuchi et al., 1983; Yamamoto et al., 1983; Bilheimer et al., 1983). When 10 patients with heterozygous FH were treated with cholestyramine alone (12 g daily) for 6 to 16 months, LDL-associated cholesterol decreased by 28%. With the addition of compactin (30 mg daily) for 12 weeks, there was a 53% decrease in LDL-cholesterol--from 263 $\pm$ 13 to 125 $\pm$ 10 mg/dl. HDL-cholesterol, which had increased during cholestyramine treatment, remained at its higher level (Mabuchi et al., 1983).

Bilheimer et al. (1983) showed that mevinolin (monacolin K) caused an increase in the FCR (fractional catabolic rate) for intravenously administered ^{131}I-LDL in FH heterozygotes and in the receptor-mediated clearance of native LDL without affecting receptor-independent clearance. These findings are consistent with the hypothesis that an increase in LDL receptors is a major mechanism for the

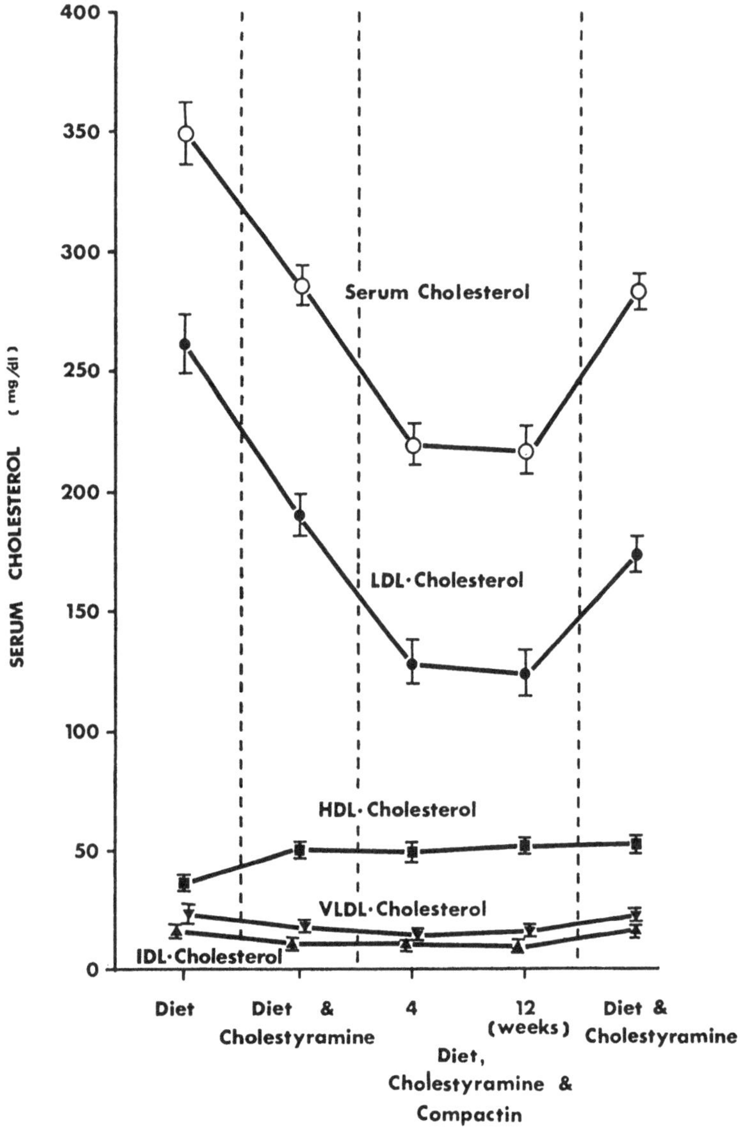

Fig. 5 Influence of cholestyramine and compactin on serum total and lipoprotein cholesterol levels in man.

effect of an HMG-CoA reductase inhibitor in diminishing plasma LDL levels in FH heterozygotes.

In FH homozygotes, compactin is less effective and higher doses are required to reduce plasma cholesterol. Of 2 FH homozygotes studied by Yamamoto et al. (Yamamoto et al., 1978; Yamamoto et al., 1980), reduction of serum cholesterol levels was as low as 14% at a daily dose of 150 mg in one patient, while no detectable changes in serum cholesterol was obtained in the other at a dose as high as 200 mg/day. In an LDL receptor-defective FH homozygote who was undergoing plasma exchange, a slight decrease in plasma cholesterol was obtained at a dose of 60 to 120 mg/day (Mabuchi et al., unpublished data).

Studies by other groups showed that compactin is much more effective in the treatment of hyperlipidemias other than FH, producing a significant reduction of plasma cholesterol levels at a daily dose of 0.1 to 0.2 mg/kg (Shigematsu et al., 1979; Hata et al., 1980; Higuchi et al., 1981).

CONCLUSION

Compactin and related compounds have already proved extremely useful in elucidating the regulatory mechanism for the synthesis of cholesterol and other isoprenoids. For example, the use of compactin to inhibit HMG-CoA reductase in cultured cells have provided new information regarding the regulatory mechanism for HMG-CoA reductase. HMG-CoA reductase, the enzyme that synthesizes mevalonate required for the synthesis of both cholesterol and other isoprenoids, appears to be regulated through a multivalent feedback mechanism. Further, evidence has been provided that one or more products derived from mevalonate, which include ubiquinone and dolichol, are essential for the growth of some cultured cells even when the cells are grown in the presence of sufficient amounts of exogenous cholesterol. Other applications of compactin include isolation of mutant cells resistant to compactin, investigation of the essential role for mevalonate-derived product in DNA replication and in cell cycle.

Compactin has been shown to be highly effective in lowering plasma LDL in many animal species as well as man. The studies with compactin have established a general principle: interference with cholesterol synthesis by a competitive inhibitor of HMG-CoA reductase can reduce LDL levels in plasma without deleting vital body stores of cholesterol. In addition to helping patients with FH, compactin offers hope to the large number of patients whose plasma cholesterol levels are in the upper range for the population and who are predisposed to atherosclerosis, yet do not have FH.

REFERENCES

Albers-Schonberg, G., Joshua, H., Lopez, M. B., Hensens, O. D., Springer, J. P., Chen, J., Ostrove, S., Hoffman, C. H., Alberts, A. W., and Pachett, A. A., 1981, J. Antibiotics, 34:507-512.

Alberts, A. W., Chen, J., Kuron, G., Hunt, V., Huff, J., Hoffman, C., Rothrock, J., Lopez, J., Joshua, H., Harris, E., Pachett, A.,

Monaghan, R., Currie, S., Stapley, E., Albers-Schonberg, G., Hensens, O., Hirschfield, J., Hoogsteen, K., Liesch, J., and Springer, J., 1980, Proc. Natl. Acad. Sci., U.S.A., 77:3957-3961.
Betterridge, D. J., Krone, W., Peckless, J. P. D., and Galton, D. J., 1978, Lancet, 1342-1343.
Bilheimer, D. W., Grundy, S. M., Brown, M. S., and Goldstein, J. L., 1983, Proc. Natl. Acad. Sci., U.S.A., 80, In Press.
Brown, M. S., Faust, J. R., Goldstein, J. L., Kaneko, I., and Endo, A., 1978, J. Biol. Chem., 253:1121-1128.
Brown, M. S., and Goldstein, J. L., 1980, J. Lipid Res., 21:505-517.
Brown, A. G., Smale, T. C., King, T. J., Hasenkamp, R., and Thompson, R. H., 1976, J. Chem. Soc. Perkin I., 1165-1170.
Carson, D. D., and Lennarz, W. J., 1979, Proc. Natl. Acad. Sci., U.S.A., 76:5709-5713.
Chin, D. J., Luskey, K. L., Anderson, R. G. W., Faust, J. R., Goldstein, J. L., and Brown, M. S., 1982a, Proc. Natl. Acad. Sci., U.S.A., 79:1185-1189.
Chin, D. J., Luskey, K. L., Faust, J. R., MacDonald, R. J., Brown, M. S., and Goldstein, J. L., 1982b, Proc. Natl. Acad. Sci., U.S.A., 79:7704-7708.
Ciegler, A., Kadis, S., and Ajl, S. J., 1971, in: "Microbial Toxins," vol. 6, Academic Press, New York.
Cohen, D. C., Massoglia, S. L., and Gospodarowicz, D., 1982a, J. Biol. Chem., 257:9429-9437.
Cohen, D. C., Massoglia, S. L., and Gospodarowicz, D., 1982b, J. Biol. Chem., 257:11106-11112.
Cuthbert, J. A. and Lipsky, P. E., 1980, J. Immunol., 124:2240-2246.
Cuthbert, J. A. and Lipsky, P. E., 1981, J. Immunol., 126:2093-2099.
Endo, A., 1979, J. Antibiotics, 32:852-854.
Endo, A., 1980, J. Antibiotics, 33:334-336.
Endo, A., 1983, J. Antibiotics, In Press.
Endo, A., and Kuroda, M., 1976, J. Antiobiotics, 29:841-843.
Endo, A., Kuroda, M., and Tanzawa, K., 1976a, FEBS Letters, 72:323-326.
Endo, A., Kuroda, M., and Tsujita, Y., 1976b, J. Antibiotics, 29:1346-1348.
Endo, A., Tsujita, Y., Kuroda, M., and Tanzawa, K., 1979, Biochim. Biophys. Acta 575:585-589.
Endo, A., Yamada, A., Takeshima, H., and Hasumi, K., 1983, J. Antiobiotics, In Press.
Endo, A., and Yamashita, H., 1983, J. Antibiotics, In Press.
Faust, J. R., Luskey, K. L., Chin, D. J., Goldstein, J. L., and Brown, M. S., 1982, Proc. Natl. Acad. Sci., U.S.A., 79:5205-5209.
Freeman, D. A., and Ascoli, M., 1982, J. Biol.Chem., 257:14231-14238.
Gibson, D. M., and Ingebritsen, T. S., 1978, Life Sci., 23:2649-2664.
Goldstein, J. L., Helgeson, J. A. S., and Brown, M. S., 1979, J. Biol. Chem., 254:5403-5409.
Haba, T., Mabuchi, H., Yoshimura, A., Watanabe, A., Wakasugi, T.,

Tatami, R., Ueda, K., Ueda, R., Kametani, T., Koizumi, J., Miyamoto, S., Takeda, R., and Takeshita, H., 1981, *J. Clin. Invest.*, 67:1532-1540.

Habenicht, A. J. R., Glomset, J. A., and Ross, R., 1980, *J. Biol. Chem.*, 255:5134-5140.

Hardeman, E. C., Endo, A., and Simoni, R. D., 1983a, *J. Biol. Chem.*, In Press.

Hardeman, E. C., Jenke, H. S., and Simoni, R. D., 1983b, *Proc. Natl. Acad. Sci.*, U.S.A., 80:1516-1520.

Hata, Y., Shigematsu, H., Oikawa, T., Yamamoto, M., Yamauchi, Y., and Goto, Y., 1980, *Geriat. Med.*, JAPAN, 17:1564-1570.

Higuchi, Y., Ishida, M., Ueda, A., Fukada, K., Fuchimoto, T., Kibata, M., and Kimura, I., 1981, *J. Japan Atherosclerosis Soc.*, 9:111-115.

James, M. J., and Kandutsch, A. A., 1979, *J. Biol. Chem.*, 254:8442-8446.

Kaneko, I., Hazama-Shimada, Y., and Endo, A., 1978, *Eur. J. Biochem.*, 87:313-321.

Kempen, H. J., Holstein, M. V., and de Lange, J., 1983, *J. Lipid Res.*, 24:316-323.

Kita, T., Brown, M. S., Watanabe, Y., and Goldstein, J. L., 1981, *Proc. Natl. Acad. Sci.*, U.S.A., 78:2268-2272.

Koizumi, J., Mabuchi, H., and Takeda, R., 1982, *Biochem. Biophys. Res. Commun.*, 108-240-246.

Kovanen, P. T., Bilheimer, D. W., Goldstein, J. L., Jaramillo, J. J., Brown, M. S., 1981, *Proc. Natl. Acad. Sci.*, U.S.A., 78:1194-1198.

Kroon, P. A., Hand, K. M., Huff, J. W., and Alberts, A. W., 1982, *Atherosclerosis*, 44:41-48.

Kuroda, M., Tanzawa, K., Tsujita, Y., and Endo, A., 1977, *Biochim. Biophys. Acta* 489:119-125.

Kuroda, M., Tsujita, Y., Tanzawa, K., and Endo, A., 1979, *Lipids*, 14:585-589.

Lam, T. Y. K., Gullo, V. P., Goegelman, R. T., Jorn, D., Huang, L., DeRiso, C., Monaghan, R. L., and Putter, L., 1981, *J. Antibiotics*, 34:614-616.

Luskey, K. J., Chin, D. J., MacDonald, R. J., Liscum, L., Goldstein, J. L., and Brown, M. S., 1982, *Proc. Nat. Acad. Sci.*, U.S.A., 79:6210-6214.

Mabuchi, H., Haba, T., Tatami, R., Miyamoto, S., Sakai, Y., Wakasugi, T., Watanabe, A., Koizumi, J., and Takeda, R., 1981, *New Engl. J. Med.*, 305:478-482.

Mabuchi, H., Sakai, T., Sakai, Y., Yoshimura, A., Watanabe, A., Wakasugi, T., Koizumi, J., and Takeda, R., 1983, *New Engl. J. Med.*, 308:609-613.

Masuda, A., Akiyama, S., and Kuwano, M., 1982, *Mol. Cell. Biol.*, 2:1354-1361.

Ness, G. C., Way, S. C., and Wickham, P. S., 1981, *Biochem. Biophys. Res. Commun.*, 102:81-85.

Nordstrom, J. L., Rodwell, V. W., and Mitschelen, J. J., 1977, *J. Biol. Chem.*, 252:8924-8934.

Oram, J. F., Albers, J. J., Cheung, M. C., and Bierman, E. L., 1981, J. Biol. Chem., 256:8348-8356.
Perkins, S. L., Leiden, S. F., and Stubbs, J. D., 1982, Biochim. Biosphys. Acta 711:83-89.
Pullinger, C., and Gibbons, G. Y., 1982, Biochim. Biophys. Acta., 713:323-332.
Rogers, D. H., and Rudney, H., 1982, J. Biol. Chem., 257:10650-10658.
Quesney-Huneeus, V., Wiley, M. H., and Siperstein, M. D., 1979, Proc. Natl. Acad. Sci., U.S.A., 76:5056-5060.
Quesney-Huneeus, V., Wiley, M. H., and Siperstein, M.D., 1980, Proc. Natl. Acad. Sci., U.S.A., 77:5842-5846.
Ryan, J., Hardeman, E. C., Endo, A., and Simoni, R. D., 1981, J. Biol. Chem., 256:6762-6769.
Savion, N., Laherty, R., Cohen, D., Lui, G. M., and Gospodarowicz, D., 1982, Endocrinology, 110:13-22.
Serizawa, N., Nakagawa, K., Hamano, K., Tsujita, Y., Terahara, A., and Kuwano, H., 1983a, J. Antibiotics, 36:604-606.
Serizawa, N., Nakagawa, K., Tsujital, Y., Terahara, A., and Kuwano, H., 1983b, J. Antibiotics, 36:608-610.
Shigematsu, H., Hata, Y., Yamamoto, M., Oikawa, T., Yamauchi, Y., Nakaya, H., Goto, Y., and Matsumura, H., 1979, Geriat. Med., Japan, 17:1564-1570.
Sinensky, M., Torget, R., and Edwards, P. A., 1981, J. Biol. Chem., 256:11774-11779.
Tanaka, R. D., Edwards, P. A., Lan, S. F., Knoeppel, E. M., and Fogelman, A. M., 1982, J. Lipid Res., 23:1026-1031.
Tanzawa, K., and Endo, A., 1979, Eur. J. Biochem., 98:195-201.
Tanzawa, K., Kuroda, M., and Endo, A., 1977, Biochim. Biophys. Acta 488:97-101.
Tanzawa, K., Shimada, Y., Kuroda, M., Tsujita, Y., Arai, M., and Watanabe, Y., 1981, FEBS Letters, 118:81-84.
Tobert, J. A., Bell, G. D., Birtwell, J., James I., Kukovetz, W. R., Pryor, J. S., Buntinx, A., Holmes, I. B., Chao, Y. S., and Bolognese, J. A., 1982, J. Clin. Invest., 69:913-919.
Tobert, J. A., Hitzenberger, G., Kukovetz, W. R., Holmes, I. B., and Jones, K. H., 1981, Atherosclerosis, 41:61-65.
Tsujita, Y., Kuroda, M., Tanzawa, K., Kitano, N., and Endo, A., 1979, Atherosclerosis, 32:307-313.
Watanabe, Y., 1980, Atherosclerosis, 36:261-268.
Watanabe, Y., Ito, T., Saeki, M., Kuroda, M., Tanzawa, K., Mochizuki, M., Tsujita, Y., and Arai, M., 1981, Atherosclerosis, 38:27-31.
Yamamoto, A., Endo, A., Kitano, Y., Okada, A., Ishikawa, K., Kuroshima, T., and Kaneko, I., 1978, Japanes. J. Med., 17:230-239.
Yamamoto, A., Sudo, H., and Endo, A., 1980, Atherosclerosis, 35:259-266.
Yamamoto, A., Yamamura, T., Yokoyama, S., Sudo, H., and Matsuzawa, Y., 1983, Inter. J. Clin. Pharmacol. Ther. Toxicol., In Press.

THE ROLE OF PHOSPHORYLATION/DEPHOSPHORYLATION IN THE REGULATION OF CHOLESTEROL 7α-HYDROXYLASE ACTIVITY

Ajit Sanghvi

Department of Pathology
University of Pittsburgh School of Medicine
Pittsburgh, Pennsylvania 15261

INTRODUCTION

The enzyme cholesterol 7α-hydroxylase catalyzes the hydroxylation of cholesterol to form 7α-hydroxycholesterol, which is the first compound in the biosynthesis of bile acids.[1] The enzyme is characterized as a mixed function oxidase which introduces one atom of a molecule of O_2 into the substrate, while the other atom is reduced to water by a reduced coenzyme, as shown in the equation:

$$RH + NADPH + H^+ + O_2 \rightarrow ROH + NADP^+ + H_2O$$

(where RH is the substrate). The enzyme consists of subunits which include a flavoprotein, NADPH cytochrome-c reductase, and a species of cytochrome-P450.[2] The evidence recently gathered in our laboratory indicates that the short-term regulation of the activity of this enzyme involves the process of phosphorylation/dephosphorylation of the enzyme molecule and that the active moiety is the phosphorylated one. This is in contrast to what is known for HMG-CoA reductase, the major enzyme in cholesterol biosynthesis, which is active when it is dephosphorylated.

A peculiar feature of cholesterol 7α-hydroxylase is that the endogenous microsomal cholesterol serves as its substrate. It has been difficult, therefore, to carry out accurate measurements of enzyme activity in a conventional manner. One of the most useful, and probably the most accurate, measures of 7α-hydroxylase activity is the measurement of the mass of 7α-hydroxycholesterol formed from the endogenous microsomal cholesterol. The results presented here were obtained using a GC/MS procedure.[3]

MATERIALS AND METHODS

Animals used in this study were male Sprague-Dawley rats weighing 200-220 g each from Hilltop Lab Animals (Scottdale, PA). Rats were kept two per cage under a strict 12-hour light-dark cycle (dark 0300-1500, light 1500-0300). The animals had free access to food and water. They were sacrificed at 0900 for each experiment. Livers were homogenized in 0.25 M sucrose containing 1 mM EDTA, pH 7.3, using 4 ml of solution per gram of liver. Cell debris and mitochondria were removed by centrifugation in the cold at 400 x g (15 minutes) and 11,000 x g (30 minutes), respectively. The supernatant was centrifuged at 300,000 x g for 20 minutes. The resulting supernatant was discarded. The microsomal pellet was gently dislodged and broken up with a glass rod with a rounded tip. It was suspended in 0.1 M potassium phosphate buffer (pH 7.4) containing 1 mM EDTA. This suspension was recentrifuged at 300,000 x g for 20 minutes, the supernatant was discarded, and appropriate buffers for particular experiments were added as indicated. After the microsomal pellet had been broken up with a glass rod, the mixture was transferred to a glass homogenizing tube, where it was mixed by using the necessary number of strokes of a hand-held Teflon pestle. Samples from this microsomal suspension were incubated under different experimental conditions as described in table legends. Also, it is this suspension of microsomes that when centrifuged at 300,000 x g for 20 minutes yielded the microsomal "supernatant" used in several experiments as referred to in the tables; for example, the supernatant obtained upon centrifugation of microsomal suspension after incubation with E. coli alkaline phosphatase or after incubation in imidazole buffer, etc. Incubation of microsomes was performed in 0.1 M potassium phosphate, 20 mM imidazole•HCl, or 20 mM Tris•HCl; each of these buffers contained 1 mM EDTA, 5 MM dithiothreitol, 0.3-0.5 mg of microsomal protein, 10 mM 2-mercaptoethylamine, two units of glucose-6-phosphate dehydrogenase, 20 mM glucose-6-phosphate, and 2 mM NADP in a total volume of 0.45 ml. The concentration of metal ions, wherever used, was 4 mM as $MgCl_2$, $Ca(OAc)_2$, or $MnCl_2$. ATP and NaF, when used, were 2 mM and 50 mM, respectively. The chemicals mentioned above were obtained from Sigma. All experiments utilized samples from combined microsomes from four or more rat livers. Microsomal protein content was determined by the method of Bradford.[4] The reaction was stopped by adding 5 ml of chloroform/methanol, 2:1 (v/v).

A gas chromatographic/mass spectrometric procedure developed in our laboratory was used to measure the 7α-hydroxycholesterol production.[3] The instrument used was a Hewlett-Packard 5986A gas chromatograph/mass spectrometer. The analyses were carried out in selected ion monitoring mode under conditions previously described.[3]

For the determination of cholesterol 7α-hydroxylase activity incubations were for short periods of time, with the cofactors described above, so that the 7α-hydroxycholesterol production was a linear function of both time and the amount of microsomal protein.

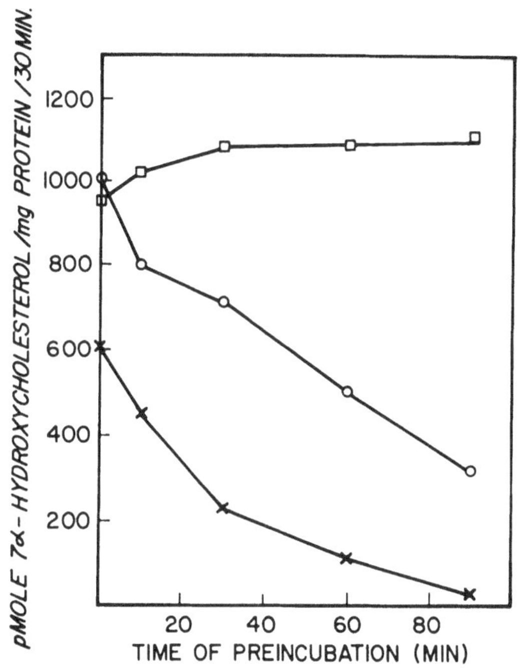

Fig. 1 Effect of preincubation of rat liver microsomes in (i) 0.2 M phosphate buffer, □—□ ; (ii) 20 mM imidazole•HCl + 5 mM DTT, X—X; and (iii) 20 mM Tris•HCl + 5 mM DTT, O—O; on 7α-hydroxycholesterol production.

Microsomes frozen in dry ice/acetone and stored at -70°C kept their activity for at least two weeks. Cholesterol 7α-hydroxylase activity was not affected adversely by refreezing and thawing microsomes, but incubation of microsomes for 60-90 minutes, followed by washing two times, resulted in 30-40% loss of enzyme activity.

RESULTS AND DISCUSSION

Since HMG-CoA reductase is shown to be active in the dephosphorylated form,[5,6] our initial thought was that 7α-hydroxylase may also be active in the dephosphorylated form. Therefore, our first experiments were carried out under dephosphorylating conditions. Accordingly, rat liver microsomes were preincubated from 0 to 90 minutes in either 0.1 M phosphate buffer or 20 mM imidazole with 5 mM dithiothreitol, or 20 mM Tris hydrocholoride with 5 mM dithiotreitol. While

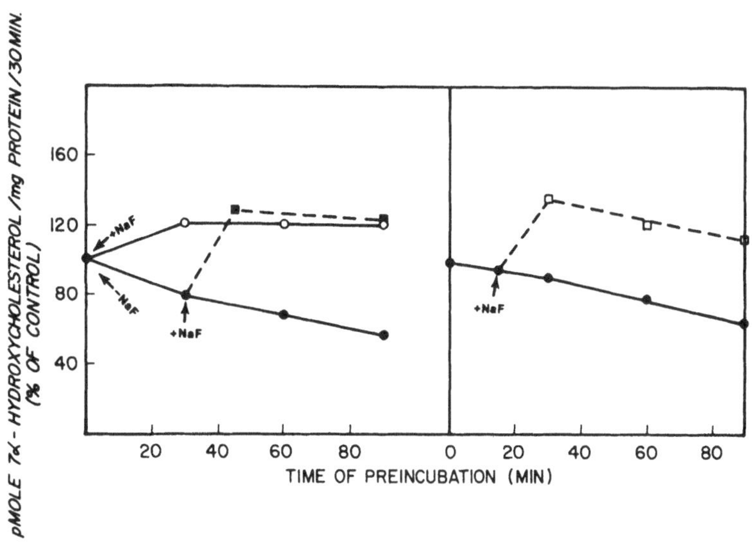

Fig. 2 7α-Hydroxylase formation in rat liver microsomes after preincubation in Tris•HCl (a) and imidazole•HCl (b) buffers. 50 mM NaF was added after 0, O—O; 15, ■—■; or 30 minutes, □—□; of preincubation as shown. ●—● is the enzyme activity in Tris•HCl or imidazole•HCl in the absence of NaF.

the activity in the phosphate buffer remained constant or even showed a slight increase with the preincubation time, the activity in either Tris buffer or the imidazole buffer declined with the preincubation time (Fig. 1). These experiments provided the first clue that the enzyme perhaps was being deactivated under dephosphorylating conditions. If this were true, then the addition of fluoride ions should be able to prevent the decline in enzyme activity. Accordingly, as shown in Fig. 2, when sodium fluoride was added either at the beginning of the preincubation or at any intermediate time during preincubation, in either Tris or imidazole buffer, the decline in 7α-hydroxylase activity was stabilized.

In order to show even more directly that the loss of 7α-hydroxylase activity was due to dephosphorylation of the enzyme, rat liver microsomes were preincubated with different amounts of E. coli alkaline phosphatase. As shown in Fig. 3, the enzyme progressively loses activity in the presence of increasing amounts of alkaline phosphatase in the incubation medium.

Having observed a loss in 7α-hydroxylase activity under dephosphorylating conditions, it was essential to demonstrate if the loss in enzyme activity could be recovered under phosphorylating conditions. Therefore, we isolated a cytosolic protein factor according

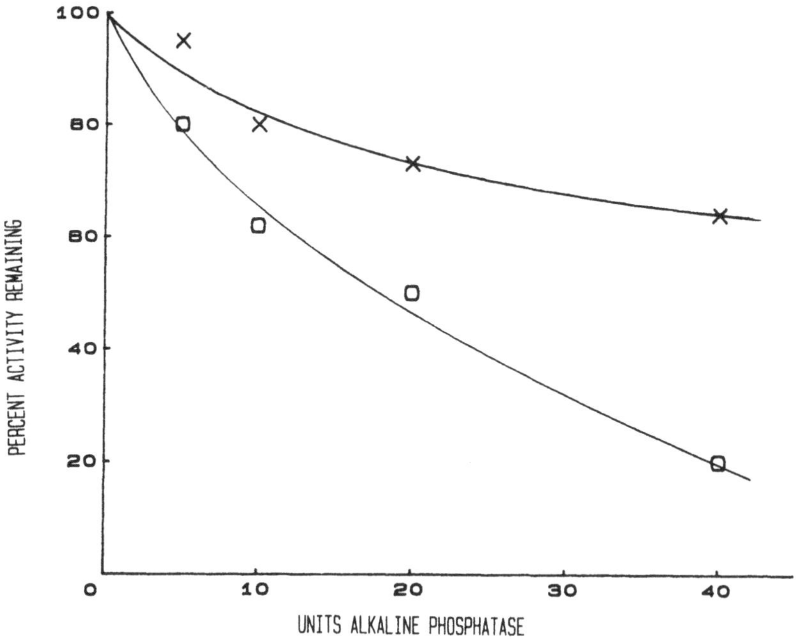

Fig. 3 Loss of cholesterol 7α-hydroxylase activity with increasing amounts of alkaline phosphatase. X and □ indicate 60- and 90-min. incubation with alkaline phosphatase, respectively.

to the method of Nordstrom et al.,[7] which had previously been shown by these authors to possess protein kinase activity and was also shown to inactivate HMG-CoA reductase in the presence of ATP. Results with microsomes preincubated in imidazole buffer for 60 minutes, followed by incubations with cofactors for 10, 30 and 60 minutes in the presence of ATP Mg and ATP Mg plus the cytosolic protein fraction showed that the rate of 7α-hydroxycholesterol formation was accelerated in the presence of ATP Mg over that in controls and that it was further enhanced upon addition of the cytosolic protein fraction, as shown in Fig. 4. Moreover, the increase in 7α-hydroxylase activity in the presence of ATP Mg alone suggested the possible presence of a microsomal kinase. Experiments discussed below further confirm this suggestion.

Results in Table 1 show that ATP Mg in the presence of cytosolic protein was able to restore 7α-hydroxylase activity in microsomes which had been incubated with alkaline phosphatase and which had lost approximately 85% of their starting activity. Under the conditions of the experiment, 65% of the original activity was recovered.

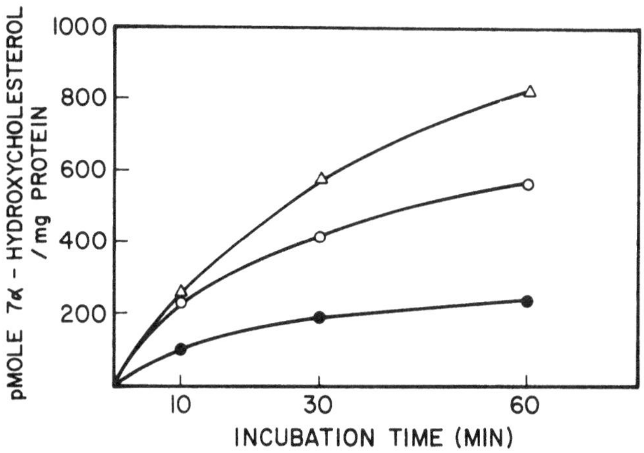

Fig. 4 Livers were homogenized in 0.25 M sucrose + 1.0 mM EDTA (pH 7.4) and microsomes preincubated for 60 minutes in 20 mM imidazole + 5 mM DTT. Following this, microsomes were incubated with 2 mM ATP + 4 mM $MgCl_2$, O—O; 2 mM ATP + 4 mM $MgCl_2$ + 120 μg cytosolic protein fraction, Δ—Δ. Controls, ●—●.

Later experiments revealed that the major part of 7α-hydroxylase activity could be recovered without the cytosolic protein. Moreover, we observed that magnesium was not only unnecessary to produce an increase in the 7α-hydroxylase activity by ATP, but could actually be deleterious to enzyme activity. Results consistent with this notion are shown in Tables 2 and 3.[8]

TABLE 1*

Experiment	pmoles/7α-hydroxycholesterol/ mg protein/30 minutes
Control	1780
+Alkaline phosphatase	300
+ATP·Mg + NaF + Cytosolic protein	1200

*Microsomes (0.3 mg protein) were preincubated for 30 minutes in 0.1 M phosphate buffer (control) followed by a 120-minute preincubation with E. coli alkaline phosphatase. After removal of phosphatase by centrifugation, microsomes were preincubated for 90 minutes in the presence of 2 mM ATP, 4 mM $MgCl_2$, 50 mM NaF, and 500 μg cytosolic protein fraction.

TABLE 2

EFFECT OF ATP AND A CYTOSOLIC PROTEIN FRACTION ON

PHOSPHATASE-INACTIVATED CHOLESTEROL 7α-HYDROXYLASE

Experiment	Activity, pmol 7α-hydroxycholesterol/mg protein per min.
Control	130
With phosphatase	56
Phosphatase removed	
With control supernatant	76
With control sup + cytosolic protein	82
With control sup + ATP	115

Microsomes were incubated for 90 min. in 0.1 M phosphate buffer alone (control) or with 25 units of E. coli alkaline phosphatase. Phosphatase was removed by centrifugation at 300,000 x g for 20 min. The resulting pellet was resuspended (i) in an equal volume of "supernatant" obtained from 300,000 x g centrifugation of control microsomal preincubation mixture called control supernatant; (ii) in control supernatant plus 150 μg of cytosolic protein fraction; or (iii) in control supernatant plus 2 mM ATP, and cholesterol 7α-hydroxylase activity was determined. No significant changes (less than 10%) in the enzyme activity were observed when incubations included cystosolic protein or cytosolic protein or cytosolic protein plus ATP.

TABLE 3

EFFECT OF ATP·Mg AND ATP ALONE

ON CHOLESTEROL 7α-HYDROXYLASE ACTIVITY

Experiment	Activity, pmol 7α-hydroxycholesterol/ mg protein
Control	246
With ATP·Mg	276
With ATP	336

Microsomes were incubated for 60 min. in 20 mM imidazole buffer. After that, 7α-hydroxycholesterol production was measured by a 30-min. incubation with the cofactors alone (control), cofactors plus 2 mM ATP and 4 mM Mg^{2+} (ATP·Mg), or cofactors plus 2 mM ATP. Liver microsomes in this experiment were from animals at the low point in their diurnal cycle.

TABLE 4

EFFECT OF Mg^{2+}, Ca^{2+}, AND Mn^{2+} ON 7α-HYDROXYCHOLESTEROL FORMATION IN DIFFERENT BUFFERS

	Activity, pmol 7α-hydroxycholesterol/mg protein			
Buffer	Control	Mg^{2+}	Ca^{2+}	Mn^{2+}
Phosphate	3194	3215	3505	3201
Tris	2782	1754	1370	325
Imidazole	2236	1216	586	ND

Microsomes were incubated for 30 min. in 0.1 M phosphate, 20 mM Tris, or 20 mM imidazole, each with 5 mM dithiothreitol, in the presence of Mg^{2+}, Ca^{2+}, or Mn^{2+} (each 4 mM). Cofactors were added and after a 30-min. incubation, the amount of 7α-hydroxycholesterol formed was measured. ND, not detectable.

TABLE 5

TIME COURSE OF INHIBITION OF CHOLESTEROL 7α-HYDROXYLASE BY METAL IONS IN IMIDAZOLE/DITHIOTHREITOL BUFFER

		Activity, pmol 7α-hydroxycholesterol/mg protein per min.			
Experiment	Preincubation time, min.	Control	Mg^{2+}	Ca^{2+}	Mn^{2+}
1	0	150	102	84	118
	5	98	35	27	7
	15	79	6	ND	ND
2	60	98	90	72	27

In experiment 1, microsomes were incubated in 20 mM imidazole plus 5 mM dithiothreitol for 0, 5, and 15 min. in the presence and absence of Mg^{2+}, Ca^{2+}, or Mn^{2+} (each 4 mM). Cofactors were added and the enzyme activity was determined. In experiment 2, microsomes were incubated for 60 min. in imidazole buffer containing 50 mM NaF and the indicated metal ions. The enzyme activity was measured as before. ND, not detectable.

The effect of bivalent cations on the 7α-hydroxylase activity was probed further. It can be seen in Table 4 that magnesium, calcium and manganese were without effect on the enzyme activity when the incubations were carried out in 0.1 M phosphate buffer. On the other hand, when the phosphate buffer was replaced with either Tris or imidazole buffer, these ions produced a significant decline in the enzyme activity. In an experiment designed to study the time course of the metal ion inhibition of 7α-hydroxylase activity, it was seen that there was significant inhibition within 5 minutes of incubation in the presence of metal ions, as shown in Table 5. It was also observed, however, that if the incubation mixture contained 50 mM sodium fluoride, the metal ions were without effect on the enzyme activity. These results strongly implied the presence of an endogenous protein phosphatase in the microsomes.

In an effort to directly detect the possible presence of such a phosphatase, we used the substrate 4-methylumbelliferyl phosphate to assay the phosphatase activity. This compound is known to be a good substrate for many phosphatases.[9,10] The results in Table 6 show that there is significant endogenous phosphatase activity which is markedly inhibited by sodium fluoride. The addition of magnesium and ATP in the presence of sodium fluoride does not reverse the inhibition. It is noteworthy that under conditions in which the endogenous

TABLE 6

ENDOGENOUS MICROSOMAL PHOSPHATASE ACTIVITY IN IMIDAZOLE BUFFER AND ITS INHIBITION BY NaF

Experiment	Phosphatase activity nmol/mg protein per hr.	Cholesterol 7α-hydroxylase activity, pmol/mg protein
Control	1094	1600
Imidazole	1060	1020
With NaF	372	1400
With NaF + Mg^{2+} + ATP	396	1650

Microsomes were incubated for 60 min. in0.1 M phosphate (control) or in 20 mM imidazole alone or containing 50 mM NaF or 50 mM NaF plus 2 mM ATP plus 4 mM Mg^{2+}. The microsomal phosphatase activity was measured with methylumbelliferyl phosphate (5.3 mM). The amount of 7α-hydroxycholesterol formed was determined after a 30-min. incubation with cofactors.

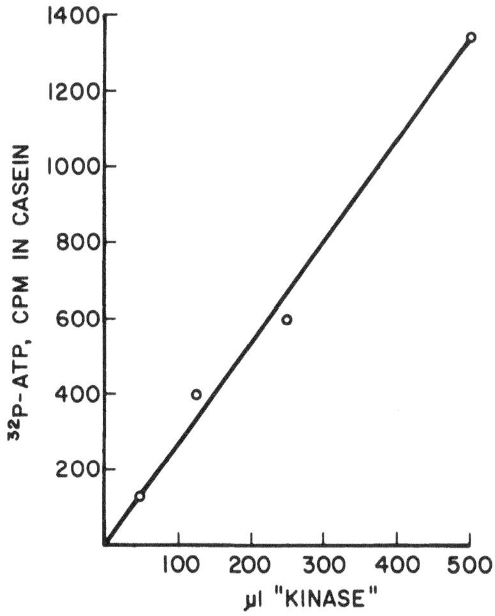

Fig. 5 Increase in 7α-hydroxylase activity in microsomes pretreated with alkaline phosphatase by the addition of ATP•Mg (O), ATP•Mg + cytosolic protein fraction (Δ). O indicates control values in phosphatase treated microsomes.

phosphatase activity is inhibited, 7α-hydroxycholesterol formation is partially restored, and when ATP is added to the incubation mixture, the activity returns to the level found in phosphate buffer.

Since the experiments with ATP indicated the possible presence of microsomal kinase, rat liver microsomes were extracted with salt solution as described by Beg et al.[6] Preliminary experiments in our laboratory, utilizing the salt extract and dephosphorylated casein, have shown that there was a linear increase in ^{32}P incorporation into casein from ^{32}P γ-labelled ATP (Fig. 5).

The additional evidence accumulated in our laboratory concerning the regulation of 7α-hydroxylase activity indicates the presence of a heat stable, dialyzable compound which appears essential for the stabilization of 7α-hydroxylase activity. When the rat liver microsomes are preincubated for 60 minutes in phosphate buffer, then centrifuged at 300,000 x g for 20 minutes, and the resulting microsomal pellet resuspended in a fresh phosphate buffer, the enzyme activity was shown to be reduced. However, if the original supernatant was added to the pellet, the enzyme activity was found to be restored to control levels. These data are shown in Table 6. This original supernatant was effective in restoring the activity even after boiling for 3 minutes. However, if the supernatant was dialyzed and then added to the microsomes, it was found to have no effect.[11] The nature of this compound is not clear at this time; however, one suggestion as to the mode of its action is that it may be an inhibitor of the endogenous microsomal phosphatase.

In summary, the evidence presented here shows that the short-term regulation of the activity of cholesterol 7α-hydroxylase can be modulated by the process of phosphorylation/dephosphorylation. Such a mechanism has been shown to be an important factor governing the activities of HMG-CoA reductase and acyl-CoA:cholesterol acyl transferase,[12] the two key enzymes concerned with the regulation of cholesterol metabolism in the liver cell. Our evidence further indicates there are components of the control system regulating the activity of 7α-hydroxylase which are associated with the rat liver microsomes. These include a phosphatase, a kinase, a dialyzable factor, and possibly a kinase-kinase similar to the one which has been postulated in the case of HMG-CoA reductase. We have recently formulated a hypothesis involving a coordinate regulation of these key enzymes--HMG-CoA reductase, cholesterol 7α-hydroxylase, and acyl-CoA:cholesterol acyltransferase--by phosphorylation/ dephosphorylation. Such a mechanism provides an elegant short-term mechanism for intracellular unesterified cholesterol homeostasis.[13]

REFERENCES

1. H. Danielsson, K. Einarsson, and G. Johansson, Europ. J. Biochem. 2:44-49 (1967).
2. N. B. Myant and K. A. Mitropoulos, J. Lipid Res. 18:135-153 (1977).
3. A. Sanghvi, E. Grassi, C. Bartman, and R. Lester, J. Lipid Res. 22:720-724 (1981).
4. M. Bradford, Anal. Biochem. 72:248-254, k2976.
5. Z. H. Beg, J. A. Stovik, and H. B. Brewer, Jr., Proc. Natl. Acad. Sci., U.S.A., 75:3678-3682 (1978).
6. Z. H. Beg, J. A. Stovik, and H. B. Brewer, Jr., Proc. Natl. Acad. Sci., U.S.A., 76:4375-4379 (1979).
7. J. L. Nordstrom, V. W. Rodwell, and J. J. Mitschelen, J. Bio. Chem. 252:8924-8934 (1977).
8. A. Sanghvi, E. Grassi, V. Warty, W. Diven, C. Wight, and R. Lester, Biochem. Biophys. Res. Commun. 103:886-892 (1981).
9. C. J. Cornish, F. C. Neall, and S. Posen, Am. J. Clin. Path. 53:68-76 (1970).
10. D. Robinson and P. Willcox, Biochim. Biophys. Acta. 191:183-186 (1969).

11. A. Sanghvi, E. Grassi, and W. Diven, Proc. Natl. Acad. Sci., U.S.A., 80:2175-2178 (1983).
12. K. L. Gavey, D. L. Trujillo, and T. J. Scallen, Proc. Natl. Acad. Sci., U.S.A., 80:2171-2174 (1983).
13. T. J. Scallen and A. Sanghvi, Proc. Natl. Acad. Sci., U.S.A., 80:2477-2480 (1983).

CALCIUM ANTAGONISTS AND ATHEROSCLEROSIS

Dieter M. Kramsch*

The Cardiovascular Institute
Boston University School of Medicine
Boston, Massachusetts 02118

INTRODUCTION

The clinically important lesion of human atherosclerosis is the fibrous atheromatous plaque which often is calcified.[1] The connective tissue changes of fibrous lesions begin to develop in the second decade of life but it usually takes decades of slow growth before they produce clinical symptoms. However, it is these connective tissue changes which threaten health and life by seriously impairing arterial function through: luminal stenoses by the raised fibrous intima, through loss of elasticity by elastica destruction and collagen accumulation, as well as through increased rigidity and brittleness by calcium mineralization. These impairments of arterial function in turn lead to insufficiency of blood flow, thrombosis, hypertension, aneurysms and vessel rupture.

Fibrous lesions are present, with rare exceptions, virtually in all individuals beyond age 35 in Western societies.[1] Moreover, there is no evidence that calcified collagenous plaques can be removed once they are established. Quite to the contrary, recent studies at Bowman-Gray School of Medicine[2] are showing that collagen accumulations of intimal plaques induced by an atherogenic diet in monkeys did not regress even after 4 years of the most drastic plasma cholesterol reduction, possible only in animals, i.e., by total withdrawal of dietary cholesterol. However, any remaining abnormal collagen deposition in the intima raises the specter of fatal thrombotic events by interaction of collagen with blood elements.[3] In view of the clinical importance of the fibrous plaque, the ultimate and critial questions appear to be: how does connective tissue accumulate and/or

*Address reprint requests to Dr. Kramsch at Merck, Sharp & Dohme Research Laboratories, P. O. Box 2000, R86-218, Rahway, NJ 07065.

become altered in the intima of plaques, and what specific measures can be taken to prevent, arrest or reverse the formation of fibrous plaques?

Several recent studies[4-6] have shown that lowering of markedly elevated serum cholesterol levels is capable of significantly reducing morbidity and mortality from coronary heart disease and, by implication, may beneficially influence atherosclerosis. However, as these studies were performed in patients with excessively high serum cholesterol concentrations, it still is not certain whether cholesterol lowering may have similar effects in subjects in whom the serum cholesterol concentrations are only mildly elevated or not at all, but who constitute the majority of coronary heart disease victims in Western societies. Furthermore, it is not known to what extent lipid lowering treatment regimens may affect the formation of fibrous plaques or their removal. It, therefore, appears to be also desirable to search for agents which are able to influence the cellular and connective tissue components of fibrous plaques directly without need to improve abnormal serum lipids or lipoproteins. Such agents could become very attractive for alternative or adjunctive treatment to lipid lowering drugs. Of all agents known to affect the arterial wall components directly, the calcium antagonists in the broadest sense of the word are furthest advanced in research. These are agents which interfere with the deposition, flux and utilization of calcium ions in the vessel wall.

ATHEROGENESIS AND THE ROLE OF CALCIUM IONS

According to the current concepts of atherogenesis depicted in Fig. 1, the main processes leading to plaque formation include: (a) increased permeability of the endothelium to macromolecules such as low density lipoproteins (LDL), as well as to blood cells: (b) migration of cells into the intima such as smooth muscle cells (SMC) from media as well as monocyte-macrophages, other white blood cells and platelets from the blood stream; (c) proliferation of these cells in the intima by mitosis; (d) synthesis and secretion by the increased SMCs of excessive amounts of collagen, elastin and other connective tissue elements; (e) increased internalization of lipids and lipoproteins by SMCs and macrophages, including by endocytosis; (f) destruction of elastica by elastolysis; and (g) gross calcium mineralization of connective tissue components in a late phase of plaque development.

As recently reviewed by Kramsch et al.,[7,8] there has been mounting evidence that localized increases in arterial calcium content in ionic form may play a key role in early atherogenesis. Some of the basic cellular and extracellular processes of atherogenesis requiring readily-available ionic calcium (Ca^{++}) also are depicted in Fig. 1.

The cellular events requiring Ca^{++} include: (a) the contraction-relaxation cycle in contractile cells such as endothelium cells (con-

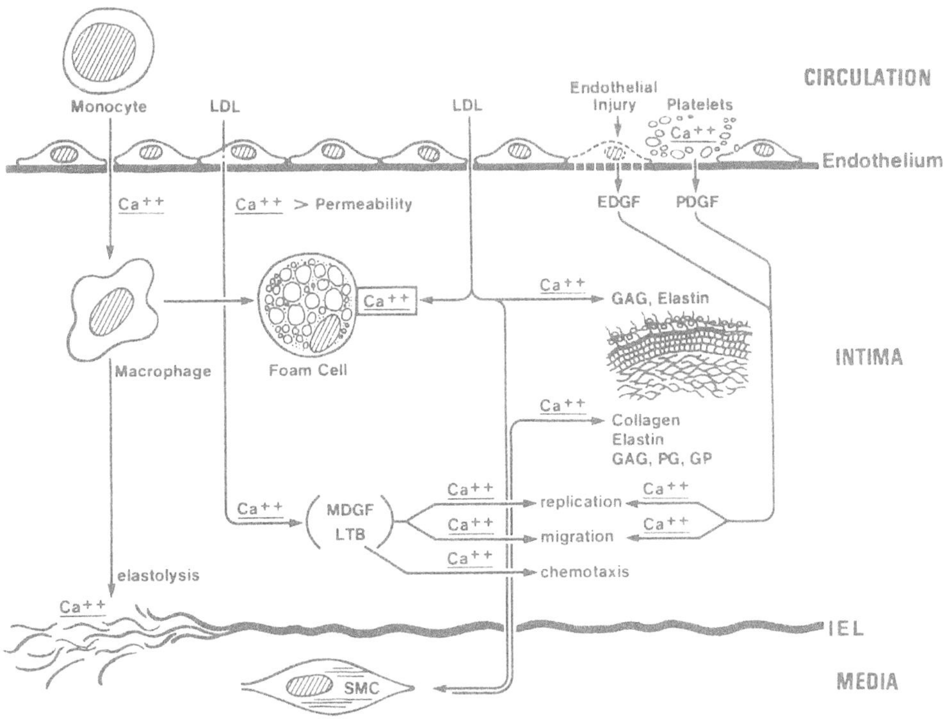

Fig. 1 Schematic representation of the current concepts of atherogenesis and the role of Ca^{++} in the main processes leading to plaque formation. Ca^{++} = ionic calcium; EDGF = endothelium-derived growth factor; GAG = glycosaminoglycans; GP = glycoprotein; IEL = internal elastic lamina; LDL = low density lipoproteins; LTB = leucotriene B; MDGF = macrophage-derived growth factor; PDGF = platelet-derived growth factor; PG = proteoglycans; SMC = smooth muscle cell.

traction leads to increased endothelial permeability) as well as SMCs, macrophage-monocytes, other blood cells and platelets (leading to migration of SMCs and blood cells and the release reaction of platelets; (b) directional movement of cells along a Ca^{++} gradient (chemotaxis); (c) the stimulus-division coupling (leading to cell replication by mitosis); (d) the stimulus secretion coupling (leading to excessive secretion by SMCs of collagen, elastin, glycosaminoglycans (GAG), proteoglycans (PG) and glycoproteins (GP), as well as by macrophages of leucotriene B (LTB) and elastase); (e) platelet function (adhesion to subendothelial collagen, aggregation and release reaction releasing platelet derived growth factor (PDGF) and proteolytic enzymes); (f) endocytosis of low density lipoprotein (LDL, leading to foam cell formation); (g) energy production from Ca^{++} dependent ATP for all of above cellular events.

The extracellular events requiring Ca^{++} include: (a) degradation of elastin (elastolysis) by macrophage elastase; (b) configurational changes of elastin causing increased absorption of cholesterol by elastin; (c) binding of extraneous proteins to elastin leading to increased binding of cholesterol esters by elastin-protein-Ca^{++} complexes; (d) complexing of lipoproteins to GAGs and PGs; (e) gross calcification (calcium apatite) of connective tissue, especially altered elastin.

PREVENTION OF FIBROUS-ATHEROMATOUS PLAQUE FORMATION BY ANTICALCIUM DRUGS

A. Experimental

We have been experimenting since 1973 with agents that have the capacity to prevent or even reverse calcium mineralization and fibrous atherosclerotic disease in rabbits and Macaca fascicular (cynomolgus) monkeys on fibrogenic atherogenic diets. These agents, which did not affect the elevated serum cholesterol levels, initially included ethane-1-hydroxy-1,1 diphosphonic acid (EHDP), an agent which is known to prevent the deposition of calcium into soft tissues, including into arteries.[9-11] Other and newer diphosphonates of similar properties[12] were later employed and included the disodium salts of amino-1-hydroxy-propane-1,1 diphosphonic acid (APDP), azacycloheptane-2,2 diphosphonic acid (AHDP) and 2-immino-pyrreolidone-5, 5 diphosphonic acid (IPDP). Successful treatment with these calcium regulating agents suggested that atherosclerosis may be beneficially influenced by regulating the availability of ionic calcium. We, therefore, treated animals on the atherogenic diet with the direct calcium ion antagonist, lanthanum, at increasing doses. Lanthanum is a calcium entry blocker of the class that operates to inhibit calcium influx to cells at receptor operated channels.[13,14] Most recently we also reported results with another anticalcium agent which inhibits the utilization of ionic tissue calcium, i.e., the cyclic AMP-phosphodiestrase inhibitor trimazosin.[15]

The fibrogenic atherogenic diet for rabbits contained 8% peanut oil and 2% cholesterol by weight;[16] that for monkeys contained 10% butter and 0.1% cholesterol.[17] The control diets were Purina Rabbit Chow and Purina Monkey Chow, respectively. Altogether, 12 groups of 10 male New Zealand White rabbits each and 6 groups, generally of 8 adult male Macaca fascicular (cynomolgus) monkeys, were fed the fibrogenic diets or the control diets: rabbits for 8 weeks, monkeys for 24 months. One group of rabbits was fed the control diet and 1 group the atherogenic diet alone, while 10 groups were given the atherogenic diet with added EHDP, APDP, AHDP, IPDP, lanthanum ($LaCl_3$, at dosage levels) and trimazosin (at 3 dosage levels), respectively. Likewise, one group of monkeys was fed the control diet and 1 group the atherogenic diet alone, while 4 groups were given the atheroge-

TABLE 1. Serum Components of Animals on Control Diets and on Atherogenic Diets With and Without Drug Treatment. Rabbits = 8 weeks; Monkeys = 24 Months; Values in mg/100 ml (Mean ± S.D.)

	Rabbits		Monkeys	
Experimental Groups	Cholesterol	Calcium	Cholesterol	Calcium
Control Diet	82 ± 23	13.2 ± 1.1	136 ± 42	11.0 ± 2.3
Atherogenic Diet, Untreated	2,573 ± 568*	13.3 ± 1.2	452 ± 163*	10.8 ± 1.8
Atherogenic Diet + EHDP	3,535 ± 738*	13.4 ± 0.6	408 ± 147*	9.7 ± 1.6
Atherogenic Diet + APDP	2,488 ± 534*	14.5 ± 0.9	512 ± 189*	9.5 ± 1.4
Atherogenic Diet + AHDP	2,283 ± 664*	14.7 ± 0.7	468 ± 133*	9.2 ± 1.9
Atherogenic Diet + IPDP	2.056 ± 845*	14.2 ± 1.3	---	---
Atherogenic Diet + $LaCl_3$(20mg)	2,431 ± 489*	14.8 ± 1.0**	---	---
Atherogenic Diet + $LaCl_3$(30mg)	2,035 ± 921*	15.3 ± 1.3*	---	---
Atherogenic Diet + $LaCl_3$(40mg)	2,537 ± 621*	16.0 ± 1.2*	397 ± 126*	9.5 ± 2.0
Atherogenic Diet+Trimazosin(20mg)	2,905 ± 331*	---	---	---
Atherogenic Diet+Trimazosin(30mg)	3,077 ± 316*	---	---	---
Atherogenic Diet+Trimazosin(80mg)	3,524 ± 300*	13.6 ± 1.3	---	---

*Highly significant changes from controls ($p < 0.01$)

**Significant changes from controls ($p < 0.05$)

nic diet with added EHDP, $LaCl_3$, APDP (4 monkeys) and AHDP (4 monkeys), respectively. The daily oral doses of drugs per kg bodyweight were: EHDP, APDP, AHDP and IPDP = 40 mg for rabbits; EHDP, APDP and AHDP for monkeys = 120 mg for the first 6 months followed by a maintenance dose of 40 mg thereafter; $LaCl_3$ = 20, 30 and 40 mg for rabbits; and for monkeys = 120 mg followed by 40 mg as with disphosphonates; trimazosin = 20, 30 and 80 mg (rabbits only). The large initial doses in monkeys were given to saturate the tissues, especially the large bone mass in the case of the diphosphonates.

B. Biochemical Findings

In all animals on the atherogenic diet, the serum cholesterol was markedly elevated to about the same level within each animal species, regardless whether or not any drugs were given (Table 1); the serum total (and ionized calcium - not shown) remained at normal values for both species, regardless of drug treatment, with the exception of either dose of $LaCl_3$, where the total calcium was elevated.

As compared to animals on the control diets, rabbits (Table 2, Fig. 2) and monkeys (Table 3) on the fibrogenic atherogenic diet revealed drastic changes in the components of aortic intima media: a marked increase in the arterial content of calcium was associated with drastic rises in the arterial content of non-lipid phosphorus, collagen, elastin and cholesterol. As noted previously,[18] the arterial elastin fraction of untreated atherogenic diet in animals of both species also was markedly altered, revealing marked increases in calcium and phosphorus as well as of polar amino acids and cholesterol (Tables 4 and 5).

In rabbits (Table 2, Fig. 2) simultaneous treatment with any of the drugs employed resulted in marked inhibition of the accumulations of aortic calcium which was associated with marked reductions in the content of the other arterial components despite continued presence of the atherogenic stimulus of unmitigated hypercholesterolemia. Best results were obtained by treatment with AHD, IPDP and $LaCl_3$ (40 mg) which completely suppressed the aortic accumulations of calcium, phosphorus, collagen and elastin; the aortic accumulations of cholesterol were drastically reduced, with the remaining lipids presumably being contained in the thin layer of intimal foam cells (Fig. 3c) that was observed as the only atherogenic alteration in these animals. The calcium, phosphorus, amino acid and cholesterol composition of elastin also was normal in rabbits treated with these 3 drugs (for $LaCl_3$-treated rabbits: Table 4). In atherogenic diet rabbits treated with the phosphodiesterase inhibitor trimazosin, the effective dose (calculated from the amount of food actually consumed per day) for maximal suppression (normalization) of the accumulations of aortic calcium, collagen and elastin was 30 mg per kg bodyweight per day (Fig. 2).

TABLE 2. Components of Intima-Media from Rabbits on Control Diets and Atherogenic Diets With and Without Treatment (Absolute Amounts in Mg/Whole Aorta Body Weight; Mean ± S.D.)

Experimental Groups	Calcium	Non-Lipid Phosphorus	Collagen	Elastin	Cholesterol
Control Diet	0.03 ± 0.007	0.04 ± 0.02	2.8 ± 0.5	10.3 ± 2.8	0.3 ± 0.2
Atherogenic Diet, Untreated	0.08 ± 0.012*	0.15 ± 0.03*	6.5 ± 1.3*	27.1 ± 1.7*	3.5 ± 1.2*
Atherogenic Diet + EHDP	0.06 ± 0.013*	0.11 ± 0.06**	4.3 ± 1.1**	21.5 ± 1.6*	1.3 ± 0.5*
Atherogenic Diet + APDP	0.06 ± 0.015**	0.13 ± 0.08	3.7 ± 0.4**	15.3 ± 1.6*	0.7 ± 0.3**
Atherogenic Diet + AHDP	0.04 ± 0.017	0.11 ± 0.05	2.9 ± 0.8	12.4 ± 1.4	0.5 ± 0.1**
Atherogenic Diet + IPDP	0.02 ± 0.009	0.06 ± 0.05	2.6 ± 0.9	7.3 ± 2.3	0.3 ± 0.3
Atherogenic Diet + $LaCl_3$(20mg)	0.04 ± 0.010**	0.06 ± 0.01**	4.2 ± 0.6*	17.3 ± 1.9*	1.9 ± 1.0*
Atherogenic Diet + $LaCl_3$(30mg)	0.03 ± 0.010	0.04 ± 0.03	3.6 ± 0.6**	14.4 ± 0.7*	1.4 ± 0.7*
Atherogenic Diet + $LaCl_3$(40mg)	0.03 ± 0.008	0.05 ± 0.02	2.9 ± 0.8	13.6 ± 4.7	0.6 ± 0.1**

*Highly significant changes from control values ($p < 0.01$)

**Significant changes from control values ($p < 0.05$)

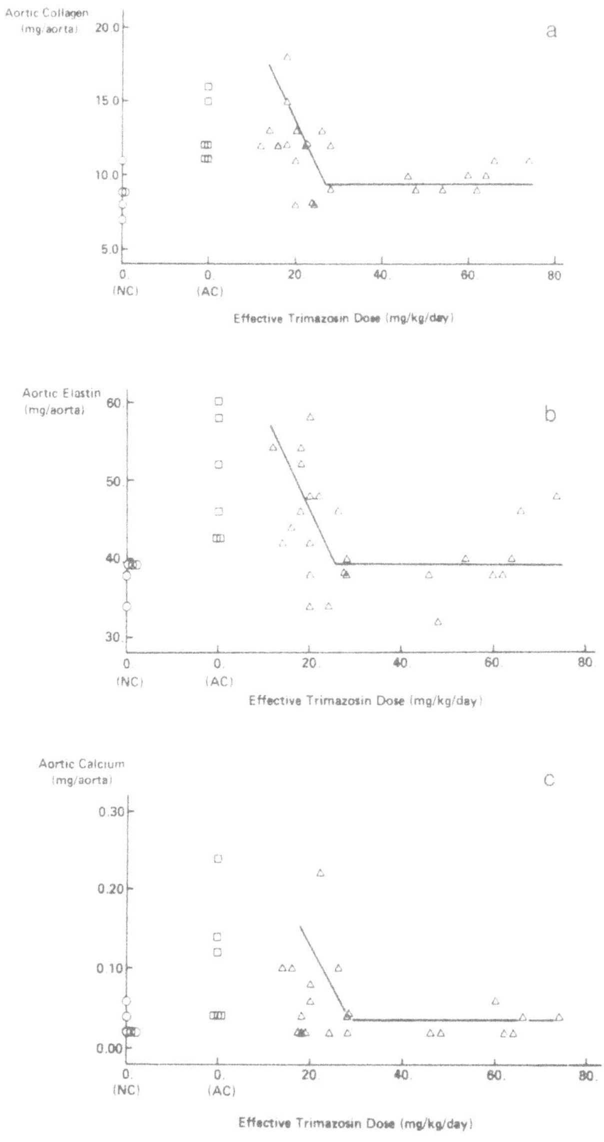

Fig. 2 (a-c) Content of collagen, elastin and calcium in intima-media of whole aorta in rabbits fed the atherogenic diet without drugs (AC = atherogenic diet controls) or with trimazosin 20 mg, 30 mg and 80 mg per kg bodyweight per day. The cumulative effective dose was calculated from the amount of food, containing the trimazosin doses, that was actually consumed per day over the eight-week study period. 2a = Aortic intimal-medial collagen vs. effective trimazosin dose; 2b = Aortic intimal-medial elastin vs. effective trimazosin dose; 2c = Aortic intimal-medial calcium vs. effective trimazosin dose.

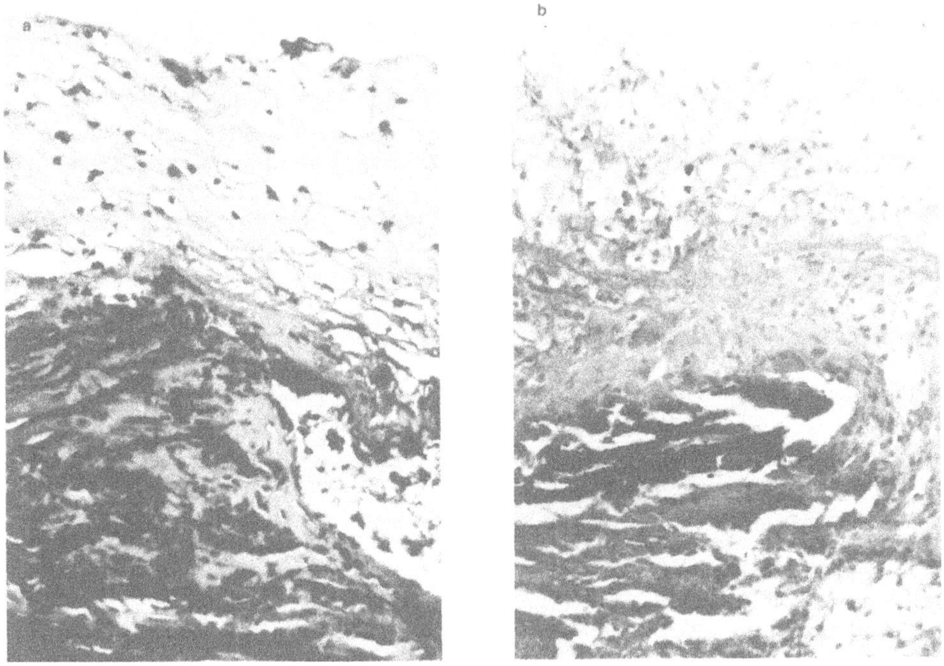

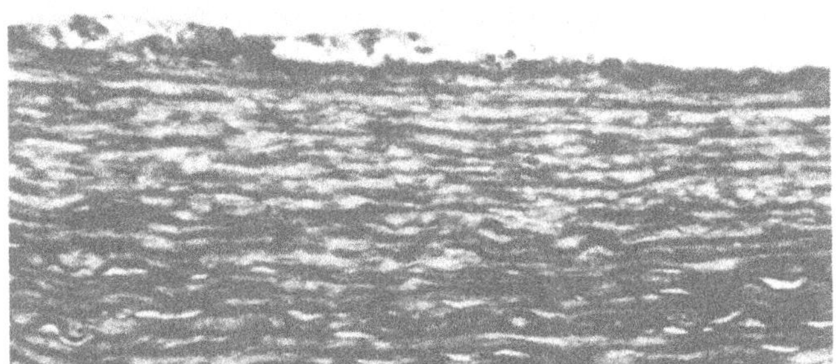

Fig. 3
(a-c)
Sections through characteristic lesions of thoracic aorta of rabbits on the fibrogenic diet for 8 weeks without drugs (a,b = sequential sections of the same lesion) or treated simultaneously with IPDP(c).
a. Note proliferation of cells and accumulation of collagen (gray) in intima and deranged elastica (black); Verhoeff's-Van Gieson, x85. b. Note deposition of calcium (black) on deranged elastica; Yasue's-light gree, x85. c. Note absence of collagen accumulation and calcium deposition, normal elastica, raising of intima by a thin layer of (lipid-rich) foam cells; Yasue's-light green, x70.

In monkeys (Table 3), treatment with lanthanum and diphosphonates resulted in similar marked reductions in the content of aortic calcium, as well as the other arterial components with the abnormalities of calcium, phosphorus, collagen and elastin being completely suppressed in abdominal aorta (and other major systemic arteries - not shown). The exception again was the arterial cholesterol content, which was greatly reduced but not to normal, with the residual lipids presumably being mainly contained in the intimal cells of the few small cellular lesions present (Fig. 4c). Treatment with EHDP and $LaCl_3$ also suppressed the atherogenic calcium and phosphorus changes in elastin of aorta as well as in other major systemic arteries of monkeys (Table 5). Arterial elastin of APDP and AHDP-treated monkeys was not analyzed but presumably would have shown similar results as with EHDP; on microscopic inspection the elastica was normal in these animals.

C. Morphological Findings

The biochemical results were in agreement with the morphological findings. Typical lesions are shown in Fig. 3a-c for rabbits and Fig. 4a-c for monkeys. In untreated rabbits, the fibrogenic atherogenic diet elicited numerous characteristic fibrous-atheromatous plagues (Fig. 3a), consisting of a markedly raised intima which contained large accumulations of collagen, many proliferated cells (some of which were lipid-filled foam cells), fragmented and deranged intimo-medial elastica as well as depositions of calcium minerals predominantly on the altered elastica (Fig. 3b). Although the lesions do not entirely resemble a human fibrous plaque, they did exhibit the same plaque ingredients. In contrast, rabbits treated simultaneously $LaCl_3$ (40 mg), EHDP, APDP, AHDP or IPDP (Fig. 3c) revealed a complete suppression of the calcium deposition, as well as marked suppression of lesion formation, leaving a few small lesions which consisted of a small aggregate of intimal foam cells on top of an otherwise normal arterial wall (especially effective: $LaCl_3$, AHDP and IPDP). Trimazosin-treated atherogenic-diet rabbits revealed similar suppressions of arterial depositions of calcium, collagen and elastin.

In untreated monkeys, the fibrogenic atherogenic diet elicited many of the same human-type fibrous plaques (Fig. 4a) as demonstrated in earlier studies.[18,19] These markedly raised plaques (here of aorta) were characterized by massive accumulations of intimal collagen, especially a fibrous cap, necroses and cholesterol clefts deep in the raised intima, derangement of intimo-medial elastica, but very

TABLE 3. Components of Aortic Intima-Media from Monkeys on Control Diets and Atherogenic Diets With and Without Treatment (μm/cm Length *In Situ*/Kg Body Weight; Mean ± S.D.)

AORTIC SEGMENT & TREATMENT	CALCIUM	NON-LIPID PHOSPHORUS	COLLAGEN	ELASTIN	CHOLESTEROL
Thoracic Aorta					
Control Diet	4 ± 2	3 ± 2	217 ± 31	544 ± 39	22 ± 8
Atherogenic Diet, Untreated	82 ± 29*	49 ± 14*	782 ± 183*	912 ± 165*	347 ± 127*
Atherogenic Diet + EHDP	5 ± 2	4 ± 2	307 ± 97	560 ± 26	136 ± 47*
Atherogenic Diet + APDP	6[a]	2[a]	392[a]	612[a]	152[a]
Atherogenic Diet + AHDP	4[a]	3[a]	302[a]	581[a]	113[a]
Atherogenic Diet + $LaCl_3$(40mg)	6 ± 1**	5 ± 1**	388 ± 112*	671 ± 199*	178 ± 83*
Abdominal Aorta					
Control Diet	2 ± 1	1 ± 1	308 ± 46	312 ± 29	10 ± 3
Atherogenic Diet, Untreated	46 ± 18*	34 ± 12*	963 ± 105*	474 ± 102*	457 ± 198*
Atherogenic Diet + EHDP	3 ± 1	3 ± 2	262 ± 88	267 ± 52	122 ± 62*
Atherogenic Diet + APDP	2[a]	1[a]	286[a]	228[a]	83[a]
Atherogenic Diet + AHDP	3[a]	2[a]	273[a]	233[a]	91[a]
Atherogenic Diet + $LaCl_3$(40mg)	2 ± 1	2 ± 1	225 ± 75	242 ± 80	143 ± 71*

*Highly significant changes from control values ($p < 0.02$)

**Signficant changes from controls ($p < 0.05$)

[a]Average values from 4 monkeys

TABLE 4. Constituents of "Elastin" from Control Rabbits and Rabbits on the Atherogenic Diet With and Without Lanthanum

Experimental groups	Total cholesterol	Total calcium	Non-lipid phosphorus	Aspartic acid[1]	Glutamic acid[1]	Lysine[1]	Arginine[1]
Control diet	10.4±2.3	0.8±0.3	0.8±0.07	2.1±0.5	13.5±1.2	4.0±0.2	5.1±0.3
Atherogenic diet without $LaCl_3$	37.4±8.5[2]	2.1±0.7[2]	1.9±0.24[2]	13.1±2.3[2]	31.1±7.6[2]	9.3±1.8[2]	8.9±0.9[2]
Atherogenic diet+ 20 mg $LaCl_3$/Kg B.W.	24.6±9.7[2]	1.5±0.3[3]	0.9±0.11[3]	4.1±0.9[2]	17.0±1.8[2]	3.8±0.3	5.8±0.4[3]
Atherogenic diet + 30 mg $LaCl_3$/Kg B.W.	11.5±1.6	1.2±0.3	0.8±0.13	2.2±0.4	14.6±0.8	3.6±0.6	5.4±0.2
Atherogenic diet + 40 mg $LaCl_3$/Kg B.W.	8.9±2.5	0.7±0.2	0.6±0.29	2.4[4]	12.6[4]	3.9[4]	5.3[4]
Control diet + 40 mg $LaCl_3$/Kg B.W.	8.5±3.7	0.9±0.1	0.5±0.30	2.4±0.3	13.9±0.7	4.2±0.4	5.5±0.3

[1] The remaining elastin amino acids were not significantly different in all groups.

[2] $p < 0.01$ compared to untreated control; [3] $p < 0.05$ compared to untreated control.

[4] Average of 3 elastin samples.

TABLE 5. Constituents of Elastin from Control Monkeys and Monkeys on the Atherogenic Diet With and Without Drugs (μg/g Elastin; Mean ± S.D.)

	CALCIUM				NON-LIPID PHOSPHORUS			
ARTERIES	Control Diet	Athero Diet	Athero & La^{3+}	Athero & EHDP	Control Diet	Athero Diet	Athero & La^{3+}	Athero & EHDP
Thorac. Aorta	3.6 ± 0.3	97.1 ± 21.3*	5.9 ± 0.4*	7.0 ± 0.5*	3.1 ± 1.5	50.7 ± 16.3*	3.5 ± 0.9	3.0 ± 1.1
Abdom. Aorta	2.8 ± 1.1	77.4 ± 19.0*	3.2 ± 1.3	4.2 ± 1.6	3.7 ± 1.3	14.0 ± 3.8*	2.2 ± 1.5	3.2 ± 0.8
Subclavian	3.9 ± 0.8	22.9 ± 6.5*	2.0 ± 1.2	5.3 ± 0.6**	2.8 ± 0.7	8.3 ± 2.2*	3.5 ± 1.4	4.5 ± 1.1
Carotid	3.7 ± 1.2	22.5 ± 7.7*	3.8 ± 0.4	5.4 ± 1.2	1.2 ± 0.4	10.2 ± 4.1*	1.2 ± 0.2	1.4 ± 0.3
Iliac	4.3 ± 1.5	16.9 ± 4.9*	3.8 ± 0.5	7.7 ± 2.6	5.3 ± 1.6	11.9 ± 2.6*	3.2 ± 1.7	5.4 ± 1.4
Femoral	2.6 ± 0.7	6.4 ± 1.8*	3.1 ± 0.6	3.9 + 1.3	-----	-----	-----	-----

*Highly significant changes from control values ($p < 0.01$)

**Significant changes from control values ($p < 0.05$)

few intimal foam cells; calcium mineralization also was present, including on deranged elastica (Fig. 4b). By contrast, no visible calcium deposits were detectable in aorta of monkeys on the same atherogenic diet for the same length of time but treated with either the calcium entry blocker lanthanum or any of the diphosphonates. In addition, the accumlations of collagen, the elastica alterations, necroses and cholesterol crystal depositions also were suppressed; the few small residual lesions consisted of a few layers of lipid-filled foam cells (Fig. 4c), giving the lesion the appearance of a mild human fatty streak, especially in monkeys treated with $LaCl_3$ and AHDP. Similar microscopic observations were made in other major systematic arteries, including coronary arteries, of untreated monkeys and monkeys treated with anticalcium agents.

It is of considerable interest in this context that other calcium entry blockers such as, nifedipine[20] and verapamil,[21] which are clinically approved for the treatment of certain other cardiovascular disorders, recently also have been shown to have antiatherogenic properties in rabbits. It is also particularly relevant that Robert, et al.[22] have demonstrated earlier that in rabbits with a certain immunogenic arterial injury, the formation of atherosclerotic connective tissue lesions can be suppressed by daily injections of the hormone thyrocalcitonin which is known to play a pivotal role in calcium homeostasis. Similarly, previous studies by ourselves[23] had shown a marked inhibition of fibrous rabbit atherosclerosis through administration of thiophenocarboxylic acid which is thought to exert a thyrocalcitonin-like effect on maintenance of calcium homeostasis.[24]

D. Mechanism of Atherogenesis Suppression by Anticalcium Agents

Taken together, the evidence from the studies in rabbits and monkeys by ourselves and others led us to formulate the ionic calcium hypothesis which states that: (a) focal increases in arterial calcium ion concentrations may facilitate excessive activation of cellular functions in response to any atherogenic stimuli (Ca^{++} as second mes-

Fig. 4 (a-c) Sections through characteristic lesions of thoracic aorta of monkeys on the fibrogenic atherogenic diet for 24 months without drugs (a,b = sequential sections through the same lesion) or treated simultaneously with AHDP(c). a. Note collagenous plaque capsule (gray) surrounding a necrotic core with cholesterol clefts; the intio-medial elastica (black) is fragmented and deranged; Verhoeff's-Van Gieson, x70. b. Note calcium deposition (black), including on intimo-medial elastica; Yasue's-light green, x70. c. The residual lesion consists of a few layers of (lipid-filled) foam cells in the intima. No connective tissue changes (or calcifications) were detectable in the lesion; Verhoeff's-Van Gieson, x70.

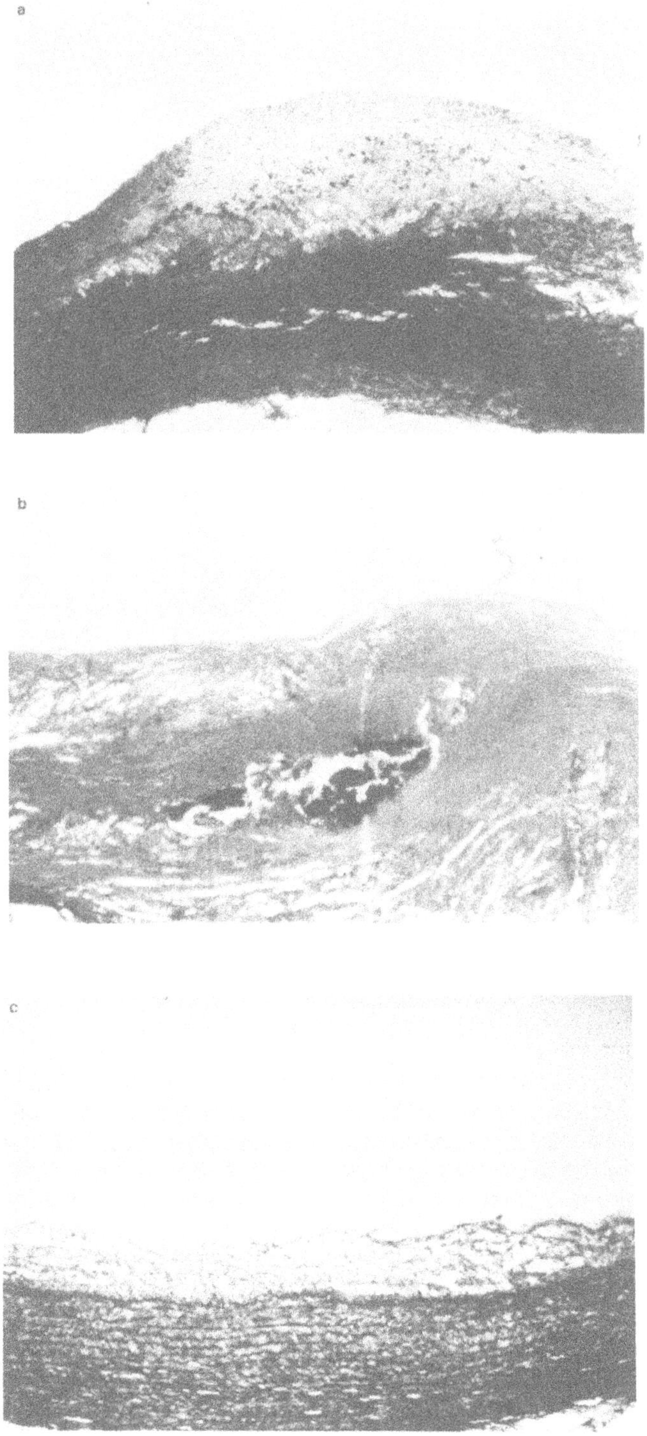
a
b
c

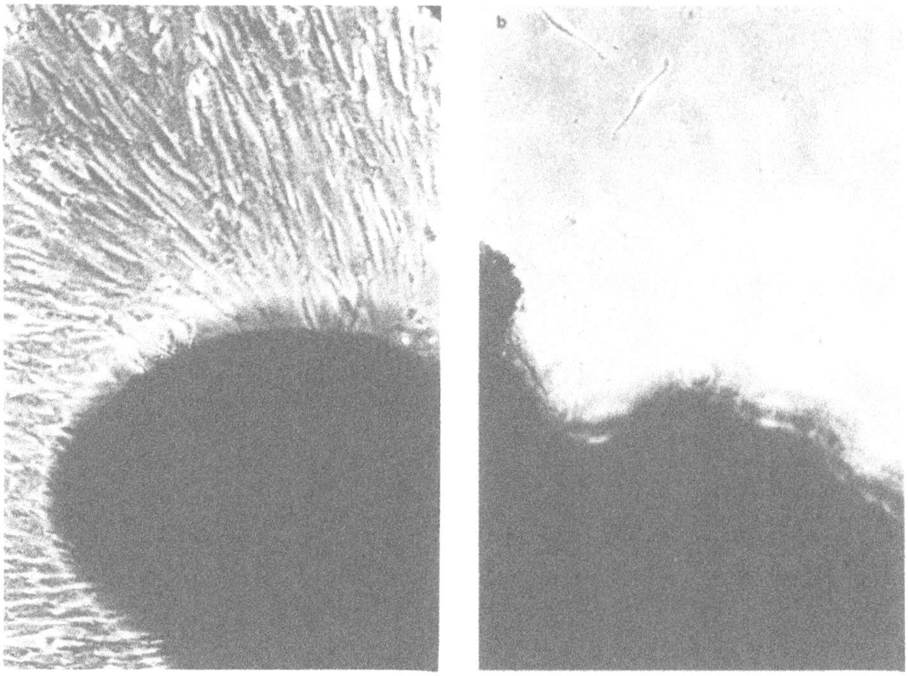

Fig. 5 (a, b) Phase contrast micrographs of smooth muscle cell cultures from aortic explants of normal rabbits fed a normal control diet without (a) and with lanthanum 40 mg per kg bodyweight (b) for 4 weeks; explants (large dark area in each micrograph) in culture for 7 days. a. Note streaming out of smooth muscle-type cells from the aortic explant of an untreated rabbit to form a confluent cell layer, x100. b. Note the paucity of cells grown out of the explants cultured for the same period of time from the aorta of rabbits treated _in vivo_ with lanthanum, x100.

senger); (b) a relative focal abundance of calcium ions in arteries also may facilitate the development of extracellular atherosclerotic abnormalities involving the connective tissue; and (c) the effects of a variety of calcium antagonists in the broad sense of the word support the concept that excessively available arterial calcium ions may play a key role in atherogenesis and that maintenance of calcium homeostasis at the arterial tissue level may be pivotal in prevention of the disorder by reducing the abundance of ionic calcium.

It noteworthy that there is experimental evidence for the direct effect of calcium entry blockers on some of the basic processes of atherogenesis. Our laboratory has treated 4 normal rabbits on control diet with 40 mg lanthanum per kg bodyweight for 4 weeks at the end of which period several aortic explants were taken from each rabbit for cultures of arterial smooth muscle cells. These cultures then were compared to similarly obtained SMC cultures from 4 untreated control rabbits. Aortic explants from untreated normal rabbits after 7 days in culture revealved normal outgrowth of SMCs (Fig. 5a). In contrast, explants from aortas of normal rabbits pretreated in vivo with lanthanum revealed a marked retardation of the cellular outgrowth at day 7 (Fig. 5b), with the slower cell growth persisting even until day 4 of the second passage. These results indicate that the calcium antagonists may affect in vivo arterial smooth muscle cell migration or mitosis or presumably both.

In another experiment (Table 6) we added lanthanum (La^{3+}) in increasing concentrations to confluent cultures of arterial SMCs from 3 untreated normal rabbits. The cultures then were pulse labeled with ^{14}C-proline and the appearance of the radiolabel was measured in the hydroxyproline fraction as an indicator of collagen biosynthesis and secretion. As indicated by the increasing reduction of the hydroxyproline radioactivity in the incubation media, increasing doses of the calcium entry blocker caused increasing inhibition of collagen secretion from the cells into the media. On the other hand, as indicated by the unchanged normal hydroxyproline radioactivity at all dosage levels in the washed cell layers, collagen synthesis in the cells appeared to be unaffected by the La^{3+} exposure. It is of interest that studies by others[25] have demonstrated that diphosphonates also inhibit secretion of collagen from collagen producing cells in vitro. These in vitro studies suggest that suppression of excessive secretion of connective tissue macromolecules by arterial SMCs may be one of the prominent beneficial effects of all calcium antagonists, supporting the in vivo treatment results with a variety of these anticalcium agents in animals with developing atherosclerosis.

REVERSAL OF PRE-ESTABLISHED FIBROUS ATHEROMATOUS PLAQUES BY ANTICALCIUM DRUGS

While a preventive effect of calcium antagonists on the development of atherosclerosis may not seem too surprising, the critical question remains as to whether these agents are capable of promoting reversal of the established disease. In some recent experiments our laboratory was able to shed some light on this question.

A. Experiment

Five groups of 10 male white New Zealand rabbits were studied for 16 weeks; one group on the control diet of Purina Rabbit Chow for the entire period and 4 groups on the fibrogenic atherogenic diet (described above for induction of atherosclerosis) for 8 weeks after

TABLE 6. Effect of Lanthanum (La^{3+}) on Collagen and Total Protein Synthesis and Secretion by Arterial SMCs (cpm x 10^4/mg N; averages of cultures from 3 rabbits)

La^{3+} Concentration in media (nMol)	Proline	OH-Proline	Inhibition (OH-Proline)	Ratio Proline/OH-Proline
		A. Incubation Media		
None	14.4	7.4	0%	2.0
0.001	9.4	4.1	-45%	2.3
0.010	5.5	2.7	-64%	2.1
0.100	4.1	1.6	-78%	2.5
		B. Cell Layer		
None	28.0	5.5	--	5.1
0.001	27.6	4.5	--	6.2
0.010	29.8	5.6	--	5.3
0.100	32.8	4.8	--	6.8

which time all 4 groups were again placed on the control diet for another 8 weeks. After cessation of the atherogenic diet, one of these 4 groups received the control diet alone while the remaining 3 groups were fed the control diet with addition of (40 mg/kg bodyweight) the diphosphonates APDP and AHDP as well as the calcium entry blocker lanthanum. These 5 groups of rabbits studied for 16 weeks were compared to one additional group of 10 rabbits which received the atherogenic diet without drug treatment for 8 weeks only (induction of atherosclerosis, atherogenic control group).

B. Biochemical Findings

In all animals on the atherogenic diet the concentrations of total serum cholesterol rose to about the same levels as described above under "Prevention of Fibrous-Atheromatous Plaques" (~2,500-3,000 mg/dl); and the serum cholesterol concentrations fell to normal control levels after cessation of the atherogenic diet.

As compared to animals receiving the control diet for the entire experimental period, rabbits on the atherogenic diet for 8 weeks and then sacrificed showed the usual marked increases in aortic collagen, elastin, cholesterol, calcium and phosphorus (Table 7, compare Table 2). After cessation of the atherogenic diet without drug treatment (Table 7), there were further substantial increases in these aortic components which is the general experience in rabbits and other animals. Treatment with APDP after the induction diet was stopped resulted in the prevention of further increases of the atherosclerotic parameters measured, indicating that APDP had an arresting effect on further progression of atherosclerosis (Table 7). In marked contrast, treatment with AHDP or lanthanum, after cessation of atherosclerosis induction resulted in complete normalization of the aortic content in collagen, elastin and phosphorus while the content in cholesterol and especially calcium were greatly reduced from atherogenic levels, albeit not to normal (Table 7). These findings suggest that both, AHDP and lanthanum, are capable of removing induced arterial calcification in addition to reversing fibrosis.

Changes in the composition of arterial elastin followed similar trends as those for atherosclerosis involvement in the experimental groups (Table 8). As compared to normal controls, elastin of rabbits receiving the atherogenic diet alone for 8 weeks showed the usual increases in calcium, phosphorus and cholesterol which still further increased after an 8-week cessation period of that diet without drug treatment. However, these additional increases were halted at atherosclerosis induction levels by treatment with APDP. In marked contrast, treatment with AHDP or lanthanum reduced the elastin content of phosphorus to normal and that of calcium to near normal levels. Likewise, the elastin cholesterol content was greatly reduced in AHDP-treated animals and was normal in the lanthanum group. The re-

TABLE 7. Components of Aortic Intima-Media from Control Rabbits and Rabbits on the Atherogenic Diet for 8 Weeks Followed by 8 Weeks on the Control Diet With and Without Drugs

Experimental Drugs	Collagen	Elastin	Cholesterol	Calcium	Phosphorus
Control Diet (16 weeks)	4.1 ± 0.8	15.6 ± 1.4	0.6 ± 0.2	0.01 ± 0.007	0.07 ± 0.03
Atherogenic Diet (8 weeks)	6.2 ± 0.7*	21.4 ± 1.6*	4.6 ± 0.9*	0.06 ± 0.013*	0.14 ± 0.03*
Atherogenic Diet followed by Control Diet without Drugs	7.5 ± 1.0*	27.5 ± 3.0*	4.8 ± 1.8*	0.10 ± 0.018*	0.26 ± 0.06*
Atherogenic Diet followed by Control Diet + APDP	5.6 ± 0.9**	19.4 ± 1.2**	5.3 ± 3.3*	0.07 ± 0.016*	0.11 ± 0.04**
Atherogenic Diet followed by Control Diet + AHDP	3.6 ± 1.2	15.1 ± 1.8	2.5 ± 1.5*	0.02 ± 0.010**	0.06 ± 0.03
Atherogenic Diet followed by Contro. Diet + LaCl3	4.2 ± 1.5	15.6 ± 2.4	1.5 ± 1.00**	0.03 ± 0.018**	0.07 ± 0.04

*Highly significant changes from control values ($p < 0.01$)

**Significant changes from control values ($p < 0.05$)

TABLE 8. Constituents of Elastin from Aortic Intima-Media of Control Rabbits and Rabbits on the Atherogenic Diet for 8 Weeks Followed by 8 Weeks on the Control Diet With and Without Drugs

Experimental Groups	Calcium	Non-Lipid Phosphorus	Total Cholesterol	% Ester Cholesterol
Control Diet (16 weeks)	0.6 ± 0.03	0.8 ± 0.07	10.4 ± 2.3	41 ± 9
Atherogenic Diet (8 weeks)	2.1 ± 0.73*	1.9 ± 0.40*	34.6 ± 6.6*	81 ± 3*
Atherogenic Diet followed by Control Diet Without Drugs	2.9 ± 0.50*	2.3 ± 0.44*	42.7 ± 8.2*	85 ± 7*
Atherogenic Diet followed by Control Diet + APDP	1.7 ± 0.68*	1.1 ± 0.06*	36.7 ± 13.2*	78 ± 9**
Atherogenic Diet followed by Control Diet & AHDP	0.8 ± 0.04**	0.7 ± 0.25	16.7 ± 6.1**	56 ± 8**
Atherogenic Diet followed by Control Diet + LaCl3	1.1 ± 0.05**	0.9 ± 0.32	14.2 ± 8.3	67 ± 9*

*Highly significant changes from control values ($p < 0.01$)

**Significant changes from control values ($p < 0.05$)

sults indicate that the elastin abnormalities also can be reversed by treatment with calcium antagonists.

C. Morphological Findings

Again, the biochemical results were in agreement with the morphological findings. Characteristic lesions of thoracic aorta after cessation of the atherosclerosis induction diet with and without drug treatment are shown in Figure 6a-c. Typically, after cessation of the atherogenic diet without drug treatment, the pre-established lesions became even more fibrotic with dense collagenous tissue in the markedly raised intima which contained essentially no foam cells; the derangement and fragmentation of the intio-medial elastica became even more pronounced (Fig. 6a, compare Fig. 3a) and, in addition, even more extensive deposition of calcium minerals were seen, especially on the severely deranged elastica (Fig. 6b, compare Fig. 3b). In marked contrast, when the animals were treated with either AHDP or lanthanum during the "regression" period, only small lesions were seen characterized by absence of collagen accumulations, repair of the intimo-medial elastica and a moderate number of intimal foam cells remaining as the only abnormality together with some minor residual calcium mineral depositions (barely visible) on the largely intact elastica (Fig. 6c).

D. Mechanism of Lesion Reversal by Anticalcium Agents

The precise mechanisms by which the diphosphonate AHDP and the calcium entry blocker lanthanum cause reversal of pre-existing calcific fibrous atherosclerosis is less clear than the mechanisms by

Fig. 6 (a-c) Sections through characteristic lesions of thoracic aorta of rabbits on the fibrogenic atherogenic diet for 8 weeks followed by 8 more weeks on the control diet without drugs (a,b = sequential sections of the same lesion) or treated simultaneously with lanthanum (c). a. Note dense accumulations of collagen (gray) in the markedly-raised intima, the extensively fragmented and deranged intimo-medial elastica (black) as well as the absence of lipid-filled foam cells; this transformation into even more fibrous plaques is typical of atherosclerotic lesions of untreated rabbits after cessation of the atherogenic diet (compare Fig. 3a), Verhoeff's-Van Gieson, x85. b. Note marked deposition of calcium (dark gray-black) on deranged elastica; Alizarin red-light green, x85. c. Note that the lesion is composed of a few layers of lipid-rich foam cells in the intima overlying an essentially normal arterial wall with absence of calcium and collagen accumulations and essentially normal elastica; Yasue's-light green, x70.

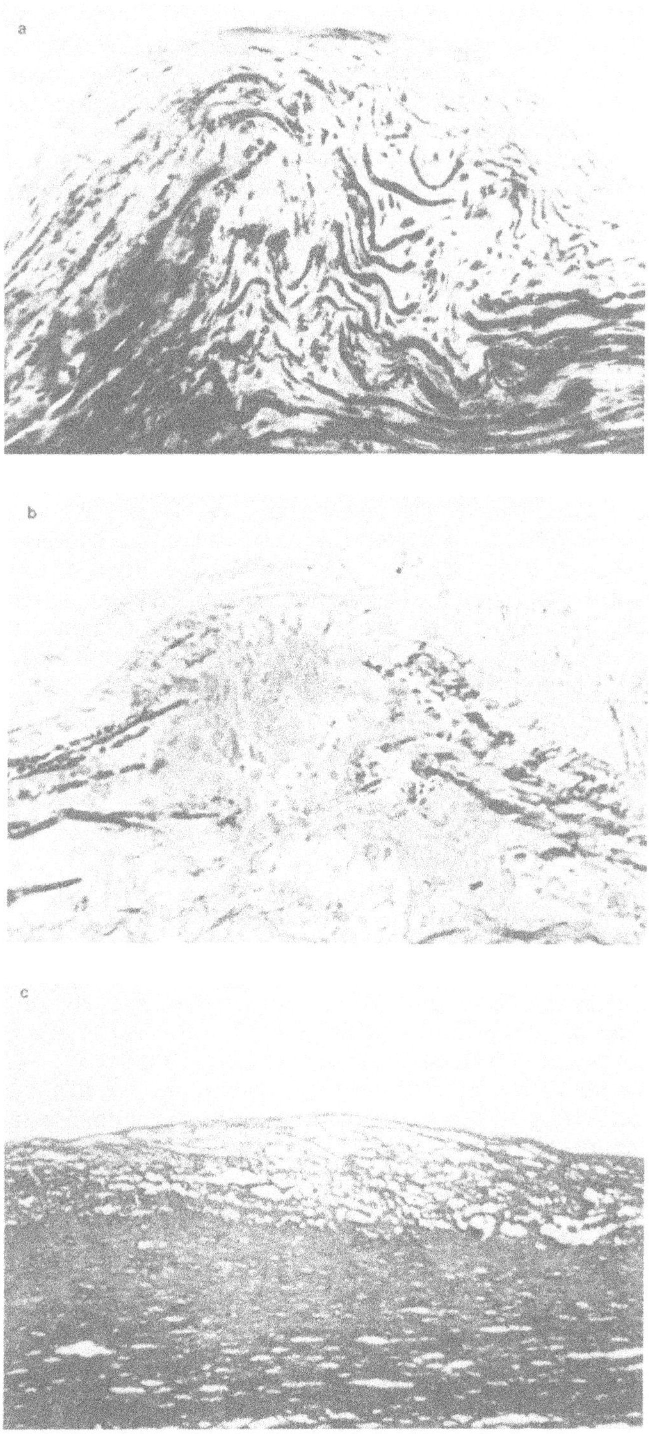

which they may operate to cause its prevention. It is possible that once the further progression of atherosclerotic lesions is arrested, the regular catabolic processes of the organism are capable of slowly restituting the diseased arterial tissue, including reversing tissue calcification. It should be recalled in this context that lanthanum is known to actually displace tissue bound calcium[13,14] as well as, like the diphosphonates,[9-11] to prevent new calcium from being bound to receptor sites.

CONCLUSION

From the results of these studies by ourselves and other workers, it is concluded that calcium antagonists capable of regulating functional calcium levels in arteries may be suitable therapeutic agents for the prevention, arrest and even reversal of the most important and most life-threatening aspect of human atherosclerosis: the calcified fibrous plaque. These agents may be useful as adjunct treatment to the treatment of atherosclerotic arterial disease with lipid-lowering drugs, or they may even be useful for such treatment by themselves as single entities. It should be emphasized again that these agents appear to exert their beneficial effects without altering unfavorable serum lipid and lipoprotein concentrations and patterns as are presumably present in most Western populations.

ACKNOWLEDGMENTS

Supported by U.S. Public Health Service Grants HL 15512 and HL 13262.

REFERENCES

1. National Heart, Lung and Blood Institute Task Force on Atherosclerosis, DHEW Publ. (NIH), 1:72-137 (1971).
2. T. B. Clarkson, Personal communication (1983).
3. J. F. Mustard, M. A. Packham, S. Moore, R. L. Kinlough-Rathbone, Thrombosis and Atherosclerosis, in: "Atherosclerosis III," G. Schettler and A. Weizel, eds., Springer-Verlag, Berlin, pp. 253-267 (1974).
4. Report from the Committee of Principal Investigators, A cooperative trial in the primary prevention of ischemic heart disease using clofibrate. Br. Heart J. 10:1069-1118 (1978).
5. The Lipid Research Clinics Coronary Primary Prevention Trial Results. I. Reduction in incidence of coronary heart disease, JAMA 251:351-364 (1984).
6. The Lipid Research Clinics Coronary Primary Prevention Trial Results. II. The relationship of the reduction in incidence of coronary heart disease to cholesterol lowering, JAMA 251: 374-375 (1984).

7. D. M. Kramsch, A. J. Aspen, and C. S. Apstein, Suppression of experimental atherosclerosis by the Ca^{++}-antagonist lanthanum, Possible role of calcium in atherogenesis, J. Clin. Invest. 65:967-981 (1980).
8. D. M. Kramsch, A. J. Aspen, and L. J. Rozler, Atherosclerosis: Prevention by agents not affecting abnormal levels of blood lipids, Science 213:1511-1512 (1981).
9. H. Fleisch, R. G. G. Russel, S. Bisaz, R. C. Muehlbauer, and D. A. Williams, The inhibitory effect of diphosphonates on the formation of calcium phosphate crystals in vitro and on aortic and kidney calcification in vivo, Europ. J. Clin. Invest. 1: 12-18 (1970).
10. I. Y. Rosenblum, L. Flora, and R. Eisenstein, The effect of sodium ethane-1-hydroxy-1,1-diphosponate (EHDP) on a rabbit model of arterio-atherosclerosis, Atherosclerosis 11:411-421 (1975).
11. W. D. Wagner and T. B. Clarkson, Slowly miscible cholesterol pools in progressing and regressing atherosclerotic aortas, Proc. Soc. Exp. Biol. Med. 143:804-809 (1973).
12. M. Potocar and M. Schmidt-Dunker, The effect of new diphosphonic acids on aortic and kidney calcifications in vivo, Atherosclerosis 30:313-320 (1978).
13. G. B. Weiss, Cellular pharmacology of lanthanum, in: "Annual Review of Pharmacology," H. W. Elliot, R. Okun, and R. George, eds., Annual Reviews, Palo Alto, 14:343-354 (1974).
14. G. B. Weiss and F. R. Goodman, Distribution of lanthanide (^{174}Pm) in vascular smooth muscle, J. Pharmacol. Ther. 198: 366-374 (1976).
15. D. M. Kramsch, A. J. Aspen, and A. C. Swindell, Trimazosin suppresses fibrosis of atherosclerosis plaques, Fed. Proc. 42:808 (1983).
16. D. Kritchevsky, S. A. Tepper, D. Vesselinovitch, and R. W. Wissler, Cholesterol vehicle in experimental atherosclerosis. Part II (peanut oil), Atherosclerosis 14:53-64 (1971).
17. D. M. Kramsch, W. Hollander, and S. Renaud, Induction of fibrous plaques vs. foam cell lesions in Macaca fascicularis by varying the composition of dietary fats, Circulation 48 (suppl. IV):41 (1973).
18. D. M. Kramsch, Biochemical changes of the arterial wall in atherosclerosis with special reference to connective tissue: Promising experimental avenues for their prevention, in: "Connective Tissue in Arterial and Pulmonary Disease," T. F. McDonald and A. B. Chandler, eds., Springer-Verlag, New York, pp. 95-151 (1981).
19. D. M. Kramsch, A. J. Aspen, B. M. Abramowitz, T. Kreimendahl, and W. B. Hood, Jr., Reduction of coronary atherosclerosis by moderate conditioning exercise in monkeys on an atherogenic diet, N. Engl. J. Med. 305:1483-1489 (1981).
20. P. D. Henry and K. I. Bentley, Suppression of atherogenesis in cholesterol-fed rabbits treated with nifedipine, J. Clin. Invest. 68:1366-1369 (1981).

21. J. L. Rouleu, W. W. Parmley, J. Stevens, J. Wilkman-Coffelt, R. Sievers, R. Mahley, and R. J. Havel, Verapamil suppresses atherosclerosis in cholesterol-fed rabbits, Amer. J. Cardiol. 49:889 (1982).
22. A. M. Robert, M. Moczar, D. Brechemier, G. Godeau, M. Miskulin, and L. Robert, Biosynthesis and degradation of matrix molecules of the arterial wall, Regulation by drug action, in: "International Symposium, State of Prevention and Therapy in Human Atherosclerosis and in Animal Models," W. H. Hauss, R. W. Wissler, and R. Lehmann, eds., Westdeutscher Verlag, Opladen, Germany, Abh. Rhein.-Westf. Akad. Wiss. 3:301-312 (1978).
23. C. T. Chan, H. Wells, and D. M. Kramsch, Suppression of fibrous-fatty plaque formation in rabbits by agents not affecting elevated serum cholesterol levels, The effect of thiophene compounds, Circ. Res. 43:115-125 (1978).
24. W. Lloyd, W. S. Fang, H. Wells, and A. H. Tashjan, 2-Thiophene carboxylic acid, A hypocalcemic, antilipolytic agent with hypocalcemic and hypophosphatemic effects in rats, Endocrinology 85:763-768 (1969).
25. C. Minkin, L. Rabadjia, and P. Goldhaber, Bone remodeling in vitro: The effects of diphosphonates on osteoid synthesis, Calcif. Tissue Res. 14:161-168 (1974).

MANAGEMENT OF ADHERENCE TO PRESCRIBED MEDICATION

William Insull, Jr.

Director, Lipid Research Clinic
Baylor College of Medicine, The Methodist Hospital
Houston, Texas 77030

"A pharmacologically effective drug may be a clinical failure because of patient nonadherence."

This paper will review the current status of our knowledge of adherence for treating lipid metabolism and will describe a comprehensive program for adherence management in small and large clinical trials adaptable to clinical practice. Our clinic has had experience with many parts of this program and has demonstrated its effectiveness.

Adherence is defined as the extent to which a person's behavior in terms of taking medication, following diets, or executing life-style changes, coincides with medical or health advice.[1] The organization of adherence into two spheres of behavior is useful for planning adherence programs, participation in prescribed clinical examinations and tests, and taking the prescribed treatment. The term adherence is preferred to the term compliance because of the latter's connotation of coercion, while the former indicates the result of free choice. Persons adhering to some selected level less than the full prescription are referred to as nonadherers. Individuals who are unable to return to the clinic and the scheduled visits are usually referred to as dropouts.

THE ADHERENCE PROBLEM

Nonadherence is a problem common to every prescribed medical treatment. While nonadherence has been recognized as a problem for many years, only since 1970 has it been systematically studied and

TABLE 1

NONADHERENCE TO PRESCRIPTIONS

Prescription	% Adherence
Short-term medication	78
Long-term medication:	
for treatment or cure	41-69
for prevention 33-69	
over one to three years	94-34
Short-term for prevention	62
Appointment keeping:	
for prevention 10-65	
for management or cure	55-84

Adapted from Sackett and Snow

methods of managing it developed. Sackett has demonstrated the wide occurrence of nonadherence and its serious implications for effective medical treatment. Serious nonadherence occurred in every prescription situation: short-term medication, long-term medication, short-term prevention, long-term prevention, and appointment keeping (See Table 1).[2]

As seen in the selected examples on Table 2, adherence is a problem in recent trials of lipid therapy for coronary heart disease trials. Small trials of efficacy and safety by Hunninghake and his collaborators experienced adherence of 92% to 95% for the active drug and comparable values for the placebo.[3] Large scale clinical trials have reported somewhat lower adherence, as in the WHO clofibrate trial (86%) and the Coronary Drug Project (approximately 85% for clofibrate, 73% for niacin and 86% for the placebo).[4] The Aspirin Myocardial Infarction Study showed 85! adherence for aspirin and 78% for placebo when assayed by three independent measures.[5] In these trials the mean adherence values cited resulted when a significant proportion of the patients took less than 80% of the drug. In the Coronary Drug Project 43% of the niacin patients, 28% of the clofibrate patients, and 26% of the placebo patients were in this category.

PURPOSE OF ADHERENCE MANAGEMENT

Important benefits result from successfully managing adherence.

TABLE 2

ADHERENCE IN RECENT LIPID-CHD TRIALS

Drug	Adherence Mean %	Assay	Study
Colestipol	90	CC	DBH[1] 1981
Clofibrate	95	CC	DBH[1] 1981
Clofibrate	86(85-95)	U	WHO 1978
Clofibrate	85	CC	CDP 1975
Niacin	73	CC	CDP 1975
Placebo	90	CC	DBH[1] 1981
Placebo	86	CC	CDP 1975
Placebo	78	CC,U,P	AMIS[2] 1982
Aspirin	81	CC,U,P	AMIS[2] 1982

CC - Capsule count, U - Urinalysis, P - Plasma
[1] - Hunninghake, [2] - Mattson

These benefits include the following:

1. Reduces sample size requirements.
2. Fulfills requirements for the trial's statistically significant outcome.
3. Assures testing effective dose of medication.
4. Avoids the costs of noncontributing participants.
5. Distinguishes biologic nonresponders from nonadherers.
6. Defines the adherence of the placebo group so that the effects of the test drug on adherence may be evaluated.

A common adherence goal is 80% of the prescribed dose. However, adherence at this level may significantly impair the therapeutic effectiveness of the drug, depending upon its pharmacologic properties. Impaired effectiveness can be demonstrated when the adherence to every prescribed dose is evaluated. Detailed observations of adherence are difficult to obtain but may provide important insight into the effect of an 80% level of adherence upon the effectiveness of the drug.

Figures 1 - 3 demonstrate different patterns of adherence observed at around 80% mean adherence.[6] These observations are from a study of patients with stable rheumatoid arthritis taking twelve tablets of medication every day for 180 days.

With drugs having short biological halflives, these different patterns of nonadherence could have different pharmacological effects. To reduce variabilities in studies, it is obviously desirable to have high adherence.

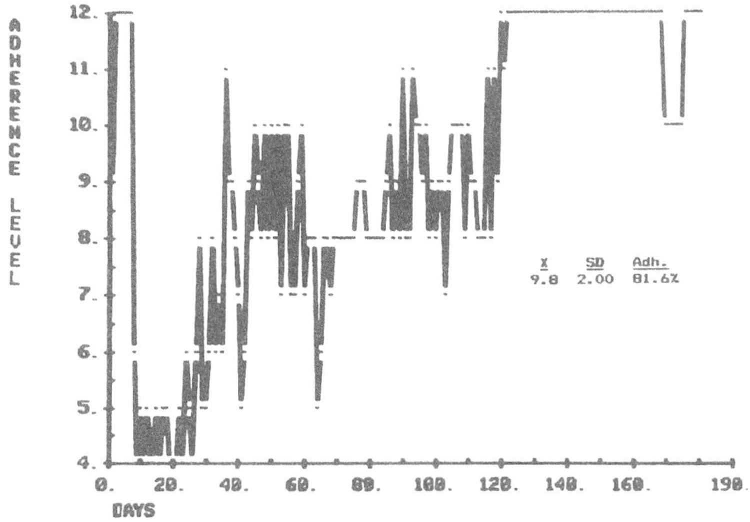

Figure 1: Patient 89 with a mean adherence of 81% or 9.8 tablets took 2/3 of the prescribed dose for approximately 1/3 of the study, 66% to 80% for a third of the study, and 100% of the prescribed dose for a third.

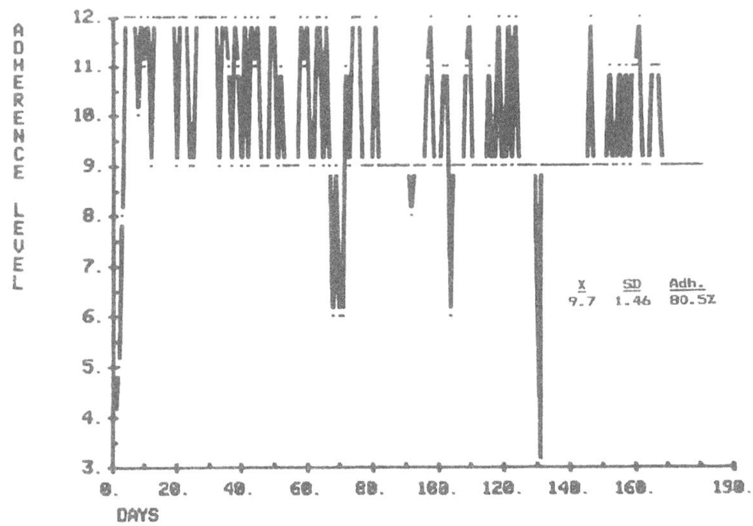

Figure 2: Patient 130 oscillated between 75% and 100% of the prescribed dose for 98% of the time.

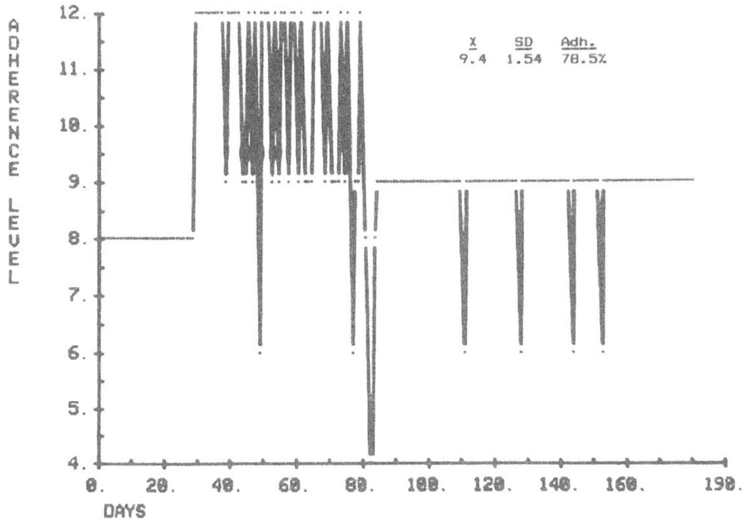

Figure 3: Patient 61 took between 75% and 100% for 1/3 of the time and approximately 75% of the dose for the remainder.

Over the past seven years, significant technologies for adherence management have been developed. However, because these technologies remained largely isolated from each other, a comprehensive program of adherence management did not evolve. Many recent large trials were initiated before nonadherence was fully described and before management techniques were developed. Adherence problems frequently appeared early in the trials, and pragmatic solutions had to be rapidly developed. Now, however, a comprehensive program for adherence management is possible. The adherence program described here is based on experiences from a number of trials and on a program of methods development undertaken in our clinic and laboratory in the last five years.

CONCEPT OF THE ADHERENCE PROBLEM

The construction of an adherence program is greatly aided by a general concept of the adherence problem. The psychological models for adherence are a matter of continued debate, as none has proven totally satisfactory.[7,8]

Table 3 summarizes the pragmatic concept that we developed on adherence to prescribed therapy. Our concept is based on analysis of the factors within the patient and the therapist which control the interaction and collaboration between them to yield adherence. The patient's risk factors for adherence include his medical knowl-

TABLE 3

CONCEPT OF ADHERENCE TO PRESCRIBED THERAPY BASED ON RISK FACTORS FOR THERAPIST AND PATIENT

THERAPIST

- Interviewing and counseling skills, possession and use

INTERACTION AND COLLABORATION → PATIENT ADHERENCE

PATIENT

- Medical knowledge
- Acceptance of diagnosis
- Habit ability
- Adherence experience
- Self debate
- Social milieu
- Job milieu
- Economic status

edge, acceptance of the medical diagnosis, capability of habit formation, his previous adherence experience, and the occurrence of chronic self debate over taking the medication.[9] The factors in the therapist are his skills needed for quality interviewing and counseling, the number of these skills possessed, and the appropriateness of their use. Achievement of adherence depends upon the clinical interaction between the patient and the therapist. Each patient presents an individually unique combination of risk factors for adherence. Adherence management requires individualized guidance and counseling for each patient in a series of counseling sessions with a one-to-one relationship between the patient and the therapist. The elements of the adherence program can be related to this conceptual framework in a practical operational sequence.

A PROGRAM FOR ADHERENCE MANAGEMENT

The comprehensive and integrated program for management of adherence consists of five major parts. From the viewpoint of administering this program, all elements are tangible and can be measured for documentation. Quality control of the program can be rational and evaluated by quantitative measures. Most elements of the program can be self monitored by the clinic staff, making practical immediate, internal quality control. These elements include: (1) Training the staff for medication adherence counseling; (2) Selecting participants by their potential for desired level of adherence; (3) Monitoring adherence objectively; (4) Managing adherence by providing participants with instructions, adherence aids, and counseling; (5) Preventing and managing nonadherers and dropouts.

Training the staff for medication adherence counseling includes three major parts. First, evaluate staff skills before and after training. Russell et al. have identified twenty-eight interviewing and counseling skills fundamental to quality counseling which can be documented objectively by review of videotaped interviews of simulated participants.[10] After acquisition and appropriate use of these twenty-eight skills, further training can be provided for advanced skills. The formal training is undertaken by didactic instruction, role playing, and critique of actual clinical interviews. Crucial aspects of staff training are to monitor the staff's counseling and to provide further training as needed. These training procedures and documentation techniques have been successfully applied in a multi-center trial to one hundred clinic staff members with various professional qualifications. These include physicians, physician assistants, nurses, registered dietitians, psychologists with master's level training, and individuals with various levels of college education.[11]

The second element is to select trial participants by their potential for desired adherence. Candidates for clinical trials are evaluated for adherence risk factors during screening: their medical knowledge, their acceptance of their medical diagnosis, the characteristics of their social and job milieu, their economic status, their capability of habit formation, their previous adherence experience, and the occurrence of chronic self debate over medication taking. Self-administered questionnaires and interviews to determine these factors are under development and are currently being tested. The risk level for nonadherence is estimated from this information. Recruitment excludes candidates whose risk level of nonadherence misses the adherence goals of the trial. The program identifies for each accepted participant the potential risk factors for nonadherence.

The third major element of the program is to monitor adherence. Adherence is measured objectively by several quick measures at regular interviews. The program promptly collates and analyzes the adherence data by computer. It identifies adherence trends of the entire treatment cohort and identifies adherence problems of individual participants by regular frequent listing of nonadherers, zero adherers, delinquents and dropouts.

Current knowledge of adherence monitoring procedures[12] includes four general types of procedures. (1) Direct measurement is done in blood, urine, saliva, or breath for the drug under study, its metabolites, physiological effects or presence of a marker co-administered with the drug. (2) Medication measurements may be undertaken by pill counting or use of a pill counting device by the participant. A recent development is a carefully labeled and cataloged blister pack which is dispensed and, after use, returned for analysis. (3) The records of filling the prescription are used. (4) Objective reports by the clinician and the patient can be used. Other techniques include direct observation of medication ingestion and evaluation of therapeutic outcome.

These various measures may be used together for evaluating consistency. The techniques most commonly used are measurement of the drug and its metabolites, pill counts, and the patient's subjective report. The most desirable technique is direct measurement. Although adherence markers are not generally available, the recent national workshop concluded that a number of substances appeared to be feasible as potential markers.

The fourth major element of the program is to manage adherence by providing participants with instructions, adherence aids, and counseling. The program should instruct all participants about the treatment rationale and study procedures by means of letters, brochures, individual conferences, group presentations, and video cassette programs in the clinic waiting room.[13,14]

The fifth element is to prevent and manage nonadherence. Procedures include maintaining efficient clinic operation for the participant, minimizing unwarranted waiting during the clinic appointment, facilitating rapid examination, and making the clinic convenient by hours and parking. Strategies are developed for groups of nonadherers who share common characteristics. The program must guide the management of individual nonadhering by case conference and by appropriate health behavior. The recovery of all dropouts and nonadherers must be attempted by specific steps.

The process of health behavior counseling consists of eight steps which require collaboration between the counselor and the patient during a series of separate counseling sessions. These steps include identifying the health behavior counseling problem, the nonadherence. The participant systematically observes his behavior. The patient and the counselor detect specific behavioral patterns, assemble a behavior profile, and analyze the influence of the social and physical environment; this procedure is a functional analysis. They then generate possible solutions. They select and implement a solution. Finally, they review the effects of the solution and revise it as needed. Collaboration between the counselor and the patient is essential for the success of these procedures. These techniques as developed by psychologists are commonly referred to as behavior modification but are most appropriately designated as applied analysis of behavior,[15] or a functional analysis.[16] These

TABLE 4

SEQUENCE OF PROCEDURES FOR DROPOUT RECOVERY#

1. Reassign dropout to physician
2. Establish and maintain contact
3. *Achieve clinic attendance
4. Obtain physical and lab data
5. Obtain medication information
6. Discuss general health problems
7. Facilitate solution for health problems
8. Obtain diet information (Trial Protocol)
9. Obtain information about study medication-taking
10. *Solve adherence problems
11. Reinstitute the study medication
12. Reintroduce the participant to adherence counseling
13. Continue problem solving and reinforce achievement

#After Probstfield et al. 1980.
*Activities producing participant resistance.

procedures of analyses, their subsequent adjustments and revisions as applied to adherence are currently undergoing significant development and refinement.

A dropout recovery program is an important element of the adherence management program. While the general opinion is that dropouts cannot be recovered to treatment, our experience has demonstrated that dropouts can be recovered and successfully re-entered into the full therapeutic regimen. The recovery program has six goals: to maintain contact with the participant, to stress the importance of the protocol completion by every participant, to convey the trial staff's genuine concern about each participant's health, to reinstate trial procedures using behavioral techniques, to emphasize the contribution made by any degree of adherence, and to reinstitute the intervention. These goals can be achieved by a sequence of certain procedures.[17] (See Table 4.)

RESULTS AND COST OF ADHERENCE MANAGEMENT

Our experience with this program has demonstrated its effectiveness on dropouts in a variety of trials of drug and diet therapy:

1. Stable mean adherence to drug and a dropout level of 1% for a cohort of 290 men for 56 consecutive months, when expecting decreasing adherence and increasing dropouts.

TABLE 5

ESTIMATED RELATIVE RISK OF NONADHERENCE FOR DRUGS AFFECTING LIPID METABOLISM

Risk	Drug	Daily Dose
Low	Dextrothyroxine	1-2 tab (4-8 mg)
	Norethindrone	1/2 - 2 tab (2.5-10 mg)
Medium	Clofibrate	2 cap 0.5 bid (2.0)
	Gemfibrozil	2 cap 0.3 bid (1.2)
	Probucol	2 tab 0.25 bid (1.0)
	Compactin	1 tab 0.03 tid (0.09)
	Nicotinic acid	4-16 tab 0.05 (2-8)
High	Cholestyramine	3-6 pkg 4.0 (12-24)
	Colestipol	3-6 pkg 5.0 (15-30)

2. Ninety percent recovery of thirty-six dropouts, absent for 10 months to four years, with low recidivism, and 70% re-establishing medication adherence.

3. Eighty-four percent of a cohort of seventy-five completed a dietary study of seven phases and nine months duration.

4. Ninety-six percent of a cohort of thirty completed a fifteen-week Phase II drug trial.

The cost of a comprehensive adherence program is about 10% of the total cost of the customary clinical trial. However, an effective program may reduce trial costs, largely by reducing the number of patients needed, the sample size, so that the net cost of the trial is reduced. The costs vary, largely depending upon the number and kind of objective tests of adherence performed. It is desirable to have at least two tests to evaluate adherence at different stages of the adherence process, e.g., pill counts and plasma levels of the drug.

ROLE OF THERAPEUTIC REGIMEN IN ADHERENCE

The nature of the therapeutic regimen can also influence adherence. By consideration of the dosing schedule, the procedures for administration, and the objective side effects, the relative risk of nonadherence among drugs can be estimated. These important factors must be considered in estimating the risks of nonadherence for any new medication.

For drugs affecting lipid metabolism, the relative risk of nonadherence was estimated by consideration of their risk factors for adherence (Table 5). Each drug was rated by four criteria: 1) the number of doses per day, 2) the number of tablets per dose per day, 3) the need for contemporary preparation of each dose, 4) the incidence and immediacy of subjective side effects. The lowest risk of nonadherence occurred with dextrothyroxine and the highest risk with the nicotinic acid and bile acid binding resins. Other agents had intermediate relative risks. The clinician's choice in prescribing lipid-lowering agents may be influenced significantly by consideration of these adherence risk factors. This complex of adherence factors must be considered by the pharmaceutical industry in the design, selection, and formulation of therapeutic agents if they are to be effective in clinical practice.

SUMMARY

Nonadherence is a major problem for long-term use of drugs affecting lipid metabolism. Effective programs for comprehensive management of aherence are available. Their administration and operation can be readily integrated within the usual operations of both large and small clinical trials. The programs are subject to quality control and, hence, can be administered effectively. The cost of a comprehensive adherence program is approximately 10% of the conventional cost of clinical trials, varies according to the nature and number of adherence tests, and is probably totally recovered through resultant economies. All of the elements of the adherence program can be adapted to private practice. The relative risks of nonadherence to drugs affecting lipid metabolism are estimated from analyses of four regimen characteristics.

REFERENCES

1. R. B. Haynes, D. W. Taylor, and D. L. Sackett, eds., Compliance in Health Care, The Johns Hopkins University Press, Baltimore, Maryland, xv-xvi (1979).
2. D. L. Sackett and J. C. Snow, The magnitude of compliance and noncompliance, in: "Compliance in Health Care," R. B. Haynes, D. W. Taylor, and D. L. Sackett, eds., The Johns Hopkins University Press, Baltimore, Maryland, pp. 11-22 (1979).
3. D. B. Hunninghake, J. L. Probstfield, L. O. Crow, and S. Isaacson, Effect of colestipol and clofibrate on plasma lipid and lipoproteins in type IIa hyperlipoproteinemia, Metabolism 30:605-609 (1981).
4. M. F. Oliver, J. A. Heady, J. N. Morris, and J. Cooper, A cooperative trial in the primary prevention of ischaemic heart disease using clofibrate, British Heart Journal 40:1069-1118 (1978).

5. Aspirin Myocardial Infarction Study Research Group: A randomized, controlled trial of aspirin in persons recovered from myocardial infarction, Journal of American Medical Association 243:661-669 (1980).
6. Unpublished observations.
7. J. M. Dunbar and A. J. Stunkard, Adherence to diet and drug regimens, in: "Nutrition, Lipids and Coronary Disease: A Global View," R. I. Levy, B. M. Rifkind, B. H. Dennis, and N. Ernst, eds., Raven Press, New York, pp. 391-423 (1979).
8. R. B. Haynes, M. E. Mattson, and T. O. Engebretson, Jr., eds., Patient compliance to prescribed antihypertensive medication regimens: A report to the National Heart, Lung and Blood Institute, pp. 7-59 (1980).
9. M. L. Russell, A. Silvers, J. L. Probstfield, and W. Insull, Jr., Self-debate: A major factor in trial participants' nonadherence to drug regimen, Controlled Clinical Trials 4(2): 150 (1983).
10. M. L. Russell, K. L. Ghee, J. L. Probstfield, and W. Insull, Jr., Development of standardized simulated patients for quality control of the clinical interview, Controlled Clinical Trials 4:197-208 (1983).
11. M. L. Russell, W. Insull, Jr., and J. L. Probstfield, Identification of varied training needs of clinical trial staff by objective demonstration of their interviewing and counseling skills, Controlled Clinical Trials 2:84 (1981).
12. M. E. Mattson and L. M. Friedman, Issues in medication adherence assessment in clinical trials of the National Heart, Lung and Blood Institute, in: "Workshop on the Development of Markers to be Used as Adherence Measures," T. P. Blaszkowski, and W. Insull, Jr., eds., In Press (1983).
13. P. W. Pace, J. C. Henske, B. J. Whitfill, S. M. Andrews, M. L. Russell, J. L. Probstfield, and W. Insull, Jr., Producing video cassette programs for diet instruction, Journal of American Dietetic Association 79:689-692 (1981).
14. P. W. Pace, J. C. Henske, B. J. Whitfill, S. M. Andrews, M. L. Russell, J. L. Probstfield, and W. Insull, Jr., Video cassette use in diet instruction, Journal of American Dietetic Association 83:166-169 (1983).
15. S. M. Zifferblatt, Increasing patient compliance through the applied analysis of behavior, Preventive Medicine 4:173-192 (1975).
16. J. M. Dunbar and A. J. Stunkard, Adherence to diet and drug regimen, in: "Nutrition, Lipids, and Coronary Heart Disease: A Global View," R. I. Levy, B. M. Rifkind, B. H. Denny, and N. Ernst, eds., Raven Press, New York, pp. 391-423 (1979).
17. J. L. Probstfield, M. L. Russell, J. C. Henske, R. Reardon, and W. Insull, Jr., A successful program for returning dropouts to a clinical trial, Controlled Clinical Trials 1:178 (1980).

MEETING SUMMARY

O. J. Pollak

9 Kings Highway
Dover, Delaware 19901

It is customary to introduce the epilogue with a prologue to start the summary with praising those responsible for the Symposium. The membership of the various committees is broad and it is impossible to recite all the names. Three names, at the poles of the Milan - Philadelphia axis, have to be mentioned, as they were at all previous symposia. They are the Scientific Directors, Doctors Paoletti and Holmes, and the Chairman of the Program Committee, Dr. Kritchevsky. The latter and his staff, especially Mrs. Nigro, his secretary, whom he generously shared with us, deserve our thanks. Having arranged a few meetings myself in the past, I am appreciative of their labors. And, thanks to all of the participants and sponsors of the Symposium. They all contributed in making the Eighth International Symposium on Drugs Affecting Lipid Metabolism a hugh success.

I recall the first symposium held in Milan in 1960. It was crowned by a memorable wine party given by Martini and Rossi on a terrace overlooking the fabled dome. I also recall the most recent meeting held in Philadelphia, in 1977, which Professor Hugh Sinclair closed with his saga of "Hiawatha's Lipid-Lowering Drug." In 1972, a symposium on nicotinic acid was enriched by "Reflections on Lipids and Atherosclerosis," a recital by composer - librettist - pianist - soloist - scientist Dave Kritchevsky. And after this year's banquet we were treated to a new edition of his witty rendition.

Those who expected a similar feast from me will be disappointed. I am better with puns in a small circle than on the stage, especially at a meeting on lipids. I am not an expert on lipids. And, after sharing with you my own definition of an expert as "an opinionated S.O.B.," you will understand why I am not keen on being called an expert. My expertise, if any, is knowledge of the bibliography. I have peeked behind the "lipid curtain" but have never stepped behind it.

The word "atherosclerosis" does not appear in the title of the program for this Symposium. Yet, it is clearly on everybody's mind. There are obvious links between hyper- and dyslipemia on one side of the ledger and atherogenesis and atherosclerosis on the other side. I am reserving the term atherogenesis for the initiation and evolution of the anatomic arterial alterations, the term atherosclerosis, for the clinical disease, the sequel of arterial changes. Derangement of plasma lipids is not the sole cause of disease. At that, hypercholesterolemia and hypertriglyceridemia play different roles at different stages. I am aware of overlaps of risks and of synergism, both within each set of risks and between the three sets listed in Table 1.

Singly, or in groups, risk factors have different weight. Atherogenesis is an episodic and a progressive phenomenon. Thus, new

TABLE 1

RISK FACTORS

A. ATHEROGENETIC RISK FACTORS*

1. Initiation of Legions

   a. Susceptible artery
   b. Trauma
   c. Hypercholesterolemia

2. Evolution of Lesions

   a. Overweight; overalimentation
   b. Hypercholesterolemia
   c. Hypertension

B. ATHEROSCLEROTIC - THROMBOGENIC RISKS**

   a. Hypertriglyceridemia
   b. Hypercoagulability
   c. Nicotine abuse
   d. Hyperestrogenemia

*A. 1., b. and c., simultaneously, or in reverse order.

**B. a., enhanced by B. c. and d.; also, by A. 2. b.

plaques are formed while older ones are undergoing evolution from fatty streaks to fibrous and on to complicated lesions. Thrombosis is not the only cause of clinical symptoms, but it is a prominent cause. A blood clot may form because of disruption of the coagulation cascade which has seventeen factors, depletion of ionized calcium which participates in five interactions or transitions of plasma factors. Yet, most attention is being paid to thrombocytes. A clot may form at a stenosis, on the surface of a lesion, or may result from a bleeding atheroma. Tabulating risks is risky; simplification is difficult. Lumping all known risk factors together is erroneous and misleading.

No matter how successful we will be in blocking or mitigating the effect of plasma lipids on the arterial wall, we cannot ignore the non-lipid risks. Many of such risks interfere with our efforts to normalize plasma lipids. Most of these risks are easier controlled than hyper- or dyslipemia.

Plasma lipids vary in all species with gender and age, in health and in disease. They undergo diurnal and seasonal variations. Study of hormonal regulation of plasma lipids has not been completed. Lipoprotein fractions fluctuate in the course of the menstrual cycle to such extent that the excursions could be used for ovulation timing. In 1925, as a medical student and an instructor in physiology, my first research assignment was the study of serology of hibernating animals, specifically, of anaphylaxy. Recalling the milky serum of moles, I think that study of the lipid metabolism of hibernating animals could prove informative.

My first criticism--maybe my second one--concerns the lack of information about factors influencing lipid metabolism and interfering with plasma lipid assays, be these performed for monitoring drug therapy or for diagnosis or prognosis. Not one of the one hundred and forty communications and papers read at the Symposium makes reference to alcohol consumption or to exercise. Only one communication states in its title that all the subjects studied were nonsmokers.

In his recording of 1972, Kritchevsky suggested repeatedly: "When you don't know what to do, measure lipids." Forty years ago, when I embarked on my first research project in atherosclerosis, I measured serum cholesterol. In 1947, at the first meeting of the American Society for the Study of Arteriosclerosis, cholesterol only was discussed. As a matter of fact, I was accused of having started a Society for the Study of Cholesterol. A year later, came the first reports on phospholipids. Soon, essays on the significance of the PL/TC ratio in patients with cerebral and coronary disease were published by Oliver and Boyd and by Davidson, Kendall, and Abell, respectively. Things have become a lot more complicated, as demonstrated in Table 2.

TABLE 2

LIPID ASSAYS: PAST, PRESENT AND FUTURE

Part 1 Cholesterol: TC, EC/TC, C-lysis, C-tolerance
Phospholipids: PL, PL/TC, PL partition
Triglycerides: TG, TG/TC, i.v. fat tolerance
Chylomicrons: count, post-prandial curve

Part 2 Lipoproteins: LP

alpha, beta, pre-beta......HDL, LDL, VLDL, $alpha_1$ (α_1), $alpha_2$ (α_2), beta très rapid (β_{tr}), beta rapid (β_r), beta lente (β_l), beta très lente (β_{tl}), beta ultra très lente (β_{utl})......VHDL, HDL_1, HDL_2, LDL_1, LDL_2, VLDL, chylomicrons

Part 3 LP Ratios: /3 LP (-C)......HDL/LDL-C

Part 4 Hyperlipoproteinemia: Type I, II, II B, III, IV, V

Part 5 Analysis of Lipids and Apolipoproteins in all the Lipoprotein Groups and Subgroups:

Ratios: (examples)

Total HDL/HDL_2
HDL_3/HDL_2
LDL/Total HDL
HDL-C/HDL-TG
HDL-PL/HDL-C
HDL-C/LDL-C + VLDL-C
LDL-C/LDL-TG
VLDL-TG/VLDL-PL

Possibilities for all Subgroups:

a) EC Partition
b) PL Partition
c) Polar/non-polar (EC, TG) lipids

Part 6 Apolipoproteins: Apoproteins, Subunits

Pro-Apo I
Apo A I, A II, A III, A Milano, A Marburg, A IV
Apo B, B 100, B 48
Apo C I, C II, C III, C III_1, C III_2, C III_0
Apo D
Apo E I, E II, E III, E III_0, E III_1, E III_2
Apo F
Apo G
Apo H

(continued)

TABLE 2 (Continued)

LIPID ASSAYS: PAST, PRESENT AND FUTURE

Ratios: (examples only)

Apo B/Apo C
Apo E/Apo C
Apo C II/Apo C III
HDL-Apo C III/LDL-Apo C III

Possibilities for All Subunits:

a) Lysine/arginine ratio
b) Numbers, types, sequence of amino acids

Part 7 Enzymes: (examples only)

LCAT
HMG/C-7α-hydrolase
Phosphohydroxylase
Lipid peroxidase
Lipase
LP-lipase
Phospholipase C, A_2

Part 8 Antibodies: (examples only)

Anti-HDL, anti-HDL, etc.
Anti-Apo A I, anti-Apo A II, etc.

There is no time for details. However, a few remarks seem in order. Calculating the PL/TC ratio may be obsolete, but should we not pay more attention to HDL-PL? Raynaud et al. separated lipoproteins into seven fractions by electrophoresis. At about the same time, Gofman et al. accomplished this by using ultracentrifugation. The French scheme never caught on. Luck went with the flotation rates. The α/β ratio, proposed by Barr et al. in 1952, was soon forgotten. Revived as the HDL-C/LDL-C ratio by Miller and Miller in 1975, it gained prompt acceptance.

Looking at my long table of tests, those performed today and those proposed for tomorrow in parts 5 to 8 of the chart, I came to believe that my secretary was correct when, in 1951, she mailed a letter to John Gofman, then head of the Department of Medical Physics at Berkeley, addressing it to the Department of Metaphysics.

Many presentations at the Symposium were based on detailed study of lipo- and apoproteins. Analysis went not always in the same direction, did not reach the same depth nor the same results. Burstein and Legmann, in their monograph on "Lipoprotein Precipitation" (S. Karger, 1982), pointed out that even seemingly minor modifications in methodology influence the results of analysis. At this Symposium, we heard that the same applies to the apoprotein assays.

Professor Wissler spoke of "splintering" of lipoproteins. Should we add to our list breakdown of LP-PL, of LP-EC, partial or complete AA analysis of apoproteins? Should we add enzyme assays and titration of anti-LP and anti-apoLP antibodies? How far can we go? How far should we go? What is feasible? What is affordable? What is practical?--for the research laboratory and for the clinical laboratory? Who will set the limits?

Normalization--assuming that we can agree on normals for all fractions, subfractions and subunits--need not extend from plasma to other body fluids, to circulating cells and to fixed tissue cells.

At present, we know of three ways by which to influence plasma lipids and, to some extent, lipid metabolism. They are, partial ileocoecal bypass, drugs and diets.

Surgical intervention, mentioned in just one communication at the Symposium, has a prompt effect. Regrettably, one of its important effects on sterol synthesis is transitory. Since atherogenesis starts early in life, the bypass should ideally be performed soon after birth. It is most doubtful that it would gain the wide acceptance of neonatal circumcision.

The main theme of the Symposium was the discussion of drugs affecting lipid metabolism. The list of drugs for lowering plasma cholesterol or plasma triglycerides proposed in the last three decades is very long, indeed. Some of the drugs never made it from the animal room to the hospital bed.

Many of once popular pharmaceuticals have been banned because of severe side effects. Often, the adverse effects were disclosed only after many years of usage. Little has been said about tolerance and about side effects of new drugs presented at the Symposium. Mostly, it was just said that a drug was "well tolerated"--by rats, that the rats did not develop hepatomegaly. In this connection, I want to single out Dr. Lageron's communication on the "Fat Overload Syndrome" as a model program for histological, histoenzymological, ultracentrifugal and biochemical work-up providing comprehensive information about the liver. To what extent could this program be used on a large scale, both for animals and for man?

Let us first look at the plasma cholesterol-lowering drugs. Of the "old" medications, Probucol (to which over twenty papers were devoted) emerged as the leading "survivor." This, in spite of the fact that its potency is not much different from that of the other cholesterol-depressents and in spite of the fact that the list of side effects of Probucol, as published in the 37th edition of "Physicians' Desk Reference" of 1983, is nearly as long as the listing for the formerly widely used Colestipol.

A new drug, Etofibrate, a derivative of niacin, with clofibrinic acid added, received much attention at a special workshop. The drug has the same broad spectrum action as nicotinic acid when given alone. Hopefully, the new drug will be tolerated better than niacin, alone.

Another newly introduced drug is Gamma-Oryzanol, a combination of phytosterols with ferulic acid. Its mode of action and its potency is ascribed to sito-, campe- and stigmasterol. Plant sterols do not cause side effects. One of the speakers at the workshop mentioned the structural similarity between ferulic acid and alpha-tocopherol. Cavete! In the last two and one-half years I came across ten reports on the effect of Vitamin E on LP fractions and subfractions. The very first report was favorable; the next nine essays reported that the results were devastating, that all the shifts were in the "wrong" directions.

In their monograph on "Sitosterol" (S. Karger, 1980) Pollak and Kritchevsky wrote that all known medications and, for that matter, all known diets, also mixed phytosterols or sitosterol alone, depress plasma cholesterol to nearly equal degree, the mean decrease amounting to a mean of 17.5 percent, with a range from 12 to 22 percent, an amount corresponding roughly to the ingested cholesterol.

Next, to plasma triglyceride-lowering drugs. The most widely used, Clofibrate, has fallen into disfavor because of its many adverse side effects. Gemfibrozil, a "survivor," and four "newcomers," Beclobrate and Clinofibrate, derivatives of Clofibrate, then, Pantethine and Mifobate, were much discussed at the Symposium. A projected slide listed the side effects of Clinofibrate and Clofibrate --in rats. The list for Clinofibrate was much shorter than that for Clofibrate; however, only about one-half of the known side effects of Clofibrate were listed.

Whereas many anti-cholesterol drugs were discarded because of low potency, this has not been true for triglyceride-depressents. All the pharmaceuticals achieve a 30 to 50 percent reduction of plasma triglycerides, exceeding the the effect of diets. Such reduction seems impressive. But, let us keep in mind that plasma triglyceride fluctuations exceed by far those of plasma cholesterol.

Cholesterol-lowering drugs have little effect on plasma triglycerides, and triglyceride-depressing drugs have even less effect on plasma cholesterol. Dual effect should not be expected since the two substances differ chemically and metabolically. Curiously, there are some who expected not only such dual effect but also a beneficial effect on thromboxanes and other substances involved in platelet aggregation and platelet adhesiveness. Any influence of lipid-lowering drugs would be indirect, based on the fact that triglycerides and also cholesterol enhance coagulation.

One report, by Dr. Yazawa, deserves notice because of simultaneous and also marked reduction of plasma cholesterol and triglycerides in rats and mice fed viable or dead cultures of *Streptococcus faecium*. Cholesterol reduction was ascribed to a protein fraction, triglyceride reduction, to a polysaccharide fraction of the microorganisms. It could be promising to experiment with purified fractions, then, to pursue the feasibility of extrapolation to humans. I recall that the field of cancer chemotherapy was initiated by using a polysaccharide from *Serratia marcescens*.

And now to the dietary approach. A widespread mistake is being made by referring to fats, proteins and carbohydrates as three separate, closed entities. Nobody ingests only fats, only proteins, etc., nor, only saturated fatty acids, only arginine, etc., only disaccharides, etc. Even a strict vegetarian diet is a mixed diet. Qualitative and quantitative variants of diets are endless. Moreover, foods change when stored, when heated, differently when cooked or when baked.

Dietary supplements, such as artichoke or avocado, are not being eaten for their effect on plasma cholesterol. No-cholesterol, low-cholesterol, high PUFA containing oils and margarines have been advertised to such extent that they have become household items in the American kitchen. Formerly exaggerated claims promising protection from heart attack have been toned down to a promise of a "statistically significant reduction of plasma cholesterol by fully 7 percent." Chemical changes, such as oxidation of cholesterol or hydrolysis of unsaturated fatty acids on heating, are never mentioned.

Diets are less costly than medications, compliance is also easier. Side effects can be avoided. The efficacy is not much lower than that of pharmaceuticals. Drugs should be used where diets fail to achieve the goal.

Not all diets are being prescribed by physicians. Many diets reflect ethnic or regional customs. Such diets are often held responsible for a high or a low incidence of ischemic heart disease. The incidence of myocardial infarction is much lower in rice-consuming populations than in countries with high consumption of potatoes. I have to add that the caloric intake of those eating rice is much lower than of those eating potatoes. Back in 1965, I stated at a meeting: "People who go barefooted do not develop atherosclerosis."

TABLE 3

DIETARY GUIDELINES

High	Low
Vegetable Proteins e.g., Soy	Animal proteins e.g., Casein
Vegetable Fats Sitosterol; PUFA	Animal Fats Cholesterol; SFA
Carbohydrates Main source: Rice	Carbohydrates Main source: Potatoes
Fiber	Caloric Intake

Epidemiologists are facing many problems. The Thai and the Sinhalese diets are similar. Both are atherogenic. Yet, myocardial infarction is rare in Thailand, frequent in Sri Lanka. Epidemiology is not stagnant. Columbus brought syphilis to America. MacArthur brought atherosclerosis to Japan. And, as I learned at this Symposium, he also brought cholelithiasis to Japan. The large number of Japanese scientists at this meeting attests to the fact that atherosclerosis has become a problem for Japan.

Twenty-five years ago, the Chinese in Hong Kong had no atherosclerosis; today, the incidence of myocardial infarction among them matches that of Westeners living in Hong Kong. The change is due to a higher caloric intake, to increased air pollution, to stressing traffic jams and, in my opinion, to the fact that organic farming has been replaced by use of phosphate fertilizers. These factors are causing a rising rate of myocardial infarction in the large cities of the Peoples' Republic of China.

Personal observations during travel and bibliographic data led me to compile the sketchy dietary guidelines for Table 3.

And now to the summation of the summary. There are three main concerns with drugs affecting lipid metabolism. They are potency, safety, i.e., tolerance and freedom from side effects, and compliance.

In the past, we were unhappy with drugs causing only a 17.5 percent reduction of plasma cholesterol, with any drug failing to depress the level below the magic 240 mg/dl mark. Many a drug has been discarded because of that. Today, many seem delirious over a decrease by 14 percent and quite happy with a decrease by 7 percent--just as long as the decrease is "statistically significant." Reduction expressed in percent loses its charm when translated into mg/dl. Statistical significance and biologic significance are not the same. Similarly, a 10 percent tax cut may have statistical and political significance. In practice, it means a lot to one whose tax bracket is high, very little to one whose income is low.

Homeostasis used to be blamed for limited success with cholesterol-lowering drugs. The term was used only twice at this Symposium: once, in passing, with reference to a drug; then, with reference to HMG-CoA reductase acting upon fibroblasts in tissue culture. Is there nothing more to be learned about homeostasis? Could there be such regulatory mechanism influencing the HDL-C/LDL-C ratio?

We heard little about the safety of newly developed and developing drugs. The lecture by Professor Walldius on nicotinic acid was a notable exception, especially as he added to discussion of tolerance and adverse effects his guidelines to safer medication. Professor Oliver, who gave two elegant talks, one at the banquet and one in the lecture hall, seemed to be the only one, besides me, expressing concern about the risks of drug therapy.

There was much concern about compliance. It presents a problem whenever a drug is being tested outside prison walls, outside an asylum or a home for the aged. It is not fair to blame failure or unexpected results on noncompliance alone. It has been known for years that it is easier to reduce a high plasma lipid level than a low one. Often, a course of drug therapy is being started after lipids have been partially reduced by dietary means. Often, drugs are being combined with a diet. Moreover, diets are not the only factors interfering with blood chemical data. A subject may be faithful to his physician's orders, yet response to medication as measured by plasma lipid assays may be unexpected. This could be due to drinking or smoking, to fasting or feasting, to jogging or resting, and so on. The caged rat lives a dull life compared to that of man.

In 1962, at a social hour closing a meeting of the Board of Directors of the American Heart Association in Scottsdale, Arizona, I was handed a telegram from Washington. It related the Surgeon General's declaration: "Smoking may be hazardous to your health." Upon reading out loud the missive, I added words of my own: "We are not to eat fat, we are not to eat meat, we are not to eat sugar, and now we can no longer smoke. The only things left are drinking, exercise and sexercise."

I have read quite a few reports on the influence of alcohol and nicotine on plasma lipoprotein fractions. I have yet to read about the influence of sex life. Anyone who would study plasma lipoproteins before and after sexual activity and would--hopefully--report an increase in HDL-C in the New England Journal of Medicine, would gain wide acclaim by the news media and become, instantly, a hero.

ABSTRACTS

Molecular Mechanics Involved in The Inhibitory Regulation of Adenylate Cyclase (AC) by Antipolytic Hormonal Factors and Nicotinic Acid

Klaus Aktories, Guenter Schultz and Karl Heinz Jakobs

Pharmakologisches Institut der Universitat Heidelberg, Germany

The antilipolytic effects of various prostaglandins, adenosine derivatives, nicotinic acid and related compounds (e.g. acipimox) are apparently mediated by a decreased intracellular cAMP level, due to inhibition of AC. Inhibition of AC by these agents depends on the presence of GTP and is largely amplified by Na^+. The antilipolytic compounds also stimulate GTP hydrolysis in adipocyte membranes. Stimulation of low K_m GTPase and inhibition of AC correlate with regard to hormone receptors involved, dose-effect relationships and GTP- and Na^+ dependencies, indicating that both processes are intimately connected. Cholera toxin (CT), which has been shown to inhibit GTPase stimulation by hormones stimulating AC, is ineffective to impair AC inhibition and GTPase stimulation by the antilipolytic compounds. In contrast, islet-activating protein (IAP), a toxin from *Bordetella pertussis*, impairs inhibition of AC and stimulation of the low K_m GTPase by the antilipolytic hormonal factors. In analogy to CT, IAP elicits these effects presumably by ADP-ribosylation of a regulatory protein of the AC system. Using ^{32}P-NAD, IAP radiolabels a 40,000 daltons protein, which is different from the CT-labeled protein in adipocyte membranes. The data suggest that the antilipolytic compounds inhibit adipocyte AC via an inhibitory GTP-binding protein, which is ADP-ribosylated by IAP and which is different from the stimulatory regulatory protein of the AC system.

The Effect of Niacin, Colestipol, and Low Fat Diet on Lipids and Apolipoproteins in Non-Smoking Men with Coronary Bypass

Petar Alaupovic, Sharon Nessim, H. P. Chin, Stanley P. Azen, and Davic H. Blankenhorn

Oklahoma Medical Research Foundation, Oklahoma City, Oklahoma and USC School of Medicine, Los Angeles, California

Apolipoprotein (Apo) B and the ratio of Apo CIII in HDL to that in LDL plus VLDL (ApoClllR) are of interest as possible risk factors in atherosclerosis. The long-term (1 year) effect of therapy by niacin and colestipol on ApoB and ApoCIIIR are studied in CLAS, an angiographic trial testing the effectiveness of aggressive cholesterol lowering therapy in atherosclerosis. Non-smoking men with coronary bypass (average cholesterol 246 mg%), prescreened on the basis of niacin and colestipol induced cholesterol reduction (at least 15%), were randomized to treatment with niacin, colestipol, and low fat diet; or, placebo and low fat diet. Of the 87 randomized, 14 drug and 15 placebo men have completed one year on treatment. The drug therapy has resulted in a large increase in ApoClllR (+136%†) and a decrease in ApoB (-31%†). Major drug related lipoprotein changes are seen in LDL (-40%†), triglycerides (-41%†), HDL (+33%†), and cholesterol (-29%†). These results demonstrate that a major perturbation of apolipoproteins, as well as lipoproteins, can be obtained with these drugs at lower lipid levels. These findings are important in view of the steep gradient of coronary heart disease risk at low cholesterol levels, which has been reported in the Framingham Study (The Lancet, Aug. 14, 1982, 734).

†p value < .01

Effect of Pantethine on Lipids, Lipoproteins and Apolipoproteins in Man

P. Avogaro, G. Bittolo Bon, and M. Fusello

General Regional Hospital and the National Research Council Sub-Project Atherosclerosis, Venice Operational Unit, Venice, Italy

The authors evaluated the hypolipemic effects on Pantethine in 19 patients with high blood lipid levels.

The study lasted 8 months, during which the patients followed continuously an isocaloric diet. From the 2nd to the 4th and from the 6th until the 8th month, they were given Pantethine 900 mg/day or oral route.

Pantethine induced a significant reduction of total cholesterol, triglycerides, LDL-C and apolipoprotein B with a concomitant rise in HDL-C and in apolipoprotein A-I, as compared with the diet-only periods.

The authors conclude that their trial confirmed, as already shown by other studies both in animals and in humans, that Pantethine, a natural important component of CoA, showed definitely effective in reducing blood lipids through a complex action involving lipids, lipoproteins and apolipoproteins.

The Effect of Probucol on Cholesterol and Lipoprotein Metabolism in Cultured Hepatocytes

J. W. Barnhart and D. L. Li

Merrell Dow Pharmaceuticals, Inc., Indianapolis, Indiana

Probucol added to cultured hepatocytes at concentrations of 10^{-5} -10^{-6}M had a significant effect on cholesterol transport. There was both increased ingress and egress but the net effect was increased cellular cholesterol. The effect on cholesterol uptake occurred whether the cholesterol was in the form of lipoprotein or a cholesterol-lecithin complex. Alpha-tocopherol acetate caused similar effects. Probucol also caused a significant reduction of incorporation of acetate but not mevalonate into sterol. Alpha-tocopherol had no effect on cholesterol synthesis. These preliminary results suggest that probucol may have some effect on cell membrane similar to that of alpha-tocopherol but that differences such as the effect on cholesterol biosynthesis distinguish the hypocholesterolemic agent from the natural antioxidant alpha-tocopherol.

Mifobate (SR-202), Profile of A New Drug Affecting Lipid Metabolism with Potential Antiatherosclerotic Activity

C. Bentzen, L. Nguyen, S. Gay, Y. Guyon and E. Niesor

SYMPHAR, S.A., Geneva, Switzerland

Mifobate [Dimethyl α - (dimethoxyphosphinyl)p-chlorobenzyl phosphate] was selected from a new series of substituted *gem*-phosphonate-phosphates as most active in clearing pre-deposited cholesterol (CHOL) from tissues of several animal species while favorably modifying the alpha/beta lipoprotein CHOL (LP-CHOL) profile. In addition, Mifobate significantly increases HDL-CHOL in normal rats, rabbits and monkeys, suggesting mediation via a common mechanism. The augmentation of HDL-CHOL in rats is dose dependent from 25 mg/kg and appears to be specifically associated with an elevation of HDL-free cholesterol and an increased CHOL turnover as observed in ^{14}C-CHOL bile and fecal elimination studies.

Normal rats treated with Mifobate for as long as one year showed persistent HDL-CHOL elevation of +78.4% ($p<0.01$) with simultaneous decrease in plasma triglycerides (TRG) of -67.7% ($p<0.001$) and body fat depots of -58.4% ($p<0.005$) with no change in food consumption compared to controls. Alterations in LP-CHOL and TRG levels have been observed in initial clinical studies in man and support the concept of a consistent mechanism of action.

Mifobate differs from classical hypolipidemic drugs by its chemical structure, physicochemical characteristics, pharmacokinetics, pharmacological mechanism of action and the absence of peroxisomal proliferation as verified by catalase activity and electron microscopic examinations.

The absence of drug deposition in tissues along with a rapid rate of elimination are consistent with the observed favorable tolerance and toxicity profiles.

In summary, the novel plasma and tissue lipid altering activity of Mifobate strongly suggests a therapeutic antiatherosclerotic potential.

Effect of Propranolol on HMGCoA Reductase Activity in Human Fibroblasts

F. Bernini, G. Cighetti, A. Corsini, G. Galli and R. Fumagalli

Inst. Pharmacology and Pharmacognosy and Department of Medical Chemistry and Biochemistry, University of Milan, Italy

We have previously described that propranolol, a widely recognized β -receptor antagonist, increases receptor-mediated catabolism of human LDL in fibroblasts cultured from normocholesterolemic subjects. Results presented here show the same effect of the drug in fibroblasts from heterozygous patients but not in those of homozygotes. These data point to a specific action of the drug on LDL receptor activity. Further, we have investigated the effect of propranolol on HMGCoA reductase activity in the same cellular systems. The enzyme activity was evaluated, measuring by multiple selected ion monitoring technique (MSIM) the amount of mevalonate formed from HMGCoA (Analytical Bioch. 110, 153, 1981). Unexpectedly propranolol (10^{-4}, 10^{-5}M) enhanced HMGCoA activity in the three tested cell lines independently from its effect on LDL receptor activity. Stimulation of HMGCoA reductase activity does not appear to be correlated to the β-blocking properties of propranolol because both enantiomers of the compound display the same effect.

Effect on Smooth Muscle Cell Proliferation and Lipid Concentration in Arterial Tissue and Blood in Cholesterol Fed Rabbits under Etofibrate Treatment

E. Betz

Physiological Institute (I), University of Tuebingen, Germany

Subendothelial smooth muscle cell proliferation in arteries of rabbits can be produced within a few days by repeated transmural electrical stimuli with D.C.-pulses. The plaques develop beneath the anode. The size of the proliferate depends on 1. strength of the electrical current, 2. duration of the single impulse, 3. duration of the stimulation period. If the rabbits receive food containing 1% or 2% cholesterol, the proliferates accumulate lipids and transform into typical atheromatous plaques. This type of plaque-production permits standardization of the stimuli and thereby a good possibility for an evaluation of drug effects on the growth of the plaques and the degree of lipid accumulation within the vessel wall. One of the drugs used was etofibrate. Six male New Zealand rabbits received for 4 weeks daily 80 mg/kg etofibrate dissolved in food containing 2% cholesterol. Six animals received the same concentration of etofibrate in food with 1% cholesterol for the same time. Twelve rabbits served as controls--6 were fed with 2% cholesterol, 6 with 1% cholesterol but without addition of drugs. One carotid artery of each animal was stimulated by means of chronically implanted graphite coated gold electrodes (4 weeks, daily 30 min. in the morning and 15 min. in the afternoon with 100 μA, 14 ms/Imp, 10 Hz). The arteries were then dissected, fixed in glutaraldehyde, cut with a cryostat, and stained with oil red. Different parts of the plaques were analysed 1. for the number of cell layers grown in the intima, 2. the degree of lipid accumulation and 3. the appearance of necrotic regions or destructions of the endothelium. Blood concentrations of cholesterol, HDL and triglycerides were also measured.

It could be seen that HDL was significantly higher in the etofibrate treated animals. A tendency for a less pronounced growth of the plaques and a smaller increase in cholesterol concentration in the blood also could be seen, whereas the lipid concentration in the plaques of animals fed with etofibrate was not different to that of the controls.

The Effect of Supplemental Vitamin E and Vitamin C Upon In Vivo Platelet Function and Serum Parameters in Human Diabetics

M. L. Bierenbaum, L. J. Machlin, H. N. Bhagavan, W. P. Maginnis, A. Stier, C. Levey, and A. Naso

Kenneth L. Jordan Cardiac Res. Gp., Montclair, New Jersey

In an earlier report on 25 diabetics given 2000 IU/day of (E) for 6 weeks, serum glucose levels were lowered significantly. Additionally vitamin C (C) has been reported to be both hypolipemic and have platelet anti-aggregatory effects. In the present study, 40 patients with adult onset diabetes mellitus were divided into 4 groups and treated for 6 months with group I receiving 800 IU of (E) daily, group II receiving 1500 mg of (C) daily, group III, 800 IU of (E) and 1500 mg of (C) daily, and group IV receiving placebo (P) only. Group I showed a significant rise in aggregation time from 433±38 to 497±34 seconds, P<.05. Peripheral blood flow was measured by the Doppler technique and group III showed a marked improvement from 3.84±.13 to 4.17±.13 units, P .025. Glycosylated hemoglobin for group I went from 8.9±.83 to 10.1±.95%, P<.05 in a direction opposite to our earlier studies. There were no other significant changes in serum cholesterol, HDL cholesterol, triglycerides, glucose, pulse or blood pressure. Additionally, there were no significant side effects noted for any treatment group. In this study, it appears that (E) beneficially effected platelet aggregability and the (E) and (C) combined can improve peripheral circulation in the diabetic. The failure to reproduce earlier noted blood sugar and lipid changes appear to be dose related. Given these findings additional studies to determine optimal dosage of (E) and (C) for the management of adult onset diabetes appear indicated.

Effect of Antilipidemic Agents and Other Drugs on The Synthesis and Secretion of Structural Macromolecules

Magdolna Bihari-Varga, Anna Kadar, Eva Csonka and H. Jellinek

Second Department of Pathology, Semmelweis Med. University, Budapest, Hungary

Endothelial and smooth muscle cell/SMC/monolayers were grown from Minnesota minipig aortas. The following compounds were added in increasing concentration / 10^{-8} - 10^{-3} / to the medium of parallel series of cultures: clofibrate /Miscleron[R]/, pyrido-1,2 pyrimidine /Chinoin-123/, glycosaminoglycans, GAG-s /hyaluronic acid,HA, chondroitin sulfate, CSA/ and proteoglycans /Rumalon[R], Recosen[R]/.

The extracellular matrix production of the cultured cells was investigated by transmission and scanning electron microscope. The synthesis and excretion of glycoconjugates, collagen and elastin was measured by biochemical methods.

Clofibrate was found to increase GAG and collagen synthesis in both types of cell cultures. CH-123 showed a dose dependent decrease in proteoglycan synthesis and secretion and an increase in collagen synthesis. Extracellularly administered GAG-s influenced the GAG synthesis of cultured cells. The internalization of CSA or HA was followed by their degradation or by the suppression of GAG synthesis within the cells.

The results obtained with Rumalon and Recosen in SMC cultures are still the subject of mathematical evaluation but will also be discussed.

Inhibition of Intestinal Lipoproteins Assembly as a New Method of Treatment of Hyperlipidemia

W. J. Bochenek, B. Kapuscinska, E. Kyriakides, J. Safarik, S. K. Peng, and J. B. Rodgers

Albany Medical College and the Veterans Administration Medical Center, Albany, New York

Existing modes of treatment of hyperlipidemia are based on methods affecting either body metabolism of lipids or inhibition of intestinal absorpition of fat in the intestinal tract. Recently hypolipemic effects of hydrophobic surfactants composed of propylene oxide and ethylene oxide polymers (Poloxalenes) were described (Atheroscleroslerosis 45:235, J. Clin. Investig., in press).

Experiments were performed in rats equipped with duodenal cannulae for infusion of lipid preparation containing triolein 12 mM, lecithin 3 mM, taurocholate 19 mM in an electrolyte/phosphate buffer, pH 6.4 (controls). Experimentals received a similar preparation containing in addition Poloxalene 2930 0.017 mM. Infusion rate for both was 2.4 ml/hr. In both groups, uptake of lipid as studied by electromicroscopy was rapid. In the controls, as early as 6 min. after infusion accumulation of chylomicrons in the Golgi stacks was noted and at 20 min., the entire Golgi apparatus area was filled with fat. In contrast, in the experimental rats, although uptake of fat was equally rapid, it did not accumulate in the Golgi apparatus but instead, was seen as large droplets in the apical positions of the enterocytes. During 7 hrs. of infusion, the quantity of lipid absorbed and transported amounted to 90 ± 2 and $47 \pm 3\%$, in the controls and experimentals, respectively ($p < .001$). After discontinuation of lipid infusion, the amount of lipid stored in the enterocytes in the experimental animals decreased exponentially, reaching a value of 6% at 180 min.

This study demonstrates that the hypolipemic effect of Poloxalene 2930 is mediated by inhibition of intestinal lipoprotein assembly. Its onset is rapid and the fat stored in the enterocytes is almost completely transported within a 3-hour period.

Hypolipidemic Profile of EMD 34 853, A New Lipid Lowering Drug Increasing Liver Lipoprotein Receptors

P. Carrara, E. Bosisio, M. Galbussera, L. Allievi, G. Galli and C. R. Sirtori

Institute of Pharmacology and Pharmacognosy, Chair of Chemotherapy, University of Milan, Italy

EMD 34 853 (2-phenyl-2-[6-ethoxy-benzothiazolyl (2)-thio]-propionic acid), a new hypolipidemic drug, neither increasing liver weight nor proliferating peroxisomes and with a mild anorectic activity, was tested in male Sprague-Dawley rats on standard and hyperlipidemic (cholesterol-cholic acid) regimens. Lipid-lipoprotein changes and the influence on liver lipoprotein receptors were examined. The two tested doses of the compound significantly lowered plasma total CHOL. and TG levels, both on a standard and cholesteremic regimen. Standard diet, 30 mg/kg: CHOL. -53%, TG -11%, 100 mg/kg: CHOL. -60%, TG -23.5%; High chol. regimen, 30 mg/kg: CHOL. -55.1%, TG -53.2%; 100 mg/kg: CHOL. -60.2%, TG -70.3%. The higher dose of the compound exhibited a mild anorectic activity. On the high chol. regimen, HDL cholesterol levels were significantly raised by EMD 34 853. CPIB (300 mg/kg), tested as the reference compound, generally exhibited a lower activity. Liver lipoprotein receptors were evaluated by the use of ^{125}I-β -VLDL from cholesterol-fed rabbits (Windler et al., J. Biol. Chem. 255, 10464, 1980). No significant changes were shown in livers from cholesterol-fed animals, where receptorial activity was suppressed. Bmax for β-VLDL in normals was 103 ng/mg protein; for rats treated with 30 mg/kg of EDM 34 853, it was raised to 366 ng/mg protein. Kd was also significantly elevated in EMD treated animals (1,769 vs. 830 ng/ml); however, the parallelism between the two lines on the Scatchard plot was not significantly modified. These findings confirm that the powerful hypolipidemic properties of EMD 34 853 may be exerted through an increased number of liver high affinity binding sites for lipoproteins.

Plasma Lipid-Lipoprotein Changes and Protection from Arterial Lesions in Cholesterol-Fed Rabbits Treated with Pantethine

P. Carrara, M. Galbussera, M. R. Lovati, C. R. Sirtori and L. Matturri

Institute of Pharmacology and Pharmacognosy, Chemotherapy Chair and Institute of Morbid Anatomy, University of Milan, Italy

The hypolipidemic and antiatherosclerotic activity of pantethine (P) was evaluated in hypercholesterolemic (HC) rabbits. P, the stable disulphate of pantetheine, major component and precursor of coenzyme A in animals, was given to New Zealand male rabbits on a 0.5% cholesterol regimen for three months (500 mg/kg/day). At the end of treatment, a significant reduction of plasma cholesterol levels was exhibited by HC animals treated with P (HC: 1033.0 ± 329.5 mg/dl; HCP+P: 368.0 ± 129.0 mg/dl, $p < 0.01$). The percentage of cholesterol associated with high density lipoproteins (HDL) was also raised in the HC+P group (HC: 7.6 ± 2.3%; HCP+P: 16.2 ± 11.2%, $p < 0.01$). Plasma total triglcerides were significantly reduced. Isolated lipoprotein fractions showed an increased protein content in HDL, both in the HC and HC+P rabbits. Apoprotein AI (determined on IEF gels) was markedly increased in the HC+P group. An interesting observation was the marked decrease of lipid content of the very low density lipoproteins, notoriously the most atherogenic fraction in rabbits, in the HC+P group. Protein content also decreased in VLDL, possibly indicating a reduction of apoprotein E.

Liver and aortic lipid compositions were not modified in HC+P rabbits, compared to the HC group; however, the total aortic area with lesions was significantly reduced in the HC+P animals. The histological examination of the aortic wall showed, in P treated rabbits, a reduced lipid infiltration and a lesser proliferation of collagen fibers. More significant changes were noted in the coronary arteries; very severe lesions were observed in rabbits on the HC regimen, whereas a clear protective effect seemed to be present in the HC+P group.

Deoxycarnitine/Carnitine Exchange in Rat Heart Slices: One to One Ratio

Mario Ciman, Lodovico Sartorelli and Noris Siliprandi

Istituto Di Chimica Biologica, Padova, Italy

The exchange between internal deoxycarnitine and external carnitine has been studied with $[C^{14}]$-deoxycarnitine. Heart slices preloaded with $[C^{14}]$ -deoxycarnitine exchange with H-carnitine present in the incubation medium. The attainment of the equilibrium was temperature dependent and totally unaffected by the inhibitors of glycolysis (NaF), oxidative phosphorylation (azide) and respiratory chain uncouplers (FCCP). Under these conditions the ratio of exchange was 1:1. The opposite exchange was also studied by preloading heart slices with $[^{3}H]$-carnitine. The ratio of ^{3}H-carnitine (in)/$[C^{14}]$-deoxycarnitine (out) was also 1:1, but the rate was dependent on the concentration of loaded carnitine. Internal L-carnitine can exchange also with external D-carnitine, acetyl-L-carnitine and L-carnitine. Since carnitine (out)/deoxycarnitine (in) exchange has a physiological meaning, the exchange ratio of 1:1 very likely reflects the presence in the sarcolemma of translocase functionally analogous to that described in the mitochondrial membrane. The above-mentioned exchanges involving carnitine are specifically inhibited by thiol reagent like NEM and Mersalyl.

Effects of 3-Hydroxy-3-Methyl-Glutaric Acid (H.M.G.) Treatment on Lipids and Lipoproteins: A Preliminary Study

Giovanni Ciuffetti, Elmo Mannarino, and Umberto Senin

Policlinico Monteluce, University of Perugia, Perugia, Italy

3-hydroxy-3-methyl-gluatric acid (H.M.G.) is a new hypolipidemic agent. Clinical experience with this substance is still insufficient, and particularly there is still a lack of information on its effect on blood lipids and on individual lipoprotein cholesterol levels. The preliminary results of a clinical trial with this substance in 10 primary hypercholesterolemic patients are here reported. After eight weeks treatment with 3-hydroxy-3-methyl-glutaric acid at the daily dosage of two grams, a reduction of both serum cholesterol and LDL-cholesterol was observed (11% and 13% respectively), while HDL-cholesterol remained substantially unaffected. The drug was always well tolerated and no side effects reported.

Effects of Guar Gum Supplementation on The Distribution of Apolipoproteins C-II and C-III Subunits in Familial Hyperlipidemic Patients

L. Cominacini, F. Ferrari, I. Zocca, U. Garbin, A. Davoli, P. DeBastiani and O. Bosello

Clinica Medica, University of Verona, C.O.C. Borgo Roma, Verona, Italy

Guar gum, a gel-forming polysaccaride seems one of the most effective fibers in eliciting changes in plasma cholesterol. The effects on triglycerides (TG) are more conflicting. The aim of the present study was to investigate the effect of guar gum diet supplementation on plasma TG and on the relative proportions of very low density lipoprotein (VLDL) apoprotein (apo) C-II and apoC-III subunits in hyperlipidemic patients. Eleven out-patients (9 men, 2 women) affected by familial combined hyperlipidemia were given 16 g/day with meals for a period of 15 days. Twelve-hours fasting blood samples were obtained before and after 15 days guar gum feeding. TG in plasma were measured by Autoanalyzer Technicon II Methodology. The isoforms of apoC were separated by polyacrylamide ultrathin-layer isoelectrofocusing. Mean total TG decreased from 181.0 $\pm$ 27.0 mg/dl to 126.0 $\pm$ 23.9 mg/dl ($p<0.01$). While apoC-III_2 as percentage of total VLDL apoC-III did not modify, apoC-III_1 increased and apoC-III_0 decreased after guar administration (respectively from 39.6 $\pm$ 5.2% to 54.0 $\pm$ 8.7%, $p<0.01$ and from 26.6 $\pm$ 5.5% to 11.9 $\pm$ 4.1%, $p<0.001$). ApoC-II as percentage of total apoC did not vary. The results indicate that the guar gum induced variation of plasma TG is associated with a change of the distribution of VLDL apoC-III subunits.

Benzodiazepines as Potential Antiatherosclerotic Drugs

B. Cuparencu, J. Horák, M. Cucuianu, C. Tomus, N. Hâncu, and Gh. Ispas

Department of Pharmacology, Medical and Pharmaceutical Institute, Cluj-Napoca, Romania

In the past years we have shown that diazepam, lorazepam, chlordiazepoxide and bipotassium chlorazepate had marked antihyperlipidaemic effects when tested in hyperlipidaemic rabbits and rats. These drugs failed to induce any changes of the serum lipids in normolipidaemic animals. We found also that these compounds brought about a significant increase of the HDL-cholesterol/total cholesterol ratio. They elevated the percentile concentration of α lipoproteins, decreasing at the same time the percentage of chylomicrons and prae β-lipoproteins. In normolipidaemic as well as in hyperlipidaemic animals, some of the benzodiazepines activated fibrinolysis. In hyperlipidaemic rats, they had an anticoagulant activity, whereas in normolipidaemic rats they had a procoagulant activity or they failed to affect blood coagulation. Plasma viscosity increased by Triton WR-1339 administration in rats was depressed by some of them. It is noteworthy that also benzodiazepine synthesis precursors had also hypolipidaemic properties. Some preliminary clinical investigations have demonstrated that also in humans diazepam and chlordiazepoxide reduced the serum lipids concentration in normolipidaemic patients. Independently of the lipid metabolism status, they activated fibrinolysis. Thus, benzodiazepines are potential antiatherosclerotic drugs.

Serum Lipoproteins and Probucol Transport

C. Dachet, M. F. Baudet, J. C. Buxtorf, B. Jacotot, and J. L. Beaumont

INSERM U 32, Henri-Mondor Hospital, Creteil Cedex, France

Changes in serum cholesterol, phospholipids and triglycerides, in the lipoprotein composition and in the distribution of Probucol in the different lipoprotein classes were studied in 12 type II patients with and without xanthomas during a 12-month treatment.

A significant decrease in serum was observed, and also in the cholesterol content of HDL measured after precipitation procedures by dextran sulfate and magnesium chloride. A smaller and unsignificant decrease in serum phospholipids was observed, but no modifications of serum triglycerides, apoproteins A and B.

All the drug was carried by lipoproteins: 6% was found in chylomicra, 25% in VLDL, 59% in LDL and 10% in HDL.

The cholesterol, triglyceride, phospholipid and protein content of the lipoproteins VLDL, LDL, and HDL obtained by ultracentrifugation was studied. The following changes were induced by a one-year treatment: for VLDL, a decrease in the protein moiety and an increase in triglyceride content; for LDL a decrease in cholesterol and phospholipid content, and an increase in triglycerides; for LDL an increase in triglyceride content, but no decrease in cholesterol.

A discrepancy was observed between the values of HDL cholesterol changes measured by precipitation technic and the ultracentrifugation, a finding which suggests modification of the HDL structure and physical properties by Probucol.

Finally, a significant decrease in serum cholesterol is induced by Probucol, a lipid-lowering drug carried by lipoproteins. Previous studies had already shown that the lipoprotein transport play an important role in the mode of action of several hypolipidemic drugs.

Influence of Antithrombotic Drugs on the Uptake of Low Density Lipoproteins by Skin Fibroblasts

Joshua S. K. David, J. P. Noval, R. M. Reichle, and F. A. Reichle

Dept. of Surgery, Presbyterian-University of Pennsylvania Medical Center, Philadelphia, Pennsylvania

Binding of low density (LDL) with receptor sites of skin fibroblasts seems to be important regulatory mechanism for the development of atherosclerosis.

In our laboratory, we have observed that normal skin fibroblasts bind LDL from diabetic peripheral vascular disease (PVD) patients less efficiently (250 ng LDL/mg of cell protein), compared to LDL from non-diabetic PVD patients (378 ng LDL/mg of cell protein), or LDL from control subjects (591 ng of normal LDL/mg of cell protein). Thus it is possible that arteriosclerosis in PVD patients is due to the difference in binding of the LDL by these normal fibroblasts. Next, we studied the influence of aspirin, persantine and dextran on the binding of LDL by the fibroblasts. We have found that aspirin increases the uptake of normal LDL by fourfold. However, aspirin tested at several concentrations did not improve the uptake of LDL by these normal skin fibroblasts. Persantine and dextran also influenced the uptake of only normal LDL but not LDL from PVD patients. These results thus indicate that aspirin, persantine and dextran can be used for prophylactic purpose in normal individuals, but may not be effective in modifying lipid metabolism in PVD patients.

Severe Hypoalphalipoproteinemia Induced by a Combination of Probucol and Clofibrate

J. Davignon, C. A. Nestruck, P. Alaupovic, D. Brossard, and D. Bouthillier

Clinical Research Institute of Montreal, Montreal, Quebec, Canada

The observation of a fall in high density lipoprotein cholesterol (HDL-C) to 5 mg/dL in a familial hypercholesterolemia (FH) patient receiving a combination of clofibrate (2 g/day) and probucol (1 g/day) prompted a review of our lipid clinic records and of the lipoprotein patterns occurring on this combination. Of 32 patients who were given this treatment for extended periods, 25 (10M, 15F) were found in whom a pre-treatment period (A), a period on either drug alone (B) and a combination period (C) could be compared. Mean age during C was 55y (41 to 66y). All subjects first treated with probucol alone in B responded with a significant fall in plasma low density lipoprotein cholesterol (LDL-C) before entering the combination period (C). In 10 subjects HDL-C was 33 ± 6 mg/dL during 84 ± 61 (20-197) weeks of C ($\bar{x}$ ± SD, range) (Group I). In 15 subjects HDL-C was reduced to 7.5 ± 1.4 mg/dL. This effect was noticeable after 29 ± 36 (4-134) weeks of C (Group II). The levels of both apo AI and AII were substantially reduced as HDL-C decreased in group II. The combination resulted in no effect or a small decrease in plasma triglycerides (TG) or very low density lipoprotein cholesterol (VLDL-C) in group I, whereas all but 2 subjects in group II had a striking rise in these parameters. Interestingly although the combination was given for up to 4 years in group II [80.5 ± 59 (15 to 218) weeks] no untoward side effects or clinical deteriorations were noticed in spite of an overall increase in the LDL/HDL ratio from 7.19 ± 1.88 in A to 32.4 ± 15.0 in C, this ratio was either lowered or unchanged in group I. In one case, xanthoma regression was recorded during period C. Until the meaning of this dramatic lowering in HDL-C is established, it is recommended that this parameter be closely monitored in subjects submitted to a combination of clofibrate and probucol.

The Role of Prostaglandins in Carcinogenic Processes

G. Sh. Davitaia, M. I. Jalyabova, K. G. Chavchanidze, M. A. Tsartsidze, and B. A. Lomsadze

Dept. of Biophysics Biology Fac., Tbilisi State University, Tbilisi, U.S.S.R.

The effect of benzo(a)pyrene (BP) on the binding of prostaglandins E and F_{2a} (PGE and PGF_{2a}) and their content has been studied, as well as its action on the quantitative changes of c-AMP, c-GMP and phospholipids of rat liver microsomes. It appeared that a BP enhances the binding of PGE_1 in rat liver microsomes and this binding is a concentration-dependent factor. At the same time, BP decreases the concentration of PGE in microsomes. Simultaneous increase of PGF_{2a} is observed. It is noteworthy that BP decreases phosphatidylcholine content in microsomes and this decrease is in accordance with the changes of PGE content. It should be noted also that BP elevates the content of c-AMP, while the concentration of c-GMP is changed insignificantly.

Possible mechanisms of the involvement of prostaglandins in experimental carcinogenesis are discussed.

The PGI_2 Enhancing Effect of Diuretics is not Correlated with a Direct Cyclooxygenase Stimulation

G. Deby-DuPont , C. Deby , R. H. Bourgain and P. Braquet .

Universite de Liege, Liege, Belgique; Laboratorium voor Fysiologie en Fysiopathologie, Vrije University, Brussel, Belgique; and IBH Research Lab., Le Plessis Robinson, France

Several diuretics are known to activate the synthesis of PGI , as demonstrated on an animal model[1] and on endothelial cell cultures[2]. In order to understand in more detail the mechanism of this activation, we studied the effect of bumetanide, piretanide, ethacrynic acid, cycletanide and its analog BN 50157, on bull seminal cyclooxygenase activity, according to a previously described technique[3]. It appears that certain drugs, exerting a strong stimulating effect on *in-vivo* PGI_2 synthesis (cycletanide and BN 50157) proved to be inhibitors of cyclooxygenase activity *in vitro*. On the other hand, drugs poorly efficient on the *in-vivo* PGI_2 synthesis, were found to be cyclooxygenase activators *in-vitro*.

Other drugs, such as ethacrynic acid, were cyclooxygenase inhibitors at 10^{-3}M, and activators at 10^{-4}M.

It may be concluded that the investigated diuretic agents stimulate PGI_2 synthesis by another mechanism than a direct effect on cylooxygenase.

These findings, together with previous observations, suggest that these diuretic agents affect the interaction of potassium transport and prostacyclin generation.

(1)DEBY et al., Winter Prostaglandins Conference, Keystone, Colorado, Jan. 4-9, 1983.

(2)BRAQUET et al., Winter Prostaglandins Conference, Keystone, Colorado, Jan. 4-9, 1983.

(3)DEBY et al., Biochem. Pharmacol. 24 : 1080, (1975).

Hypertriglyceridemia and Atherosclerosis: Reversal of Abnormal Lipoprotein Profiles with Bezafibrate Treatment

Shlomo Eisenberg

Department of Medicine B, Hadassah University Hospital, Jerusalem, Israel

Because arterioclerosis is common in hypertriglyceridemia (H) but is not due to triglyceride (TG) molecules, the plasma lipoproteins in H were searched for the presence of atherogenic lipoproteins and for the possible effects of bezafibrate (B) treatment on such lipoproteins. H-VLDL is a TG-poor, cholesterol ester (CE)-rich lipoprotein with CE/protein (C/P) ratio of 1.18 (n=0.76) that is highly correlated with plasma TG level (r=0.72). H-LDL is composed of multiple TG-rich fractions, with a main peak that is denser and of smaller size than N-LDL. C/P ratios in H-LDL are 1.0 or less (n=2.0), and estimated density of LDL is negatively correlated with plasma TG level (r=0.85). H-HDL is also denser than N-HDL, is enriched with TG and poor in CE. All these abnormalities can be ascribed to prolonged exposure of the plasma lipoprotein to lipid transfer reactions, predominantly CE-TG transfers. Because H-LDL and H-HDL are CE-poor, they clear from plasma sub-normal amounts of cholesterol that can be as low as 50% of normals. The other 50% of plasma CE is cleared with abnormal CE-rich VLDL via catabolic pathways that bypass LDL (non-LDL pathways). Such pathways are potentially atherogenic. B treatment increases lipoprotein lipase activity, decreases plasma TG levels and is associated with reversal toward normal of all lipoprotein abnormalities.

A Lipomobilizing Thioxanthine with a Negative Inotropic and Chronotropic Effect

G. Fassina, F. Carpenedo, R. M. Gaion, and L. Perissinotto

Dept. of Pharmacology, Padua University, Padua, Italy

The effects of 6-thiocaffeine (S-Caff) and theophylline (Th) were compared in different experimental systems, i.e., adipose tissue lipolysis, fat cell and heart cAMP-phosphodiesterase activities as well as contractility of isolated atria. In rat adipose tissue S-Caff was less potent than Th in stimulating lipolysis directly, but more effective in potentiating norepinephrine-induced lipolysis. S-Caff and Th had similar potencies as competitive inhibitors of cAMP-PDEases isolated from adipocytes. Thus PDEase inhibition does not seem to be strictly related to the lipolytic activity of these compounds. In spontaneously beating guinea-pig atria equimolar concentrations of S-Caff and Th elicited opposite effects. S-Caff caused a dose-dependent decrease of the contractile tension (IC_{50} 0.5 mM) associated with a low chronotropic effect. Again S-Caff and Th were equipotent as inhibitors of calf heart PDEases (IC_{50} 0.15 mM) and their action was not Ca^{2+} dependent. Thus, if the positive inotropic effect of Th is mediated by cAMP-PDEase inhibition, this mechanism is in contradiction with the negative inotropic action of S-Caff.

Apart from the mechanism by which S-Caff affects lipolysis and heart inotropism, the present results indicate that this xanthine derivative potentiates lipomobilization induced by sympathetic neurotransmitter without stimulating the heart. If found to have similar effects in vivo, it might be useful in obesity.

Effects of L-Acetylcarnitine on Fatty Acid and Ceramide Metabolism in Brain

A. Fiumara, M. C. Morale, F. Guerrera, and V. Rizza

Dept. of Pharmacology and Biochemistry, University of Catania Medical School, Catania, Italy

The role of L-carnitine (4-N-trimethylammonium-3-hydroxy-butyric acid) in fatty acid oxidation has been extensively documented. It is generally recognized that L-carnitine is necessary for transport of long chain fatty acid across mitochondrial membranes and plays an important role in striated and cardiac muscle where it is known that fatty acids are preferred substrates for oxidative metabolism in these tissues.

The function of L-carnitine or acetylcarnitine in the nerous tissue has been receiving considerable attention in recent times. We have compared the effects of L-carnitine and acetylcarnitine in brain lipid metabolism after intraventricular administration of ^{3}H stearic acid or ^{3}H oleoylsphingosine. The results show marked differences with time in the distribution of radioactivity in brain phospholipids, cerebrosides and sulfatides. These effects were more prominent with acetylcarnitine as compared to carnitine. These observations pose intriguing possibilities regarding brain fatty acid metabolism as well as turnover of complex lipids associated with membrane structure.

Effect of Mucopolysaccharides (MPS) on Plasma Lipids and Lipoprotein Lipase Activity in Man

C. Fragiacomo, R. Cairoli, L. Margon, E. Massera, P. L. Bernasconi, and G. Noseda

Ospedale Beata Vergine, Mendrisio, Switzerland

The effect of MPS (a new purified Ateroid®) on plasma lipids and lipoprotein lipase activity (LPL) was studied in 12 healthy volunteers with different doses of the drug and different pharmaceutical administration.

a) IV administration of 1 mg/kg, 0.25 mg/kg, 0.0625 mg/kg in 4 subjects: an important increase of LPL with 1 mg/kg (from 0.03 to 1.63 mmol F.F.A.) and with 0.25 mg/kg (from 0.16 to 1.59 mmol F.F.A.) was noted with a simultaneous reduction of plasma triglycerides (from 83.67 to 42.33 mg/dl and respectively from 125.67 to 102.00 mg/dl). Plasma cho lesterol remained unchanged.

b) Peroral administration of 20,000 LRU in 4 subjects: LPL increased from 0.15 to 1.31 mmol F.F.A. (maximum value after 6 h) with a biphasic type of response, together with a reduction of plasma triglycerides from 64 to 54 mg/dl and no change in plasma cholesterol values.

c) Peroral administration of 5000 LRU in 4 subjects: LPL increased from 0.08 to 1.93 mmol F.F.A. (after 6 h) with a subsequent very slow reduc tion of the values which were not completely restored to the basal levels after 8 hours.

d) Peroral administration of 3000 LRU during 14 days in 10 subjects: the increase of LPL levels was confirmed to be statistically significant ($p<0.05$) after 7 and 14 days of treatment (from 0.10 to 0.57, resp. 0.49 mmol F.F.A.) with no change in plasma cholesterol and triglyceri des values.

A further investigation of cholesterol fractions showed after 14 days higher levels of HDL with an increased ratio HDL/LDL+VLDL. These results may suggest that the employed MPS could possibly have a protective effect on vessels as a consequence of stimulation of LPL, activation of the catabolism of LDL and VLDL and increase of HDL.

Clinical Investigation on Antihyperlipidemic Effects of Clinofibrate

Iwao Fukui

Central Laboratory for Clinical Investigation, Kyoto Prefectural University of Medicine, Kyoto, Japan

In order to determine the optimal dose in clinical application, antihyperlipidemic potency of clinofibrate was investigated between the daily dose of 300 mg and 600 mg. The reduction of serum cholesterol by clinofibrate was dose-related, whereas the reduction of serum triglyceride was the similar level over 20% at both doses. As to serum lipoproteins, clinofibrate produced a significant increase of HDL_2 cholesterol together with a significant reduction of cholesterol and triglycerides in VLDL and LDL. This drug also caused a significant increase of plasma apoprotein A-I but did not influence the level of apoprotein A-II. Inhibitory effect of clinofibrate on platelets aggregation was observed in patients with diabetes mellitus. These results suggest that clinofibrate at 600 mg/day is useful in the therapy of hyperlipidemia and hyperlipidemic diabetes.

Lecithinated Soy Protein Lowers Cholesterolemia and Exerts A "Normalizing" Activity on HDL-Cholesterol Levels

A. Gaddi, G. C. Descovich, G. Noseda, C. Fragiacomo, F. S. Feruglio, L. Cattin, E. Gatti, A. Strano, G. Weber, M. Sirtori, and C. R. Sirtori

Collaborating Clinics from Bologna, Milan, Trieste, Siena, Mendrisio, and Palermo (Italy and Switzerland), c/o Center E. Grossi Paoletti, University of Milan, Italy

Substitution of animal proteins with textured soy proteins has been repeatedly shown to remarkably reduce cholesterolemia in type II patients. In the majority of the studies, however, reductions of total cholesterolemia were not accompanied by significant changes in high density lipoprotein (HDL) cholesterol (CHOL) levels (Descovich et al., Lancet ii, 704, 1980). A new textured soy product (CHOLSOY L), containing 6% by weight of lecithin, was tested in 65 patients (29 M and 36 F) with plasma CHOL in excess of 300 mg/dl, previously kept for at least 3 months on a standard low lipid-low cholesterol regimen. The experiment was carried out in four phases, each of 4-week duration: I. traditional hypocholesterolemic regimen; II. total substitution of animal proteins with lecithinated soy proteins; III. same as phase I.; IV. partial substitution (40-50%) of the animal proteins. During phase I of the study, plasma CHOL was reduced only 2.4% in males and 5.1% in females, whereas after phase II (total substitution) the reduction was 22.4% in males and 20.27% in females, both $p<0.001$. During phase III, a slow return to baseline was noted in all patients, whereas phase IV (partial substitution) was accompanied by a reduction of 14.4% in males and 12.2% in females. LDL-CHOL levels paralleled the change in total cholesterol, whereas an increase of HDL-CHOL was noted during the phase II of the study (+7.6% in males and +8.9% in females), followed by a modest reduction during phase III and an increase during phase IV, thus making the overall change highly significant. By dividing patients into those with low, intermediate or high HDL-CHOL levels, only in the two lower tertiles, was a significant increase noted with the regimen. A significant beneficial effect on HDL cholesterolemia may be exerted by lecithinated soy proteins in patients with low starting HDL-CHOL levels.

Dietary Intervention Studies, Serum Lipids and Platelet Thromboxane I. North Karelia Study

C. Galli , E. Tremoli , A. Petroni , R. Dougherty , P. Puska and J. Iacono

Institute of Pharmacology and Pharmacognosy, University of Milan, Italy; Beltsville (USA) and Helsinki, Finland

A dietary intervention study was carried out in Liperi, North Karelia. After a two-week baseline period (B), 30 normal couples consumed for a six-week period (I), a diet with a lower content of total fat, saturated fat and cholesterol, and a higher content of polyunsaturated fat (higher P/S) in respect to the usual diet. A six-week switch back period (SB) followed. During B and SB, the subjects consumed the usual diet. Serum lipids (T-Ch, LDL-Ch, HDL-Ch, TG) (Table 1), and TxB_2 formation in collagen-stimulated platelets (Table 2) were measured at the end of each period.

(SEE TABLE)

Conclusions: Dietary intervention significantly reduced serum T-Ch, LDL and HDL-Ch in both sexes. In females, HDL/LDL-Ch increased more than in males, during I, and remained elevated during SB. TxB_2 production was reduced only in males, during I, and was unexpectly reduced in females during SB. Correlations between dietary fat, serum lipids and platelet TxB_2 are discussed.

- Supported by USDA

Table I. Serum Lipid Levels (mg/dl)

	MALES			FEMALES		
	B	I	SB	B	I	SB
T-Ch	263	201+	259	239	188+	231
LDL-Ch	185	137+	183	164	125+	156
HDL-Ch	54	44+	55	56	47+	60
HDL/LDL-Ch	0.29	0.32	0.30	0.34	0.38	0.38
TG	124	96	99	91	76	76

+Different from B and SB.

Table II. TxB_2 (pg/10^9 Platelets)[1]

MALES			FEMALES		
B	I	SB	B	I	SB
449°	367°	388	397	441°	335°

[1]2 min. after 10 /ug/ml collagen.
°Different from each other.

Dietary Intervention Studies, Serum Lipids and Platelet Thromboxane. II. South Italy Study.

C. Galli , E. Tremoli , A. Socini , P. Maderna , S. Colli , A. Ferro-Luzzi, M. Mancini, and J. Iacono

Inst. of Pharmacology and Pharmacognosy, University of Milan; Rome; Naples; and Beltsville (USA).

A dietary intervention study was carried out in Pollica, South Italy. After a two-week baseline period (B), 28 normal couples consumed, for a six-week period (I), a diet with a higher content of total fat, saturated fat (lower P/S) and cholesterol in respect to the usual diet. A six-week switch back period (SB) followed. During the B and SB periods, the subjects consumed the usual diet. Serum lipids (T-Ch, LDL-Ch, HDL-Ch, TG) (Table 1) and TxB_2 formation in collagen stimulated platelets (Table 2) were measured at the end of each period.

(SEE TABLE)

<u>Conclusions</u>: Dietary intervention significantly raised T-Ch and LDL-Ch in both sexes, but HDL-Ch was raised only in females. HDL/LDL-Ch was reduced only in males. During SB, T-Ch and LDL-Ch returned to B values in both sexes. HDL/LDL-Ch did not change in females. TxB_2 production was decreased in males during SB and remained unchanged in females in all periods.

Combined studies show: a) different response of HDL-Ch to dietary fats in males and females, b) TxB_2 production is more affected in males especially when dietary P/S ratio is increased (I in North Karelia, SB in Italy).

- Supported by USDA

Table 1. Serum Lipid Levels (mg/dl)

	MALE			FEMALE		
	B	I	SB	B	I	SB
T-Ch	207	246+	190	177	206+	172
LDL-Ch	148	188+	133	124	146+	120
HDL-Ch	40	41	42	43	51+	42
HDL/LDL-Ch	0.27	0.22	0.32	0.35	0.35	0.35
TG	137	166	151	91	97	98

+Different from B and SB.

Table 2. TxB_2 (pg/10^9 Platelets)[1]

MALE			FEMALE		
B	I	SB	B	I	SB
366	400	253°	390	370	328

[1] 2 min.after 10 /ug/ml collagen.
°$p < 0.05$ from B and I.

Pharmacokinetics and Metabolism of L 44 (2-*tert*-butyl-4-cyclohexyl-phenyl Nicotinate) in Rats

G. Galli, E. Bosisio, and W. Schatton

Inst. Pharmacology and Pharmacognosy, University of Milan, Italy, and Merz & Co., Research Dept., Frankfurt/Main, Germany

The pharmacokinetics and metabolism of [^{14}C] labelled L 44 (2-*tert*-butyl-4-cyclo-hexyl-[U-^{14}C] phenylnicotinate) were studied in rats after i.v. and oral administration of 0.2 mg of [^{14}C] L 44 (26.5 uC/mg). Radioactivity was evaluated in serum, urines, feces and tissues.

From the decay of radioactivity in serum of i.v. treated animals, the half-lives of the distribution and elimination phases and the area under the plasma curve (AUC) were calculated according to a two compartment open model.

The half-lives of and phases were 10.7 min. and 7.4 hrs., respectively. AUC was 406 700 DPM ml $^{-1}$. hr., and the recovery of radioactivity in urines and feces 24 hrs. after administration was 11.7 $\pm$ 4.9% and 15.4 $\pm$ 6.2%, respectively (mean $\pm$ S.E.). When [^{14}C] L 44 was administered orally, the elimination half-life was 15.2 hrs., and the recovery of radioactivity in urines and feces 24 hrs. after administration was 11.6 $\pm$ 2.8 and 36.1 $\pm$ 3.5, respectively (mean $\pm$ S.E.).

The radioactivity in plasma was associated with L 44 and its metabolite L 44 phenol (2-*tert*-butyl-4-cyclohexylphenol). In urines, radioactivity was associated with a polar metabolite which structure is under investigation. In feces both the L 44 phenol and the polar metabolite were present. The amount of L 44 phenol was 60% and 40% of the radioactivity recovered in feces after i.v. and oral treatment, respectively.

The Soybean Protein Diet Maintains A Normal Number of Liver Lipoprotein Receptors During A Dietary Cholesterol Challenge

G. Galli, C. R. Sirtori, E. Bosisio, P. Carrara, and M. Galli-Kienle

Institute of Pharmacology and Pharmacognosy and Dept. of Medical Chemistry and Biochemistry, University of Milan, Milan, Italy

The soybean protein diet lowers cholesterolemia in most animal species fed cholesterol. Similarly, in man, only patients with significant hypercholesterolemia appear to respond. Among the different mechanisms, those related to the aminoacid composition (arginine richness, low lysine/arginine ratio) have received the most support. Based on recent evidence for a regulatory role of liver lipoprotein receptors in lowering cholesterolemia (Kovanen et al., J. Biol. Chem. 254, 11367, 1979), Sprague Dawley female rats received a cholesteremic regimen, specifically designed to cause a moderate hypercholesterolemia without fatty liver (Terpstra et al., Atherosclerosis 42, 85, 1982), with either soybean (S) protein or casein (C). Plasma lipid-lipoproteins and liver lipids were monitored, together with determination of the liver affinity binding curve for ^{125}I-β-VLDL from CHOL. fed rabbits. Finally, enzyme activities of the liver lipoprotein receptor pathway were analyzed. Plasma CHOL. levels were raised approximately 70% by C, compared to controls, and brought back to the normal range by S; major changes occurred in VLDL-lipids, almost 10-fold higher with the C diet and normal with S. A 50% lowering of the Bmax for rabbit β-VLDL was noted in the C group; Bmax was normal in the S treated animals; Kd did not change with either regimen. A significant depression of liver HMG CoA reductase activity was noted in C treated animals, whereas S treated rats only showed a slight decrease. ACAT activity was markedly elevated in the C group and normal in S; similarly cholesterol 7 α-hydroxylase rose with C and was normal with S diet. These findings suggest that the S diet, even in the presence of a dietary cholesterol challenge, maintains a normal receptorial activity in the liver, avoiding the down-regulation exerted by C.

HCG 497, An Effective Novel Class Lipoprotein Regulator

E. Granzer, K. Mueller, and H.-J. Lang

HOECHST AG, Frankfurt/Main, Germany and CIBA-GEIGY AG, Basle, Switzerland

Hoechst-Ciba-Geigy 497 (HCG 497), 2-chloro-N, N-dimethyl-5-[3-methyl-2-(phenyl-imino)-4-thiazolin-yl]-benzenesulfonamide, is a lipoprotein regulator which effectively lowers the atherogenic lipoprotein fractions in animals without affecting HDL. Notably, HCG 497 is free of side effects which is particularly important with respect to the liver. In normal rats and pigs, it decreases LDL. In rats it also decreases VLDL.

Male rats 7 days p.o. 10 [30]mg/kg: LDL-C -29 [-43%], VLDL-TG -23 [-36%]

male miniature swine 14 days p.o. 20 [60]mg/kg: LDL-C -27 [-27]%, LDL-Prot. -19 [-34]%

HCG 497 also lowers increased concentrations of LDL and VLDL in genetically hypercholesterolemic rat strains.

Male RICO-rats 7 days p.o. 10 [30]mg/kg: LCL-C -23 [-49]% male HBC-rats 7 days p.o. 30[100]mg/kg: LDL-C -24 [-43]%

Furthermore, HCG 497 displays hypolipidemic activity in various forms of experimentally induced hyperlipidemias: fructose or triton® induced hypertriglyceridemia of rats, hypercholesterolemia induced by dietetic cholesterol supplementation in rats and rabbits.

The overall pharmacological investigations did not reveal any undesired or adverse effects which would preclude the further development of HCG 497. HCG 497 is non-toxic in rats and mice (LD_{50} p.o.>4g/kg). In a 4-week tolerability study in rats at 3 and 30 mg/kg/day, p.o. HCG 497 was well tolerated.

Clinical Pharmacology of etofibrate

A. Gustafson

Med. Dept., University of Lund, Lund, Sweden

The results obtained with etofibrate in a decade of clinical atherosclerosis research are presented in survey form.

Etofibrate effectively lowers cholesterol and triglycerides. This is largely attributable to a reduction of the vasoaggressive LDL and its precursors, the VLDL. Inversely, the protective HDL are elevated. This results in a reduction of the atherogenic index, a direct indicator of the atherosclerotic risk.

Etofibrate promotes the conditions necessary for the degradation of accumulated triglyceride-rich lipoproteins by elevating the LPL activity and its apoprotein C II and simultaneously lowering the inhibitory C III peptides.

As a result of the inhibition of the HMG-CoA-reductase activity, the reduction of plasma cholesterol can be intensified by administering etofibrate in the evening.

The reduction of the prostaglandin derivative thromboxane and the elevation of prostacyclin observed under etofibrate would lead to an inhibition of the platelet aggregation and to improvements in vessel reactivity as well as in blood pressure.

The treatment of the concomitant diseases that frequently accompany hyperlipoproteinaemias - diabetes mellitus, hyperuricaemia, and hypertension - is supported under the influence of etofibrate by reduction of the blood sugar, the blood pressure, and the uric acid.

Etofibrate therefore affects nearly all the important processes involved in the pathogenesis of atherosclerosis and is thus excellently suited for the prevention and treatment of atherosclerosis and cardiovascular diseases in particular.

It is hoped that substances such as etofibrate with broad action spectra would be used to an increasing extent for the treatment of atherosclerosis.

Effects of Pantethine on Serum Lipids and Lipoproteins - A Collaborative Study on 871 Patients with Dyslipidemias

Yoshiya Hata

Dept. of Medicine, Keio University School of Medicine, Tokyo, Japan

To elucidate the clinical utility of pantethine for the treatment of dyslipidemias, a collaborative study was performed with 124 doctors from 107 institutions and hospitals. A daily dose level of 600 mg was given for 12 weeks to 936 patients with dyslipidemias. Forty-four cases (5%) who did not meet the entry criteria were omitted from the study, and 21 subjects (3%) dropped out. The remaining 871 patients, 428 male and 443 female, were subjected to evaluation for the clinical utility of the drug.

Pantethine decreased on an average of 19 mg/dl (7%) of total cholesterol, 26 mg/dl (6%) of triglycerides, and increased 4 mg/dl (12%) of HDL-cholesterol. All of these changes were statitically significant at the level of 0.1% when compared with the initial levels. The unit dose effect, e.g., the change in lipids caused by 100 mg of pantethine, turned out to be 3.5 mg/dl for total cholesterol, 5.8 mg/dl for triglycerides, and 0.7 mg/dl for HDL-cholesterol. The effective response rates, the ratio of the number of cases whose unit dose effect was positive over that of negative ones were 84% for total cholesterol, 79% for triglycerides and 85% for HDL-cholesterol.

The adverse symptoms and signs observed in this study were 19 cases (2%). The global utility rate judged by the participant doctors was 50%. This data was a little lower than that observed in the double blind study, but a large number of patients supported the clinical utility of pantethine.

Probucol Inhibits The Calcium-Dependent Potasssium Channel in Human Erythrocytes

J. L. Howland and J. N. Daughety

Committee on Biochemistry, Bowdoin College, Brunswick, Maine

Erythrocytes from many mammalian species exhibit a potassium conductance which depends upon the calcium concentration in the cell interior. The operational definition of this channel is the dramatic increase in potassium efflux that occurs when cells or ghosts are treated with calcium plus the ionophore, A23187 (the "Gardos effect"). This channel, which appears to occur in a wide variety of excitable cells, as well, is also defined by its sensitivity to quinine and its isomers, compounds which also exhibit antiarrythmic activity. We have estimated the _in vitro_ flux through the channel by following potassium exit from washed erythrocytes with a potassium-sensitive electrode after treatment with 1 mM calcium chloride plus 4.0 μM A23187. We find that Probucol, recently said to produce quinine-like effects upon heart conduction, also blocks the calcium-sensitive potassium flux with 50% inhibition at a concentration of about 250 μM.

Efficacy of Mevinolin Plus Colestipol in the Treatment of Severe Heterozygous Familial Hypercholesterolemia

D. Roger Illingworth

Division of Endocrinology, Metabolism, and Clinical Nutrition, Dept. of Medicine, Oregon Health Sciences University, Portland, Oregon

Eight patients with severe heterozygous familial hypercholesterolemia, in whom other hypolipidemic drugs had failed to lower serum cholesterol values below 300 mg/dl, were sequentially treated with mevinolin (a specific inhibitor of HMG CoA reductase, the rate-limiting enzyme in cholesterol biosynthesis) and colestipol. Concentrations of plasma cholesterol decreased from 462 $\pm$ 40 mg/dl on diet only to 322 $\pm$ 47 mg/dl on mevinolin (20-40 mg twice daily) and fell to 260 $\pm$ 39 mg/dl with subsequent addition of colestipol (15-30 gm/day). These changes were reflected by decreases in the concentrations of LDL cholesterol which declined 36% on mevinolin. Subsequent addition of colestipol resulted in a further 29% decrease so that values on the combined regimen were 54% below those on diet only. Concentrations of triglycerides of HDL cholesterol did not change significantly on either the single or combined drug regimens. The regimen has been well tolerated by all patients and no consistent biochemical abnormalities have been noted during 5-8 months of therapy. If long-term safety can be established, specific inhibitors of HMG CoA reductase, used in combination with a bile acid binding resin, offer considerable promise in the therapy of heterozygous familial hypercholesterolemia.

The Effect of Clinofibrate on the Apo C Subspecies and Lipids Composition in Very Low Density Lipoprotein

T. Ishikawa, H. Nakamura, N. Tada, N. Suzuki, K. Kondo, N. Fidge and P. J. Nestel

Jikei University, Aoto Hospital, Katsushika, Tokyo, Japan and Baker Medical Research Institute, Melbourne, Australia

Forty hyperlipidemic patients (Type IIa:17, IIb:11, and Type IV:12) were administered 600mg of Clinofibrate [2,2'-(4,4'-cyclohexylidenediphenoxy)-2,2'-dimethyldibutyric acid] daily for 4 weeks.

After the administration of Clinofibrate, plasma triglyceride decreased significantly in all groups and HDL-cholesterol and HDL-cholesterol/(VLDL+LDL)-cholesterol ratio increased significantly in type IV groups.

VLDL-TG, VLDL-PL and VLDL-TG/VLDL-protein ratio decreased after the administration.

Analysis of the distribution in apoprotein C subspecies of VLDL by isoelectric focusing showed the increase in apo CII and the decrease in apo $CIII_0$, and the increase in apo CII/apo CIII ratio ($P<0.02$). These changes were similar to those observed during the accelerated removal of TG rich lipoprotein by the administration of heparin.

Apolipoprotein AI, AII, B and E have been measured.

These results support the hypothesis that one of the main mechanisms of Clinofibrate in lowering plasma lipids is the acceleration of the removal of VLDL.

The Effect of Clinofibrate on Serum Lipids and Lipoproteins in Hyperlipoproteinemias

Hiroshige Itakura, Tatsuhiko Kodama, Takashi Moriyama, Toshio Murase, and Fumimaro Takaku

The Third Dept. of Internal Medicine, Faculty of Medicine, University of Tokyo, Hongo, Tokyo, Japan

The effect of clinofibrate on serum lipids, lipoprotein fractions and lipoproteins have been investigated in hyperlipoproteinemias. The patients received clinofibrate at a dosage of 600 mg per day divided into three times. The subjects were ambulant and blood analysis were performed monthly.

Cholesterol and triglycerides were measured by enzymatic methods in whole serum and in the individual lipoprotein fractions, very low density lipoprotein (VLDL), low density lipoprotein (LDL) and high density lipoprotein (HDL_2 and HDL_3), after sequential ultracentrifugation. Measurement of apo-AI, apo-AII and apo-B were performed on commercial plates (Daiichi Pure Chemical and Behringwerke).

The administration of clinofibrate of hyperlipoproteinemic patients resulted in significant decreased triglyceride concentrations. The tendency of decrease of serum total cholesterol and increase of HDL cholesterol were observed. In the majority of cases, the ratio of VLDL+LDL cholesterol to HDL cholesterol were decreased after treatment with clinofibrate. Significant changes were noted in the ratio of HDL cholesterol to apo-AI and the ratio of VLDL+LDL cholesterol to apo-B. The ratio of HDL cholesterol to apo-AI was increased and the ratio of VLDL+LDL cholesterol to apo-B was decreased in most cases.

These changes of cholesterol distribution among lipoprotein fractions may be beneficial for prevention of atherosclerosis. Side effects were minimal. Clinofibrate appears to be a safe and effective hypolipidemic agent.

Effects of Probucol on Serum Lipoprotein Levels and Very Low Density Apolipoprotein Compositions in Heterozygous Patients with Familial Hypercholesterolemia

Hideaki Ito, Hiroshi Mabuchi, and Ryoyu Takeda

The Second Department of Internal Medicine, Kanazawa University School of Medicine, Ishikawa, Japan

We studied the effects of probucol on serum lipoprotein levels and very low density apolipoprotein compositions in ten heterozygous patients with familial hypercholesterolemia. During the eight weeks' treatment with probucol at the dose of 1.0 g per day, serum cholesterol decreased from 313 ± 15 to 270 ± 19 mg/dl, (mean ± S.E.M.; $p<0.001$). Intermediate density lipoprotein (IDL) and high density lipoprotein (HDL) cholesterol decreased from 19 ± 4 to 14 ± 2, ($p<0.05$) and 54 ± 4 to 39 ± 2, ($p<0.01$), respectively. Serum triglyceride slightly decreased, while low density lipoprotein (LDL) triglyceride decreased significantly, ($p<0.05$). On isoelectric focusing patterns of apo-VLDL, the ratio of apoprotein CII to apoprotein CIII increased from 0.22 ± 0.03 to 0.34 ± 0.03 and the ratio of apoprotein E to apoprotein C decreased significantly from 0.56 ± 0.11 to 0.30 ± 0.04, ($p<0.05$). These results suggest that probucol not only lowers serum cholesterol levels, but also changes compositions of apo-VLDL.

Effect of Long Term Treatment by Probucol on Xanthomas and Skin Cholesterol

B. Jacotot, J. L. Beaumont, J. C. Buxtorf, V. Beaumont, and L. Edouard

Inserm U 32, Hopital Henri Mondor, Creteil Cedex, France

Thirty patients having Type II hyperlipoproteinemia with tendinous xanthomas or xanthelasmas, were treated by probucol (1g/day) during 1 to 5 years. The mean serum lipid levels before treatment were: cholesterol 10.6±0.50 mmol/l; HDL cholesterol 1.20±0.10 mmol/l; triglycerides 1.70± 0.90 mmol/l. After 1 year of treatment the following changes were observed: total cholesterol -12.25 percent ($P<0.001$); HDL cholesterol -34 percent ($P<0.001$); triglycerides 6.7 percent (N.S.).

Tendinous xanthomas were noted in 28 subjects. Their evolution was recorded by photographs and by echographs of the Achilles tendons. A regression was observed in 20 cases, generally as early as the first year of treatment, but became really obvious only after 18 months to 2 years of treatment. There were tuberous xanthomas in 4 cases and they decreased markedly in all cases. A xanthelasma was present in 8 subjects and it decreased or completely disappeared in 6 cases.

Skin biopsies were taken from 10 subjects to measure cutaneous free cholesterol (FC) and cholesterol esters (CE). The mean skin free cholesterol level was 3.59±0.57 mg/g of dry tissue before treatment and it increased by 8 percent after 1 year of treatment with probucol. The mean skin cholesterol ester level was 1.39±0.35 mg/g of dry tissue before treatment and increased by 23 percent after treatment. The esterification ratio of the skin cholesterol (CE/TC) was 0.28 before treatment and increased by 28 percent after probucol.

In some subjects the measures of skin cholesterol were made after 2 and 3 years of treatment. In these cases there was a marked decrease in free cholesterol, while cholesterol esters decreased only weakly, so that the CE/TC ratio continued to increase, reaching 0.50 after 2 years of probucol.

In conclusion, it is obvious that long-term treatment by probucol induces a strong regression of xanthomas and xanthelasmas in most subjects having a Type II hyperlipoproteinemia with cutaneous or tendinous lipid deposition. In addition, this treatment brings about a change in the skin cholesterol, mainly an increase of the CE/TC ratio, which is perhaps associated with the favourable effect of the drug on the tissue cholesterol deposition.

Effect Of A Novel Hypocholesterolemic Agent, Poloxalene 2930, On Cholesterol And Protein Lipoprotein Distribution

B. Kapuscinska, W. J. Bochenek, E. Kyriakides, S. Friday, and J. B. Rodgers

Albany Medical College, Dept. of Medicine, Albany, New York

We have previously shown that hydrophobic non-ionic surfactants can prevent the development of atherosclerosis in animals, inhibit intestinal fat absorption and lower serum cholesterol level. We now report on the effects of one of these surfactants, Poloxalene 2930, on serum lipoproteins in rabbits.

Three groups of animals were fed one of the following diets: Gp A -regular rabbit chow, Gp B - atherogenic diet containing 5% neutral fat and 0.5% cholesterol, Gp C - atherogenic diet plus 1% Poloxalene 2930. After 10 weeks serum cholesterol (mg%) and its distribution (% of total) among lipoproteins was as follows:

(SEE TABLE)

Protein levels in all three lipoproteins in general paralleled the changes in cholesterol levels, with the exception of VLDL in Gp B where the cholesterol/protein ratio was higher than in the other groups.

It is concluded that Poloxalene 2930 is capable of preventing hypercholesterolemia induced by diet, and in the treated animals HDL becomes the major cholesterol carrying lipoprotein.

Table I.

p	Total Cholestrerol	VLDL	LDL	HDL
A	65.1 ± 22.1	15.8 ± 9.5	55.6 ± 19.4	28.6 ± 6.1
B	912.2 ± 221.4	49.6 ± 20.2	45.6 ± 19.3	4.8 ± 1.6
C	59.5 ± 16.1*	21.0 ± 6.6*	36.0 ± 10.6	43.0 ± 12.5*

* $p < 0.05$ C vs. B   # $p < 0.05$ C vs. A

Effect of Probucol (4'4-isopropylidenedithiobis) (2-6-di-t-butylphenol) and Etofibrate on HDL-composition in Patients with Hyperlipoproteinemia

G. Klose, B. Gniesmer, W. Daerr, E. Steinhagen-Thiessen, and H. Greten

Universitatskrankenhaus Hamburg-Eppendorf, Medizinische Kernklinik und Poliklinik, Hamburg, Germany

The lipid-lowering effect of clofibrate and related compounds may be accompanied by even elevated plasma HDL-cholesterol concentrations. Following Probucol (P) administration, however, not only a decrease of LDL-cholesterol levels could be observed, but also HDL-cholesterol fell significantly. Despite the evidence about the prognostic significiance of elevated HDL-cholesterol from epidemiological studies, the clinical response to P in patients with FH (xanthoma regression) might suggest a possible effect as an antiatherosclerotic agent.

This study was designed to evaluate the effect of P on plasma lipoproteins with special emphasis on HDL composition. Thirty patients with primary hyperlipoproteinemia (Phenotype IIa/IIb) were randomized to 3 months of treatment with either P or Etofibrate (E) following an 8-week dietary period. Total and LDL-cholesterol was reduced with P (-14% and -7%, respectively) and E (-7% and -3%, respectively) in addition to diet, but an increase could be observed during further treatment. HDL-cholesterol and Apo AI decreased in all subjects (-26% and 32.5%, respectively) after P, but were found increased after E.

HDL_2 as measured by zonal centrifugation showed a 99% decrease. Triglycerides, VLDL and HDL_3-trends were variable. The mean QT_c-interval was elevated under P, but this was also true following the administration of the clofibrate derivative.

It is concluded that P is a well tolerated cholesterol lowering agent that reduces LDL-cholesterol and Apo B. The clinical significance of the concomitant fall of the HDL due to a decrease of apoprotein AI, AII and HDL_2 remains to be determined.

Influence of Dehydroepiandrosterone (DHEA) on Cholesterol Metabolism in Rats

David M. Klurfeld[1], Shirley A. Tepper[1], David Kritchevsky[1], and Arthur G. Schwartz[2]

DHEA has been reported to reduce triglyceridemia and weight gain in mice; to inhibit cholesterol synthesis in guinea pig mammary tissue; and not to affect cholesterolemia in normal rats.

We have fed DHEA (0.5%) to male Wistar rats maintained on a semipurified diet containing 54% sucrose (53.4% of calories), 25% casein (24.5% of calories), 10% corn oil (22.1% of calories), 5% salt mix, 5% cellulose and 1% mineral mix. Control rats received an additional 0.5% sucrose.

In the first experiment, the rats (7 per group) were also fed 0.5% cholesterol (replacing the same amount of corn oil). The duration of feeding was 14 days. DHEA significantly reduced weight gain but increased relative liver size. Serum cholesterol was elevated in the DHEA-treated rats (122 $\pm$ 8 vs. 70 $\pm$ 4 mg/dl), but liver triglyceride levels were reduced (196 $\pm$ 42 vs. 507 $\pm$ 95 mg/100 g). Cholesterol absorption was 29% lower in the DHEA-fed rats ($p<0.05$).

In a second experiment, dietary cholesterol was deleted. Weight gain was again significantly reduced in the treated rats, and serum cholesterol levels were elevated (131 vs. 99 mg/dl). Both liver cholesterol and triglyceride levels were reduced significantly in the rats fed DHEA. Liver slices from treated rats converted more radioacetate to cholesterol than did slices from control rats, but there were no differences in cholesterogenesis from labeled mevalonic acid.

DHEA increases serum cholesterol levels despite the fact that it reduces cholesterol absorption and increases the excretion of neutral steroids in the feces. The findings suggest that the effects of DHEA on cholesterol metabolism may be mediated at the level of transport or exchange with tissue cholesterol.

(Supported, in part, by NIH grants HL-03299, CA-14661, and AG-00368 and Research Career Award HL-00734.)

[1]Wistar Institute, Philadelphia, PA [2]Temple University, Philadelphia, PA

Effects of Unmodified and Time-Release Forms of Niacin on Lipoproteins in Hyperlipidemic Subjects

Robert H. Knopp, James T. Ogilvie, G. Russell Warnick, and John J. Albers

Northwest Lipid Research Clinic, Seattle, Washington

The effects of unmodified vs. time-release niacin (Nicolar vs. Nicobid, Armour) on drug adherence, side effects, triglyceride (TG), low density lipoprotein cholesterol (LDL), high density lipoprotein cholesterol (HDL), HDL_2 and HDL_3 and apoproteins A_I and A_{II} has been examined in a 6-month randomized, diet-controlled study of 71 hypercholesterolemic and hypertriglyceridemic subjects (>90th percentile). Subjects randomized to Nicolar and Nicobid matched closely on anthropomorphic and lipid variables. At a target dose of 3 g/day, adherence to Nicolar was 90.2% but only 63.8% to Nicobid, because Nicobid has more adverse gastrointestinal side effects despite less symptomatic flushing than Nicolar. Comparing Nicolar vs. Nicobid, TG was reduced 27% vs. 8%, LDL was reduced 21% vs. 13%, and HDL was increased 26% vs. 9%. In both groups, HDL_3 increased 30%, apo A_I 12%, and apo A_{II} was unchanged. HDL_2 increased significantly (37%) only in the Nicolar group. We conclude that Nicolar can be more successfully taken than Nicobid and that the greater efficacy of Nicolar on TG, whole HDL and HDL_2 levels cannot be wholly explained by differences in drug adherence. Also, Niacin and Nicobid differed in their effect on TG, LDL, HDL and HDL_2. Therefore, the mechanisms by which Nicobid and Nicolar act on lipids and lipoproteins appear to differ.

Probucol and Colestipol Treatment of Patients with Familial Hypercholesterolemia

P. T. Kuo and A. C. Wilson

University of Medicine and Dentistry of New Jersey, Rutgers Medical School, New Brunswick, New Jersey

In this study, the effects of probucol and colestipol alone and in combination were assessed. Forty-four FH patients with toal cholesterol (TC) $\leq$280 mg/dl, low density lipoprotein-cholesterol (LDL-C) $\leq$190 mg/dl entered the study. Following an 8-week therapeutic diet period, the patients were randomly assigned to either probucol (1 gm), or colestipol (30 gm), per day. After 5 months, all of the patients were given the combined two-drug/diet therapy which will be continued for 7 months.

(SEE TABLE)

The therapeutic diet alone lowered TC and LDL-C only slightly. Supplementation of the diet with either drug significantly reduced TC and LDL-C from the baseline vaules. Probucol treatment also reduced HDL-C an average of 30.1%, while colestipol treatment had no effect.

Three months of the combined two-drug/diet treatment markedly lowered the LDL-C, compared with the mean baseline values, but also resulted in decreased HDL. Follow-up study suggests a more definitive additive effect existing between the long-term use of two-drug treatment. Serial quantitative arteriograms are needed to determine the anti-atherosclerotic value of the proposed therapy.

Table I.

CHOLESTEROL AND TRIGLYCERIDE: Group Mean % Changes From Visit 1

Treatment	Total C	LDL-C	HDL-C	Total TG
Diet Only	- 6.9	- 7.9	+ 1.6	+ 6.9
Diet + Probucol	-30.9	-19.9	-30.1	+ 3.6
Diet + Colestipol	-31.6	-32.5	- 2.0	+ 8.8
Diet + Probucol + Colestipol	-34.3	-40.6	-35.1	+16.0

Effect of Glycyrrhizin on Lysosomal Enzymes in Rat Arterial Wall

Akira Kumagai, Yasuko Shiki, Kohji Shirai, and Yasushi Saito

The Second Dept. of Internal Medicine, Chiba University School of Medicine, Chiba, and Toyama Medical-Pharmaceutical University, Japan

It has been reported that Glycyrrhizin inhibits the elevation of plasma total cholesterol level and reduces the formation of atheroma in the lanolin-loaded rabbits. To clarify the mechanisms of the antiatherosclerotic action of Glycyrrhizin, the effects of Glycyrrhizin on lysosomal enzyme activities, which were involved in the lipid metabolism of rat arterial wall, were investigated.

Glycyrrhizin did not affect the uptake and the hydrolysis of cholesteryl [^{14}C]oleate-labelled LDL in smooth muscle cells. Acid cholesterol esterase (acid CEase) activity was decreased by the addition of 0.25 mM Glycyrrhizin. Glycyrrhetinic acid which is the aglicone from Glycyrrhizin did not change acid CEase activity. Phospholipase A_2 (PLase A_2) activity increased in hypercholesterolemic rat arterial wall. PLase A_2-treatment of arterial lysosomal fraction increased the releases of acid phosphatase (AcPase) and acid CEase from the lysosome. By the addition of Glycyrrhizin to PLase A_2-treatment of lysosomal fraction, the release of AcPase from the lysosome was suppressed.

From these results, it was suggested that Glycyrrhizin may stabilize the lysosome by inhibiting PLase A_2 activity.

Fat Overloaded Syndrome: Clinical, Histoenzymological and Biochemical Data

A. Lageron, M. Beaugrand, and P. Callard

INSERM U9, Paris, France

Total parenteral nutrition (TPN) was administered concurrently to a 60-year old woman and a 26-year old man. Mrs. A had a sub-occlusive syndrome following radiotherapy for cervix carcinoma; Mr. K was also suffering from a sub-occlusion as an episode of Crohn disease. Both patients received identical TPN: one flask daily composed of 2000 ml of 10% glucose, 500 ml of Azonutril 25, 125 ml of 20% Intralipid, electrolytes, and vitamins. Six weeks later hepatic dysfunction appeared with an increase in transaminases, alkaline phosphatases, γ GT and bilirubin. Histological, histoenzymological, ultrastructural (1 case) and biochemical (1 case) data led to the diagnosis of fat overload syndrome and the identification of its lipid components. The main change in these livers occurred in the reticulo endothelial system. Kupffer cells were enlarged and filled with free fatty acids (FFA) stained by oil red, Sudan black and Holczinger's reaction, blue with Nile Blue, black-brown with OTAN but disappearing after mild alkaline hydrolysis. The unsaturated form of these FFA suggested by the positive peracetic-Schiff was confirmed with GLC of the FFA isolated in TLC of the liver lipid extract showing an increase of 183.2% of linoleic acid. Ultrastructure revealed some Kupffer filled with rounded, homogeneous $\pm$ osmiophilic inclusions. Lysosomal enzymes were hyperactive in all macrophages. In hepatocytes, the increase of numerous enzymatic activities indicated hypermetabolism. Many hepatocytes in centrolobular areas were overloaded with brownish pigments containing phospholipids (Baker's reaction) and triglycerides (Adams-). In lipid extract, phospholipids were slightly increased (22%). Some large and clarified hepatocytes in portal areas showed a mild glycolipid overload (PAS diastase resistant). All the abnormalities disappeared 1 year later. The relationship between stored liver lipids and Intralipid compounds needs to be discussed. Might the batch of Intralipid used be implicated in the fat overload syndrome observed in 2 adults treated at the same period?

Influence of Bezafibrate on the Glomerular Filtration Rate

C. Luley, H. Botsch, W. Schwartzkopff, F. Llach, and H. U. Kloer

Fett und Stoffwechselambulanz, Klinikum Charlottenburg, Free University, Berlin, Germany

Treatment with clofibrate and its analogs, such as etofibrate, fenofibrate and bezafibrate (BF), has been shown to cause a slight but significant increase in serum creatinine (SCr). In order to evaluate whether this increase is due to an alteration of the glomerular filtration rate (GRF), a randomized, double blind, cross-over study was carried out in 22 patients with hyperlipoproteinemia (type IIa, IIb and IV) treated with BF. Eight patients had normal SCr (<1.3 mg/dl, group "SCr-N"), while 14 showed pathological levels between 1.3 and 2.8 mg/dl (group "SCr-P"). Group "SCr-N" received 3 x 200 mg bezafibrate per day, while "SCr-P" patients were treated with 2 x 200 mg/day (SCr between 1.3 and 2.0 mg/dl) or 1 x 200 mg/day (SCr>.0 mg/dl). Treatment periods were 6 weeks for both BF and placebo. At the end of each period SCr values (Jaffe and an enzymatic method), GFR (creatinine - and ^{51}Cr-EDTA-clearance), BF levels (gas chromatography) and other laboratory parameters were measured. After 6 weeks on bezafibrate, a significant decrease in GFR was noted both by creatinine (from 86 to 65 ml/min) and by ^{51}Cr-EDTA clearance (from 69 to 62 ml/min). This effect was more apparent in the "SCr-N" than in the "SCr-P" group. In parallel with a reduction in GFR, SCr values increased significantly by 0.27 mg/dl (Jaffe method). BF levels were significantly higher in "SCr-P" than in "SCr-N" patients (2.1 vs. 0.6 µg/ml.

Our results seem to indicate that the administration of clofibrate analogs, such as bezafibrate, may lead to a mild impairment of kidney function. Therefore, patients with renal disease and hyperlipidemia should not be treated with these compounds.

Lipids, Apoproteins and Coagulation Parameters Remain Unchanged Under Therapy With Dried Garlic

C. Luley, W. Schwartzkoff, W. Lehmann-Leo, B. Mueller, and T. Martin

Klinikum Charlottenburg, Free University, Berlin, Germany

The intake of garlic has been claimed to have some anti-atherosclerotic effect by causing changes in cholesterol levels and blood coagulation. In order to assess these potential effects, we carried out 2 studies in which the impact of 2 different dosages of dried garlic in coated tablets (3 x 198 mg or 3 x 450 mg/day, respectively) on blood lipids, apolipoproteins and coagulation parameters were investigated. The randomized, double blind, cross-over studies comprised garlic and placebo treatment periods of six weeks' duration each. In the first study, 34 patients with hyperlipoproteinemia type IIa, IIb and IV received the lower dosage, while in the second study 51 patients were treated with the higher dosage. In both studies, the following serum parameters were measured every 3 weeks: total cholesterol, HDL- and LDL-cholesterol, triglycerides and several safety parameters. In addition, apolipoproteins A and B, euglobulin time, fibrin split products, prothrombin time, bleeding time and fibrinogen levels were determined in the second study only.

The results indicated that neither dosage of dried garlic showed any significant effect on any of the parameters measured. It is therefore concluded that, if there is any effect of garlic on the parameters measured, it is not apparent when using a dried preparation.

Carnitine Antagonizes Ethionine Induced Liver Metabolic Disturbances in The Rat

F. Maccari, A. Arseni, M. T. Ramacci, and L. Angelucci

Sigma Tau S.p.A., Biological Research Laboratories, Pomezia and Institute of Pharmacology II, Faculty of Medicine, University of Rome, Italy

Repeated administration of L-Carnitine, 250 mg/kg per os, antagonizes in the fasting female Wistar rats the acute metabolic disturbances induced by ethionine, 1 g/kg per os. The accumulation of triglycerides in the liver and the modification in the plasma lipoprotein pattern are opposed. These effects are accompanied by the restoration of liver Acetyl- and Acyl-Carnitine normal levels by the exogenous L-Carnitine. Apparently, ethionine-induced liver metabolic disturbances are produced via an interference with some essential steps in the utilization of Carnitine in the lipid metabolism.

Carnitine Opposes Dietary Hyperlipidemia and Promotes Renal Excretion of Acyl-carnitines

F. Maccari, P. Pessotto, M. T. Ramacci, and L. Angelucci

Sigma Tau S.p.A., Biological Research Laboratories, Pomezia and Institute of Pharmacology II, Faculty of Medicine, University of Rome, Italy

L-Carnitine, 500 mg/kg per os, strongly antagonizes the increase in plasma triglycerides (TG) and in free fatty acids produced by feeding male Wistar rats with a 25% olive oil-enriched diet.

The myocardial and liver TG increase is also opposed.

In the same time, exogenous carnitine normalizes the liver and myocardium Carnitie, Acetyl- and Acyl-carnitine levels, as well as the myocardium neutral lipase activity, with no changes occurring in the myocardial and adipose tissue lipoprotein lipase activity.

The exogenous L-Carnitine effects above are concomitant to a marked increase in renal excretion of Acetyl- and long Acyl-carnitines, which are present in urine only in traces, both in basal conditions and in presence of a fat-enriched feeding.

Pharmacological Effects of A New Nicotinic Acid Derivative: L 44

F. M. Maggi, G. F. Caselli, M. R. Accomazzo, W. Schatton, and L. Puglisi

Inst. Pharmacology and Pharmacognosy, University of Milan, Italy and Merz & Co., Research Dept., Frankfurt/Main, Germany

L 44 is the 2-tert-butyl-4-cyclo-hexyl-phenyl ester of nicotinic acid.

The antilipolytic activity of this drug together to the effect on arachidonic acid metabolism on the artery irrorating the epididimal adipose tissue (EAT) was investigated in rats. L 44 inhibits stimulated as well as unstimulated free fatty acid (FFA) mobilization after a single dose of 200 mg/kg p.o.

In the EAT artery, the arachidonate metabolism appears to be correlated with the activity of the adipocytes since an increased FFA mobilization leads to an enhanced formation of prostacyclin by endothelial cells in the adipose tissue. L 44, inhibiting lipolysis, normalizes also the production of an important physiological modulator of the functional vasodilatation.

The antilipolytic effect of the drug can explain its ability to counteract the ethanol-induced hypertriglyceridemia as well as alterations of lipid metabolism in streptozotocin-diabetic rats. On the other hand, L 44 is not able to antagonize the hypertriglyceridemia due to a high carbohydrate intake. It has been shown that fructose activates many enzymes involved in neutral lipid synthesis. Our results suggest that L 44 does not directly interfere, at enzymatic level, with the formation of triglycerides in the liver.

Lipoprotein Induced Histamine Release from Mast Cells

Vesa Manninen, Jorma Kokkonen and Marjatta Mälkönen

First Dept. of Medicine, University of Helsinki, Helsinki, Finland

Several attempts have been made to establish a correlation between changes in mast cell numbers in the cardiovascular system and the severity of atherosclerosis. However, results have been contradictory and difficult to interpret in the absence of any direct measurement of parameters indicating mast cell function. Our alternative approach was to investigate whether lipoproteins would stimulate mast cells *in vitro*. It was found that chylomicrons and VLDL induce concentration-dependent histamine release from both rat peritoneal cell suspensions and isolated mast cells. Maximum histamine release was 16.9% and 13.6% for chylomicrons and VLDL, respectively, in response to lipoprotein concentrations of 2.0 and 1.0 mmol/l (expressed as triglyceride content). Histamine release was completed in 1 min. and required no extracellular calcium. ^{35}S-labelled mast cells released histamine almost exclusively, indicating that histamine release is not accompanied by granule extrusion and heparin release. Sodium cromoglycate (10^{-2} - 10^{-5} M) inhibited in a concentration-dependent manner the release of histamine (up to 63%). The results suggest that lipoproteins are physiological and non-immunological releasers of histamine from mast cells.

Effect of Clinofibrate (Lipoclin[R]) on Lipid Metabolism in High Cholesterol Diet Fed Rats

Nobuo Matsuoka, Yoh Ishikawa, Toshio Nishide, Norihiro Sasaki, Shunichi Murano, Kohji Shirai, Yasushi Saito and Akira Kumagai

Kawasaki Steel Hospital, Chiba and Toyama Medical-Pharmaceutical University, Toyama, Japan

Atherosclerotic lesions were observed in the aorta of rats fed a diet containing propylthiouracil (PTU), vitamin D_2) and high cholesterol for 8 weeks. Clinofibrate significantly decreased the high plasma cholesterol level of atherosclerotic rats and the reduction was due to the reduction of very low density lipoprotein (VLDL). Heparin releasable lipoprotein lipase activity in epididymal adipose tissue, post heparin lipolytic activity and VLDL triglyceride hydrolysing activity in adipose tissue stromal vessels were higher in clinofibrate-treated rats than in atherosclerotic rats. Acid cholesterol esterase activity was decreased in atherosclerotic rats and clinofibrate treatment increased this activity, the ratio of acyl-CoA cholesterol acyl transferase activity (ACA) to neutral cholesterol esterase activity was higher in atherosclerotic rats than in control rats and was lower in clinofibrate-treated rats than in atherosclerotic rats. From these results, it is concluded that clinofibrate reduces the cholesterol ester content of the arterial wall and lowers the plasma VLDL and LDL cholesterol levels.

Effect of Elastase on Lipid Metabolism in the High Cholestrol Fed Rabbit Arterial Wall

N. Matsuoka, K. Shirai, N. Sasaki, S. Murano, Y. Ishikawa, T. Nishide, Y. Saito, A. Kumagai, A. Miyazaki, Y. Masuda, Y. Inagaki, J. Tamaru, and I. Iwasaki

The Second Dept. of Internal Medicine; The Third Dept. of Internal Medicine; The First Dept. of Pathology, School of Medicine, Chiba University, Chiba; and Toyama Medical-Pharmaceutical University, Toyama, Japan

Administration of porcine pancreatic elastase (Ela.) is reported to have antiatherosclerotic effect. To clarify the precise mechanism, effects of Ela. on lipid metabolism in rabbit arterial wall were studied. Three groups of rabbits were kept for 4 months as follows: first group was fed normal diets, second group was fed 1% cholesterol, and third group was fed 1% cholesterol diet and was injected with Ela. 5 mg/kg/day intraperitoneally.

Total cholesterol content in the arterial wall was lower in group III than in group II. Serum cholesterol and triglyceride levels were lower in group III than in group II, and those contents in VLDL and LDL fractions were decreased in group III comparing with group II. Acid cholesterol esterase, neutral cholesterol esterase and acyl CoA cholesterol acyl transferase activity in the arterial wall in group III were not significantly different from those in group II. The binding of cholesterol [1-^{14}C]oleate-labelled LDL to 800 x g pellet fraction of arterial wall homogenate in group II was increased comparing with that in group I. When cholesterol-loaded aorta was treated with Ela., the binding of LDL to the 800 x g pellet fraction was decreased. These results may suggest that Ela. had antiatherosclerotic effect by reducing serum VLDL and LDL levels, and decreasing the binding of LDL to the arterial wall.

Differences in Size and Chemical Composition of Lipoproteins Between $ApoE_3$ Deficiency and Familial Hypercholesterolemia Showing the Phenotype of Type III

Yuji Matsuzawa, Shuichi Nozaki, Kaoru Kameda, Masaharu Kubo, Seiichiro Tarui, Akira Yamamoto, Ichiro Hara, and Mitsuyo Okazaki

The Second Dept. of Internal Medicine, Osaka University Medical School, Osaka, Japan

The lipoprotein analysis of 5 subjects of Type III hyperlipoproteinemia with $ApoE_3$ deficiency was performed by high performance liquid chromatography (HPLC) in addition to ultracentrifugation and PAG-disc electrophoresis, and the results were compared with those of 4 subjects with familial hypercholesterolemia showing the phenotype of Type III (FH-Type III) classified by β-migrating VLDL and the increase of IDL but without $ApoE_3$ deficiency. VLDL subfraction contained increased concentration of cholesterol and triglyceride and were relatively rich in cholesterol in both classical Type III and FH-Type III. LDL subfraction in classical Type III was poor and the ratio of cholesterol to triglyceride was very low even before treatment when total cholesterol level was high, while FH-Type III had high level of LDL-cholesterol. HPLC for lipoproteins revealed no lipoprotein eluted at the regular LDL position and elution position of major component shifted to the position of larger particle size than LDL. In FH-Type III major fraction was eluted at the exact position of normal LDL, although PAG-disc electrophoresis showed broad β pattern similar to classical Type III. Clofibrate treatment decreased cholesterol and triglyceride level to normal ranges, although no change was seen in electrophoretic pattern and elution pattern of HPLC in classical Type III. However, in FH-Type III broad β pattern disappeared and was converted to typical Type IIa by clofibrate treatment, while LDL-cholesterol tended to increase after treatment. From the data above, we conclude that the mechanism of the appearance of Type III phenotype was clearly different between classical Type III with $ApoE_3$ deficiency and the others, and it is possible even without ApoE analysis to diagnose classical Type III (E2/2) by lipoprotein analysis using HPLC and by the mode of responses to clofibrate treatment.

The QT Interval After Probucol

Donald McCaughan

V. A. Outpatient Clinic, Worcester, Massachusetts

Two groups of male patients treated with probucol for hypercholesterolemia were studied by electrocardiogram (ECG) before and during long-term therapy. Group I consisted of 45 patients who had Frank orthogonal ECGs recorded simultaneously on F.M. tape. The records were analysed by digital computer. The QT interval was measured from the earliest onset of the QRS in any lead to the last deflection of the T wave in any lead. Five to ten beats were measured and averaged, and the QT corrected (QTc) by Bazett's formula (QTc/ $\sqrt{R-R}$), using the proceed R-R interval as reference.

The QTc rose from 390 ± 29 mS (range 333-450) before treatment to 412 ± 23 mS (370-470) after 1 or 2 years of probucol therapy ($p<0.05$). The normal range of the QTc by this method is 410 ± 27 mS (340-520). The lengthening of the QTc by 22 mS on average, though significant, is not readily apparent on the ECG. In two cases, the QTc lengthened to 470 mS at 1-2 years, but in subsequent tracings reverted to previous values on continuing therapy.

Standard 12 lead ECGs were done pre treatment and annually in another 45 patients. In these patients, plasma probucol levels were measured. No correlation was observed between QTc and plasma probucol level ($r=0.03$).

In twelve years of observation, no serious ventricular arrhythmias were encountered. Numerous exercise tests did not provoke arrhythmias. Probucol may lengthen the QT by acting on the automatic innervation or by showing conduction in the fast channel, a quinidine-like effect.

Clofibrate Improves Glucose Tolerance Through The Changes of Insulin Receptors

K. Murakami, S. Nambu, H. Koh, M. Tsushima, Y. Nishioheda, M. Kobayashi, S. Ohgaku, and Y. Shigeta

The Third Department of Medicine, Shiga University of Medical Science, Shiga, Japan

Although the recognized effect of clofibrate on glucose tolerance, its glucose-lowering mechanism is not well known, we administered, therefore, 1500 mg of clofibrate daily for one month to 15 non-insulin dependent diabetics who were treated with diet alone. 75 g oral glucose tolerance test (75 g GTT) and insulin tolerance test (ITT) was carried out before and after the treatment. Fasting plasma glucose values were decreased from 168.1 ± 9.5 to 136.5 ± 6.0 mg/dl (mean $\pm$ SE) ($p<0.01$), and fasting IRI levels were decreased from 13.8 ± 1.7 to 10.1 ± 1.5 μ U/ml ($p<0.05$) in spite of the stable body weight. However, insulinogenic index and ΣIRI/Σ glucose ratio during 75 g GTT were not changed. Enhanced glucose fall in ITT was also observed.

As these results suggested the enhanced tissue sensitivity to insulin, we examined the insulin receptors using erythrocytes before and after three months' treatment. Insulin binding were increased from 3.41 ± 0.17% to 4.11 ± 0.20% at 1 ng/ml of exogenous insulin ($p<0.01$). The Scatchard analysis showed an increased affinity without a change in the number of insulin receptors.

These results suggest that improved glucose tolerance by clofibrate might be derived from the enhanced tissue sensitivity to insulin, probably through the enhanced affinity of insulin receptors.

Effect of Clinofibrate (Lipoclin^{R}) on Lipid Composition of Serum Lipoprotein in Hyperlipidemic Patients

Shunichi Murano, Masako Otabe, Yoh Ishikawa, Toshio Nishide, Norihiro Sasaki, Kohji Shirai, Nobuo Matsuoka, Yasushi Saito, Yasuhiro Kobayashi, and Akira Kumagai

Dept. of Internal Medicine and Central Laboratory for Clinical Investigation, Kawatetsu-Chiba Hospital, Chiba; The Second Dept. of Internal Medicine, School of Medicine, Chiba University; Dept. of Internal Medicine, Tohgane Hospital, Chiba; and Toyama Medical and Pharmaceutical University, Toyama

In this study, 600 mg/day or 1200 mg/day of Clinofibrate (Lipoclin^{R}) was orally administered to 42 hyperlipidemic patients during three months. Clinofibrate decreased serum triglyceride about 32% by 600 mg/day and 48% by 1200 mg/day. It decreased serum cholesterol 5% by 600 mg/day and 7% by 1200 mg/day. The patients were classified to 28 Type IIb, 9 Type IIa and 5 Type IV hyperlipidemics according to the WHO pheno-types of hyperlipidemia. The lipid lowering effect in each lipoprotein fraction was studied. The lipoproteins were fractionated by ultracentrifugation using Beckman Lp-42 Ti rotor. In Type IIb hyperlipidemics, 600 mg/day of Clinofibrate lowered VLDL and LDL cholesterol and VLDL triglyceride and increased HDL cholesterol. However, 1200 mg/day of Clinofibrate lowered VLDL cholesterol and triglyceride but increased LDL cholesterol, slightly. Clinofibrate was known to increase lipoprotein lipase activity in peripheral adipose tissue. So, this difference between 600 mg/day and 1200 mg/day might be due to the amount of VLDL catabolized by lipoprotein lipase. The clinical usefulness of 1200 mg/day administration of Clinofibrate was partly confirmed and must be studied in the case administered for longer trial. At last, no adverse reaction was observed in this trial.

The Effect of Probucol Treatment Upon Plasma Lecithin:Cholesterol Acyltransferase of Cynomolgus Monkeys

Linda H. Myers, Robin T. Zon, and Ben J. Cerimele

Merrell Dow Pharmaceuticals, Inc., Indianapolis, Indiana

The present study examined the effects of probucol treatment upon lecithin:cholesterol acyltransferase (LCAT) and upon the LCAT-substrate characteristics of high density lipoproteins (HDL) in cynomolgus monkeys. Fractional esterification rates (FER's) of free cholesterol (FC) and molar LCAT activities, the product of FER and FC concentrations, were determined. Probucol treatment increased the FER's of plasma FC but decreased plasma FC concentrations. Plasma molar LCAT activities were unchanged by probucol treatment. When $d > 1.21$ g/mL plasma fractions from individual monkeys were used as sources of LCAT to react with a common HDL substrate pool, neither FER's nor LCAT activities were affected by probucol treatment. When HDL from probucol-treated or control animals were reacted with the same LCAT pool, the FER's of HDL from treated animals were greater than controls ($p=0.056$), an increase independent of changes in HDL-FC concentrations. Molar LCAT activities were unchanged. The HDL of probucol-treated monkeys had similar FC/phospholipid but larger FC/cholesteryl ester ratios than the HDL of control animals. The results indicate that the increased plasma FER's of probucol-treated monkeys were likely due to probucol-induced compositional changes in HDL and were unrelated to any direct effect of probucol upon the enzyme LCAT.

Further Reduction of Plasma Lipids by a Combined Treatment of Clinofibrate and Melinamide

H. Nakamura, T. Ishikawa, N. Tada, N. Suzuki, K. Kondo, and K. Kimura

Jikei University, Aoto Hospital, Katsushika, Tokyo and Sumitomo Chemical Company, Ltd., Osaka, Japan

It has been generally observed that elevated VLDL can be lowered by Clinofibrate (2,2'-(4,4'-cyclohexylidene-diphenoxy)-2,2'-dimethyldibutyric acid) alone and increased LDL can be reduced by Melinamide (N-(α-methylbenzyl) linoleamide). The aim of the present study is to assess the accelerated reduction of plasma lipids by Clinofibrate plus Melinamide.

In experimental normal rats, plasma cholesterol and triglyceride decreased further by a combined administration of both agents compared with the results obtained by each single administration. In cholesterol-fed rats, this reduction was also apparent on a combined treatment. Total bile acid excretion was more increased and neutral sterol was excreted less relatively in the bile. Therefore, lithogenic index was markedly reduced on this treatment.

Similarly, the accelerated reduction of LDL and VLDL was confirmed in hyperlipidemic human subjects. This combined treatment of these two agents seems to be more favorable for the control against hyperlipidemia.

Pharmacokinetics and Metabolism of Mifobate (SR-202) in Human Plasma

L. Nguyen, A. Rougemont, J. Orlando, E. Niesor, and C. Bentzen

SYMPHAR, S.A., Geneva, Switzerland

Mifobate [Dimethyl α-(dimethoxyphosphinyl)p-chlorobenzyl phosphate] is a potential antiatherosclerotic agent structurally unrelated to the clofibrate analogs.

Pharmacokinetic studies in rat, dog and human using Mifobate labeled with ^{14}C at the α-position have shown that the drug is rapidly absorbed and quantitatively excreted (>85%). In all three species the parent compound is similarly biotransformed in plasma into one major metabolite which is present in urine as the principal excretion form of the drug.

A specific reversed-phase HPLC method was developed for the quantification of non-labeled Mifobate in human plasma. Ten healthy volunteers were administered single oral doses of Mifobate (400 and 600 mg capsules). Study results showed that at least 90 to 95% of the drug is eliminated from plasma after 24 hours. Plasma peak concentrations of Mifobate were reached within 1-2 hours, ranging from ca 10 to 14 and 11 to 18 μg/ml respectively, and appeared to be dose-dependent. Drug half-life ranged from 3.2 to 5.8 hours and total body clearance from 4.3 to 6.1 l/h. In addition, several other analytical methods including HPLC have permitted the identification of the metabolite as a monodemethylated derivative of Mifobate.

A subsequent clinical study conducted with doses of 50 mg t.i.d. established that after 28 days of treatment, plasma peak levels of Mifobate did not exceed a value of 1.5 μg/ml which was predicted on the basis of the single dose pharmacokinetic study.

In summary, the detection and quantification of plasma levels of Mifobate in the therapeutic range have been made possible by an HPLC method. These results confirm the metabolic and pharmacokinetic studies performed with radiolabeled drug.

Mechanism of Action of Mifobate (SR-202) on Tissue-Plasma Cholesterol Mobilization and Elimination

E. Niesor, J. R. Rossier, K. Kalathakis, and C. Bentzen

SYMPHAR, S.A., Geneva, Switzerland

The lipid mobilizing activity of Mifobate was studied in rats by simultaneously analyzing plasma, tissue and bile lipids.

A rapid, dose-dependent, choleretic effect was produced by doses from 25 to 200 mg/kg (i.d.) with bile flow increasing from +15% to +120% within 30 min. At 2 and 5 hours following a single oral dose of 200 mg/kg, total plasma cholesterol (CHOL) - mainly from the beta-CHOL fraction - and triglycerides (TRG) dropped significantly by 30% and 51%, respectively. At 2 hours the plasma free/toal CHOL ratio increased markedly (+65%). Changes in liver lipids were observed only in TRG (-25%) and FFA (-39%, $p<0.05$) 5 hours post dose. Analysis of the biliary content of the small intestine revealed a higher concentration of lecithin (+64%), bile acids (+175%, $p<0.05$) and CHOL (+52%) 5 hours post dose. Thus, a rapid mobilization of plasma TRG and CHOL made available for liver catabolism and bile elimination, characterizes the initial activity of Mifobate.

Similar experiments using red blood cells and lipoproteins labeled with ^{14}C-CHOL confirm that Mifobate is a potent tissue and plasma CHOL mobilizing drug.

Four oral doses of drug (200 mg/kg) to rats fed a normal diet significantly increased plasma α-lipoproteins (+50%, $p<0.05$), as well as bile flow (+74%, $p<0.05$), and bile acids secretion (+26%). In addition, simultaneous feeding of a CHOL-cholic acid rich diet and drug administration produced changes in bile flow (+53%, $p<0.05$), bile CHOL (+31%, $p<0.01$) and bile acid (+40%, $p<0.05$) elimination, thus confirming that treated rats are more actively eliminating CHOL and bile acids.

These results and the changes in plasma lipoproteins also observed in monkey and man strongly suggest that Mifobate positively alters liver activity, therefore resulting in increased tissue cholesterol mobilization.

Cholesterol and LDL Metabolism By Blood Mononuclear Cells Following Partial Ileal By-Pass Surgery in Familial Hypercholesterolemia

Karin Nilausen and Hans Meinertz

Dept. of Anatomy C, University of Copenhagen, and Dept. of Medicine B, Rigshospital, Copenhagen, Denmark

Since the cholesterol requirements of peripheral cells are met largely by uptake and degradation of circulating low density lipoprotein (LDL), therapeutic lowering of elevated cholesterol levels in familial hypercholesterolemia might affect cellular LDL and sterol metabolism. Partial ileal by-pass surgery lowered LDL-cholesterol from a preoperative level of 354 ± 86 mg% (Av±SD, n=8) by 32% 10 days postoperatively, by 43% after 28 days and by 44% after 2 months and more. Sterol synthesis by freshly isolated mononuclear cells, measured by incorporation of labeled acetate, increased from a preoperative level of 18 ± 4.8 pmoles per 5 x 10^6 cells and per 2 hours, by 77% ($p < .01$) after 10 days postoperatively and by 47% ($p < .05$) after 28 days, but after 60 days or more the rates were back to preoperative levels ($p > .10$). Incorporation of octanoate and mevalonate labels likewise increased significantly 10 days postoperatively. Separation of the mononuclear cell mixture into lymphocytes and monocytes showed that both cell types participated in the postoperative increase in sterol synthesis. Degradation of radio-labeled LDL via the LDL-receptor pathway was increased by a factor of 3.4 ($p < .02$) and by the receptorindependent pathway by a factor 4 ($p < .02$) in the immediate postoperative period. Thus, LDL-lowering by ileal by-pass surgery has profound effects on cellular lipoprotein and sterol metabolism, but the effects appear to be transient and limited to the first few postoperative weeks.

This work was supported by the Danish Heart Foundation.

Inhibitory Action of Soluble Elastin on Thromboxane B_2 Formation in Blood Platelets

Hiromichi Okuda and Keizo Sekiya

Dept. of Medical Biochemistry, School of Medicine, Ehime University, Ehime, Japan

Soluble elastin was prepared from insoluble elastin by oxalic acid or elastase hydrolysis. The soluble elastin was found to inhibit the formation of thromboxane B_2 (TXB_2) both from exogenously supplied [1-^{14}C] arachidonic acid in washed platelets and from [1- C] arachidonic acid prelabeled platelets stimulated by thrombin. In contrast to TXB_2, the formation of 12-hydroxy-5,8,10,14-eicosatetraenoic acid (12-HETE) was accelerated in both cases.

The formation of TXB_2 from exogenously supplied arachidonic acid was inhibited 21% by 1 mg/ml soluble elastin and 59% by 10 mg/ml. In prelabeled platelets, the formation of TXB stimulated by thrombin was inhibited 44% by 1 mg/ml soluble elastin and 94% by 10 mg/ml. The formation of 12-HETE from exogenously supplied arachidonic acid was increased about 3.4 and 7.3 times by 1 and 10 mg/ml soluble elastin, respectively. In prelabeled platelets, the formation of 12-HETE stimulated by thrombin was increased about 1.3 and 2.8 times by 1 and 10 mg/ml soluble elastin, respectively.

This inhibitory action of elastin did not have to be replaced by desmosine.

The level of cAMP in platelets was not affected by the soluble elastin.

These results suggested that soluble elastin exert its inhibitory action against platelet aggregation by inhibiting thromboxane A_2 formation, especially from endogenous arachidonic acid.

The Urinary 6-keto-PGF$_1\alpha$ Level is Augmented in the Early Nicotinic Acid Treatment of Hyperlipidaemia

Anders G. Olsson, Erik Änggård, Carlo Patrono, and Lars A. Carlson

King Gustaf V Research Institute and Dept. of Alcohol and Drug Addiction Research, Karolinska Institute, Stockholm, Sweden and Dept. of Pharmacology, Catholic University, Rome, Italy

The 24 h urinary excretion of prostaglandin F$_2\alpha$ and of 6-keto-PGF$_1\alpha$ were determined during stay in metabolic ward in 8 female subjects with hyperlipidaemia. Determinations were made before and after 48 h and after 28 days of nicotinic acid treatment in the dose of 1 g 4 times daily.

(SEE TABLE)

The excretion of 6-keto-PGF$_1$ α increased significantly during the initial phase of nicotinic acid treatment, coinciding with the well-known flushing effect of the drug. During continued treatment excretion declined to pretreatment levels concomitant with the disappearance of the tachyphylaxis for the flush during nicotinic acid treatment.

Conclusion: The flush during the initial phase of nicotinic acid is probably caused by an increased production of prostacyclin. As the production decreases during continued treatment, we do not believe that this effect is responsible for the lowered mortality observed during secondary prevention of ischaemic heart disease with nicotinic acid. This effect is probably mediated through decreased atherogenic serum lipoprotein concentrations.

<u>Results</u>: Mean $\pm$ SEM.

	<u>Before</u>	<u>48 h</u>	<u>28 h</u>
6-keto-PGF_1, ng/24 h	84 $\pm$ 8	130 $\pm$ 30^1	101 $\pm$ 21^2
PGF_2, g/24 h	2.2 $\pm$ 0.4	2.9 $\pm$ 0.7	2.9 $\pm$ 0.7

1 = significant difference ($p<0.05$) from before treatment.
2 = significant difference ($p<0.01$) from 48 h.

Effects of Eicosapentaenoic Acid (EPA) and Docosahexaenoic Acid (DHA) on Platelet Aggregation and Composition of Fatty Acid in Man - A Cross Over Study

Hajime Orimo, Yuzo Nagakawa, and Michiyoshi Harasawa

Dept. of Geriatrics, Faculty of Medicine, University of Tokyo, Japan

The aim of this report is to investigate the effects of EPA and docosahexaenoic acid (DHA) on platelet aggregation and composition of fatty acid in plasma and platelet. Twelve volunteers (mean age, 63.5 ± 12.1 years) were subjected to the cross-over study comparing the effect of EPA with that of DHA. They were divided into 2 groups: group A in which EPA 2g/day was given for 4 weeks and after 4 weeks off treatment, DHA 2g/day was given for the subsequent 4 weeks and group B in which DHA was given first followed by EPA treatment. Significant decrease in platelet aggregation was observed following the treatment with 2g of DHA, but platelet aggregation tended to increase after the treatment with 2g of EPA. Platelet aggregation tended to decrease following the treatment with 2g of EPA, but it was increased after the treatment with 2g of DHA. The content of EPA and DHA in plasma and platelet was increased following the treatment of EPA and DHA respectively. DHA thus appears to be more potent than EPA in inhibiting platelet aggregation. However, this inhibitory effect was blunted by the prior administration of EPA or DHA.

Effect of Streptococcus Avium on the Serum Cholesterol and Triglyceride Level

Yoshiaki Oshida, Tetsuya Suga, and Yasuo Kawai

The effect of the administration of *Streptococcus avium* on the serum cholesterol and triglyceride levels was examined. The oral administration (10^{10} viable cells/animal) of *Streptococcus avium* lowered the serum cholesterol and triglyceride levels by 20% and 78%, respectively, in the ex-germfree mice. The oral administration of the dead cells of *Streptococcus avium* 10^{10}(day/animal for 4 weeks lowered the serum cholesterol and triglyceride levels by 40% and 36%, respectively, in conventional mice. When high cholesterol diet (1% cholesterol + 0.5% sodium cholate) was given, the serum cholesterol and triglyceride were lowered by 30% and 52%, respectively, by the streptococcal administration in conventional rats. The effective constituent was extracted with aqueous solvent, and the effective substance, like polysaccharides, obtained from the extract gave a single band detected by toluidine blue on the electrophoretic film. This effective substance lowered the serum cholesterol and triglyeride levels by about 30% and 40%, respectively, by the oral administration (20 mg/day/animal) into rats for 2 weeks.

Effects of an Anti-Oestrogen (Tamoxifen) on Serum Lipoproteins in Patients After Breast Cancer Surgery

Stephen Roessner and Arne Wallgren

King Gustaf V Research Institute and Radiumhemmet, Karolinska Hospital, Stockholm, Sweden

Several studies indicate that ostrogens increase the concentrations of VLDL and HDL, probably because of a stimulated secretion from the liver. LDL is often lowered. Tamoxifen is an anti-oestrogen with a weak intrinsic oestrogenic activity, which is now widely used in treatment of breast cancer. No studies on the possible effects on lipoprotein metabolism of this compound seem to have been published. We studied 21 females after surgery for breast cancer. They were in a stable clinical condition after the operation. They were randomly divided into two groups. One served as a control group, the other received tamoxifen 40 mg daily. Serum lipoproteins were determined before and after two months of therapy.

Data from all cancer patients were compared with Stockholm data for a group of randomly selected healthy women in the same age. In cancer patients the HDL-cholesterol concentration (2.11 mmol/l) was 14% higher than in controls.

In controls, no lipoprotein changes with time were observed. In patients treated with tamoxifen, LDL-TG increased from 0.46 $\pm$ 0.13 to 0.56 $\pm$ 0.20 mmol/l ($p<0.01$) and LDL-cholesterol decreased from 5.11 $\pm$ 1.16 to 4.10 $\pm$ 1.07 mmol/1 ($p<0.001$). The LDL TG/cholesterol ratio increased from 0.09 to 0.14. No other significant changes were found. The study extends previous observations that HDL-concentrations may be elevated in breast cancer patients. The antioestrogen tamoxifen only partly acted as a weak oestrogen by selectively influencing the lipid composition of the LDL fraction.

Effects of Mifobate (SR-202) on Liver and Hepatic Enzymes Affecting Cholesterol Metabolism in the Rat

A. Rougemont, B. Mitha, E. Niesor, and C. Bentzen

SYMPHAR, S.A., Geneva, Switzerland

Mifobate produces a pharmacological response associated with an increase in HDL-cholesterol and enhanced cholesterol elimination in several species with definitely different pre-existing plasma lipoprotein profiles.

In the rat, comparative Mifobate/Pentobarbital/Fenofibrate biochemical and electron microscopic studies have clearly demonstrated that the dose-dependent hepatomegaly caused by Mifobate is characterized by an increase in smooth endoplasmic reticulum mass and related microsomal mixed-function oxygenase activities, without effect on peroxisomal mass and catalase acitivity.

Oral administration of a single 200 mg/kg dose to normal rats resulted in a significant increase in hepatic ACAT and cholesterol 7α-hydroxylase activities after 2 hours, with a concomitant drop in plasma cholesterol, phospholipid and triglyceride levels. These data indicate that Mifobate, unlike Clofibrate and analogs, alters plasma lipid levels without changes in peroxisomal activities; unlike barbiturates, its primary action is not correlated with changes in microsomal activities. In addition, comparative Mifobate/Triparanol studies have shown that the observed alterations in plasma and tissue cholesterol contents are not related to changes in desmosterol concentrations.

These results show that in the rat Mifobate influences hepatic functions in a unique manner different from classical hypolipidemic agents; furthermore, the single-dose data strongly support the concept of an original primary mechanism of action involving increased hepatic lipoprotein catabolism with a consequent enhancement of tissue cholesterol mobilization.

Effect of Pantethine (Pantosin^R) on Lipid Metabolism in Vessel Wall from the Point of View of Atherosclerosis

Yasushi Saito, Akira Kumagai, and Masanao Ishihara

The Second Dept. of Internal Medicine, Chiba University, Chiba; Toyama Medical and Pharmacological College, Toyama; and Daiichi Seiyaku Co., Ltd., Tokyo, Japan

Experiments were carried out to clarify the effects of pantethine on vascular injury including atherosclerosis from the point of view of lipid metabolism in vessel wall. Pantethine reduced the cholesterol ester (CE) synthesis from free fatty acid (FFA), increased the acid cholesterol esterase and reduced the ratio of CE synthesizing activity to neutral cholesterol esterase in high cholesterol diet-fed rat arterial wall. These results suggest that pantethine has a preventive effect for foam cell formation. We already reported that FFA oxidation was inhibited in brain microvessel of hypertensive rat and that caused the angionecrosis. Reduction of FFA oxidation was prevented in pantethine administered spontaneous hypertensive rats brain microvessels. The mechanism of action of pantethine and the electron microscopic studies on the mitochondrial structure in brain microvessels will be shown.

Mechanism of Action of Gemfibrozil in Increasing HDL and Lowering Triglycerides

K. Saku, B. A. Hynd, P. S. Gartside, and M. L. Kashyap

Lipid Research Division, University of Cincinnati Medical Center, Cincinnati, Ohio

Gemfibrozil increases plasma high density lipoprotein (HDL) cholesterol and lowers triglycerides in hypertriglyceridemic patients. However, its mechanisms of action in man is unclear. Four patients with endogenous hypertriglyceridemia with fasting chylomicronemia (type V phenotype) and subnormal HDL cholesterol (hypoalpha-lipoproteinemia) levels were treated initially by diet and once stabilized, were given gemfibrozil for 8 weeks. The following studies were done before and following gemfibrozil treatment: 1. Kinetics of apolipoproteins (apo) AI and AII (major proteins of HDL) metabolism were assessed by analysis of the specific activity decay curve after injection of autologous HDL labeled with ^{125}I; 2. Hepatic triglyceride lipase (H-TgL) and extra hepatic lipoprotein lipase (LpL) were assessed after intravenous injection of heparin; 3. HDL_2 and HDL_3 were assessed by rate zonal, gradient gel electrophoresis and preparative ultracentrifugation.

<u>RESULTS</u>: 1. An increase in absolute synthetic rate of both apo AI (by 22 $\pm$ 8%) and AII (by 27 $\pm$ 6%) was found, and there was no appreciable change in the fractional catabolic rates; 2. LpL increased and H-TgL decreased; 3. Both HDL_2 and HDL_3 cholesterol concentrations increased, but HDL_2 cholesterol increased to a greater extent than HDL_3.

<u>CONCLUSIONS</u>. In these patients, Gemfibrozil raised HDL by stimulation of apo AI and AII synthesis, and by depressing H-TgL, an enzyme which catabolizes HDL. It decreased total plasma TG by stimulating extra hepatic LpL, which catabolizes very low density lipoproteins that transport plasma TG.

Inhibition of Rat Liver Cholesterol 7α-Hydroxylase and Acyl CoA:Cholesterol Acyl Transferase Activities by Enterodiol and Enterolactone

A. Sanghvi, W. F. Diven, H. Seltman, V. Warty, M. Rizk, D. Kritchevsky, and K. D. R. Setchell

Dept. of Pathology, University of Pittsburgh School of Medicine, Pittsburgh, Pennsylvania; The Wistar Institute, Philadelphia, Pennsylvania and Division of Clinical Chemistry, Clinical Research Center, Harrow, Middlesex, United Kingdom

Enterodiol and enterolactone are lignans formed by microbial action on precursor lignans of plant origin present as constituents of mammalian diet. They are excreted in urine and bile predominantly as glucuronide conjugates. We have tested the ability of enterodiol and enterolactone to modulate the in-vitro activities of HMG-CoA reductase, cholesterol 7α-hydroxylase, and acyl CoA:cholesterol acyl transferase (ACAT) in rat liver microsomes. Both lignans were found to inhibit cholesterol 7α-hydroxylase and ACAT activities in a dose-dependent fashion. Enterolactone was the more potent inhibitor of the two. In contrast, HMG-CoA reductase activity was not significantly affected by either of the lignans, even at 400 μg/tube of assay mixture. At this concentration, cholesterol 7α-hydroxylase and ACAT activities were 30 and 50 percent, respectively, in the presence of diol and about 10 percent in the presence of lactone, of the activities measured in the absence of lignans. The mechanism of inhibition of the activities of these two enzymes by enterodiol and enterolactone is not clear, but it does not seem to involve a change in the state of phosphorylation of the enzymes.

The Role of Phosphorylation/Dephosphorylation in the Regulation of Cholesterol 7α-Hydroxylase Activity

A. Sanghvi

Department of Pathology, University of Pittsburgh School of Medicine, Pittsburgh, Pennsylvania

The enzyme, cholesterol 7α-hydroxylase, catalyzes the hydroxylation of cholesterol to form 7α-hydroxycholesterol, which is the first compound in the biosynthesis of bile acids. Bile acid biosynthesis is believed to be critically regulated by alterations in the level of cholesterol 7α-hydroxylase activity. Our recent studies using a GC/MS procedure indicate that the short-term regulation of cholesterol 7α-hydroxylase activity involves the process of phosphorylation/dephosphorylation of the enzyme molecule and that the active moiety is the phosphorylated one. Thus, dephosphorylating conditions, such as incubations in imidazole buffer or with E. coli alkaline phosphatase, significantly reduced 7α-hydroxylase activity. The activity was restored to control levels by incubation with ATP Mg and a cytosolic fraction with protein kinase activity. Later studies showed the presence of a metal ion sensitive microsomal phosphatase which could deactivate 7α-hydroxylase under proper conditions. Activity of this endogenous phosphatase could be prevented by NaF. Also, a dialyzable microsomal factor appears essential for stabilizing the enzyme because dialysis of a microsomal suspension results in a considerable loss of enzyme activity.

Decreased Concentration of High Density Lipoprotein Cholesterol in Schizophrenic Patients Treated with Phenothiazines

Jun Sasaki, Koji Kitajima, and Kikuo Arakawa

Dept. of Internal Medicine, Fukuoka University, Fukuoka, Japan

In chronic schizophrenic patients treated with phenothiazines for long term (n=29, average 9 yrs.), the high density lipoprotein cholesterol (HDL-C) levels were significantly low (30 ± 10mg/dl) compared to normal controls (50 ± 11mg/dl) and patients not treated with phenothiazines (59 ± 18mg/dl). The triglycerides (TG) and low density lipoprotein cholesterol (LDL-C) levels were significantly higher in patients treated with phenothiazines than controls and patients not treated with phenothiazines. No significant difference in total cholesterol (TC), TG, HDL-C and LDL-C was found between users and non-users of benzodiazepine in schizophrenic patients receiving phenothiazines. In addition to chronic schizophrenia, eight new patients with schizophrenia were studied. The HDL-C level in patients with schizophrenia prior to phenothiazine administration was 59 ± 18mg/dl, then decreased significantly to 48 ± 10mg/dl following administration of phenothiazines. No significant differences were found in TC and TG levels for 15 weeks after initiation of phenothiazines administration. Aluminium-clofibrate was administered to individuals treated with phenothiazines for short and long term. In both groups, the concentration of HDL-C was significantly increased and TG levels were significantly decreased following administration of Aluminium-clofibrate. These results suggest direct correlation of phenothiazines to low serum HDL-C level in schizophrenic patients and possible beneficial effect of Aluminium-clofibrate.

Betaxolol, Lipids and Lipoproteins. A Long Term Study in Hypertensive Patients

J. P. Sauvanet, J. Jaillard, J. Rouffy, and B. Orofiamma

Clin.Res.,LERS-SYNTHELABO, Paris; Int.Med.,C.H.R.,Lille and Int.Med. Hosp. St.-Louis, Paris

Betaxolol, a long-acting selective β -blocker was given during 12 months to 26 patients with essential hypertension. Twenty-two patients were normolipidemic, 6 were affected by HLP (2 type IIa, 4 type IV) normalized prior to the inclusion, due to an individual controlled diet maintained throughout the study. Betaxolol was given once daily (10 - 60 mg/day).

Weight was stable (69.6 ± 1.9 kg before and 68.0 ± 1.7 kg after 12 months' therapy).

Mean blood pressure was reduced significantly ($p < 0.001$) during betaxolol therapy (from 193/107 mmHg to 151/83 mmHg after 6 months, and to 148/80 mmHg after 12 months). Heart rate was also reduced from 78 to 58 beats/min. after 12 months ($p < 0.001$).

Lipids and lipoproteins determinations were performed initially and after 3, 6 and 12 months of betaxolol. No significant changes were observed in total cholesterol, LDL and VLDL-cholesterol. HDL-cholesterol decreased slightly after 12 months of betaxolol (from 1.21 ± 0.05 to 1.16 ± 0.04 mmol/l, $p < 0.05$).

A moderate increase was seen in total triglycerides after 12 months (+ 10%, $p < 0.01$); this change was related to an increase in VLDL-triglycerides (from 0.68 ± 0.07 to 0.88 ± 0.09 mmol/l, $p < 0.001$) and a decrease in LDL-triglycerides (from 0.67 ± 0.04 to 0.57 ± 0.05 mmol/l, $p < 0.01$).

Apoproteins B remained unchanged.

In this study, changes in lipids and lipoproteins appear delayed (only after 12 months) and remained always slight. These variations, moderate in comparison with data from the literature, are possibly related to the individual controlled diet in this population, so as to a possible influence of the liposolubility of betaxolol, unusual for a selective β-blocker.

Phospholipids and Stroke

H. Sekimoto, M. Nakanishi, T. Nakano, Y. Matsutani, O. Shimada, and O. Katayama

Dept. of Gerontology, Kanazawa Medical University, Ishikawa-ken, Japan

Effects of phospholipids on cerebral hemorrhage in experimental animals were investigated. The hemorrhage was induced by constriction of renal arteries or infusion of Habu venom into carotid arteries of rabbits. Scanning electron microscopic observation of cerebral arteries demonstrated that the microvilli and marginal folds of the endothelium had disappeared, and there were craters found along the marginal folds. Red blood cells and other components in the blood were considered to extravasate through the craters. Pre-treatment of animals with essential phospholipids prevented the ultrastructural damages of endothelial cells.

On the other hand, in the patients who had suffered stroke, the serum levels of HDL-phospholipids were significantly lower than control. Also, it was shown that the serum phospholipids level in spontaneous hypertensive rats was lower than in Wistar Kyoto rats. These results suggested that phospholipids are able to protect the cerebral hemorrhage and that phospholipids may be of clinical use in the treatment of stroke.

The Role of Modified High Density Lipoproteins with Polyenphosphatidylcholine vesicles

Kohji Shirai, Yasushi Saito, and Akira Kumagai

The Second Dept. of Internal Medicine, School of Medicine, Chiba University, Chiba and Toyama Medical-Pharmaceutical University, Toyama, Japan

High density lipoproteins are known to have a function to remove cholesterol from the peripheral tissues. To study the mechanism of cholesterol removal by HDL, and to multiply the function of HDL, modified HDL were prepared with polyenphosphatidylcholine vesicles (soya bean lecithin = dilinoleyl phosphatidylcholine 60%, deoxycholic acid 30%, EPL®) and their functions were studied. PPC vesicles increased the release of [^{3}H]cholesterol from [^{3}H]cholesterol-laden periotoneal macrophages of rats and was much more efficient than dipalmitoyl phosphatidylcholine vesicles. Apolipoprotein AI, CI and CIII alone did not enhance the release of [^{3}H]cholesterol, but in the presence of PPC vesicles, these apolipoproteins augumented the releases of [^{3}H]cholesterol from macrophages. Incubation of PPC vesicles with HDL formed new complexes. These complexes eluted at density from 1.14 to 1.28 in zonal ultracentrifugation and were poor in apolipoprotein AI and AII (2.5% or 25% of those in native HDL) and rich in phospholipid. The addition of modified HDL to macrophages which were preincubated with [^{3}H]cholesterol or [^{3}H]cholesterol oleate-labeled acetylated low density lipoprotein, increased the release of [^{3}H]cholesterol from the cells. Their releasing activities were greater than native HDL, when the releasing activity was expressed as a function per protein concentration of HDL or modified HDL. These results suggest that removal of [^{3}H]cholesterol from the macrophages may be multiplied by modifying HDL with PPC vesicles.

Controlled Evaluation Of Panthethine, A Natural Hypolipidemic Compound, In Patients With Different Forms Of Hyperlipoproteinemia

C. R. Sirtori, G. Montanari, A. Gaddi, G. C. Descovich, G. Noseda, C. Fragiacomo, L. Colombo, and A. Craveri

Lipid Clinics from Milan (Center E. Grossi Paoletti and S. Paolo Hospital) and Bologna (II Medical Clinic of the University), Italy; and Beata Vergine Hospital, Mendrisio, Switzerland

The hypolipidemic activity of pantethine, the stable disulphate of pantethine, major component and precursor of coenzyme A, was tested in 29 patients, 11 with type IIB hyperlipoproteinemia, 15 with type IV, and 3 with an isolated reduction of high density lipoprotein cholesterol (HDL-C) levels, in a double blind protocol with a cross-over design (8 weeks for pantethine or for a corresponding placebo). In type IIB patients, pantethine (P, 300 mg bid) significantly lowered plasma total and low density lipoprotein (LDL) cholesterol (-13.5% for both parameters, P <0.01). HDL-C increased about 10% at the end of treatment in the same patients (p <0.05). Both in type IIB and type IV patients, plasma triglyceride levels were reduced around 30%, when P was given as the first treatment; when P was preceded by placebo, the reduction was less striking. HDL-C levels were not increased by P in type IV and in the patients with low HDL cholesterolemia. In type IV, LDL cholesterol levels showed a variable response to P: they tended to increase when below 132 mg/dl prior to treatment, and to be reduced when above this level. The reported study provides objective evidence for a significant, although not dramatic, hypocholesterolemic activity of P, a natural compound free of side effects; the compound may also raise HDL-C levels in type IIB patients, while moderately reducing triglyceridemia.

Treatment Of Primary Hypercholesterolemia With A Multiple Drug, Low Dose Regimen

E. A. Stein, M. Mellies, M. Yates, and C. McNerney

University of Cincinnati Medical Center, Cincinnati, Ohio

Fifteen patients (10 female) with primary hypercholesterolemia were enrolled in a study consisting of four 3-month phases: diet only; diet and colestipol (CTPL) 10 gm or probucol (PBL) 1 gm; diet, CTPL, and PBL; diet, CTPL, PBL, plus niacin 1.5 gm/day. Monthly visits assessed clinical status, drug compliance by packet/pill count, and fasting plasma was drawn for vcholesterol, triglycerides, HDL-C, LDL-C, HDL_2 and HDL_3 (by ultracentrifugation), and apolipoprotein AI and B.

(SEE TABLE)

The reductions in total and LDL-C of 159 mg/dl (40%) and 141 mg/dl (45%) as compared to diet treated values are dramatic considering the relatively low doses of medication. The fall in HDL-C, HDL_2-C, HDL_3-C and Apo AI was associated with the use of PBL and was not reversed by niacin. The therapeutic regimen was extremely well tolerated, as reflected by the high drug compliance and no study drop-outs.

		Diet Only	CTPL/PBL	CTPL and PBL	CTPL, PBL, & Niacin
Cholesterol (mg/dl)		398 $\pm$ 82	337 $\pm$ 70	291 $\pm$ 59	239 $\pm$ 56
Triglyceride (mg/dl)		140 $\pm$ 56	142 $\pm$ 61	143 $\pm$ 73	140 $\pm$ 85
HDL-C (mg/dl)		49 $\pm$ 13	42 $\pm$ 18	32 $\pm$ 10	29 $\pm$ 9
LDL-C (mg/dl)		322 $\pm$ 83	267 $\pm$ 74	231 $\pm$ 60	181 $\pm$ 52
LDL/HDL Ratio		7.2 $\pm$ 3.7	9.7 $\pm$ 10	8.6 $\pm$ 5.5	8.3 $\pm$ 7.0
HDL_2-C (mg/dl)		26 $\pm$ 11	22 $\pm$ 10	17 $\pm$ 8	15 $\pm$ 7
HDL_3-C (mg/dl)		26 $\pm$ 5.8	23 $\pm$ 7.8	18 $\pm$ 5.3	17 $\pm$ 4.8
Apo AI (mg/dl)		101 $\pm$ 22	91 $\pm$ 35	77 $\pm$ 26	73 $\pm$ 23
Apo B (mg/dl)		309 $\pm$ 69	247 $\pm$ 36	231 $\pm$ 45	203 $\pm$ 46
Drug Compliance*	Colestid		97.6 $\pm$ 3.9	92.6 $\pm$ 7.6	92 $\pm$ 7.7
	Probucol		90.1 $\pm$ 9.5	92.2 $\pm$ 7.6	90.6 $\pm$ 8.5
	Niacin		---	---	78.6 $\pm$ 15.6

*$\frac{\text{Dose Taken}}{\text{Dose Prescribed}} \times \frac{100}{1} = \%$ (all as mean $\pm$ S.D.)

Acipimox (A), A New Lipid Lowering Drug, Compared With Clofibrate (C)

P. M. J. Stuyt, A. F. H. Stalenhoef, P. N. M. Demacker, and A. van 't Laar

Dept. of Medicine, University Hospital St. Radboud, Nijmegen, The Netherlands

Ten patients with type III and 10 with type IV hyperlipoproteinemia (HLP) participated in a comparative open cross-over study of the effect of C (2x 1 gram) and of A (3x 250 mg) (at random each during 6 weeks) on the lipoproteins. Two type III patients complained of flushing during A, resulting in one drop-out. In type III, HLP serum cholesterol (chol) decreased 24% during C and 30% during A and serum triglycerides (TG) 34% and 48%, respectively (see table). In type IV, HLP chol remained unchanged and TG decreased 35% during C and 34% during A. HDL-chol increased with both drugs in both groups. There were no or slight changes in HDL_2, HDL_3, apo A_I, A_{II} and B, but their significance is unknown.

(SEE TABLE)

Conclusion: A has in type III and type IV HLP a similar hypolipidemic affect as C.

Type III	Before	3 wk. C	6 wk. C	Before	3 wk. A	6 wk. A
Chol	8.88 ±1.95	6.76** ±1.66	6.72** ±1.15	10.00 ±3.19	8.08** ±2.07	7.05** ±1.04
TG	5.57 ±2.39	3.67** ±1.43	3.68** ±1.61	7.99 ±6.30	4.51** ±1.73	4.15** ±1.51
HDL-Chol	0.93 ±0.17	1.07* ±0.26	1.02* ±0.24	0.91 ±0.24	1.04** ±0.25	0.97 ±0.22
Type IV						
Chol	6.28 ±0.94	6.11 ±1.08	6.15 ±0.81	6.55 ±1.40	6.26 ±1.03	6.07 ±0.88
TG	5.14 ±2.45	3.57** ±2.07	3.36** ±1.77	5.95 ±5.77	4.29 ±2.59	3.95* ±2.30
HDL-Chol	0.79 ±0.16	0.86 ±0.18	0.88* ±0.20	0.81 ±0.18	0.86 ±0.13	0.90* ±0.21

mean ± SD *$p < 0.05$, **$p < 0.01$

Activities of Phospholipase C, Diglyceride Lipase and Phospholipase A_2 in Platelets from Several Mammalian Species

C. A. Sutherland, C. Whyzmuzis, D. Amin, and A. Khandwala

Dept. of Biochemical Research, R&D Div. of Revlon Health Care Group, Tuckahoe, New York

The relative PLA_2 activities (arbitrary units, AU) in platelets from some commonly studied mammals were 245:87:47:3:1:0.9:0 for the rat, horse, rabbit, dog, human, cat and guinea pig (GP), respectively. The corresponding relative diglyceride lipase (DGL) activities (AU) were 23:17::10:8:4.3:3.4:1 for GP, dog, rat, cat, horse, human and rabbit, respectively. Phospholipase C (PLC) activity was comparable in platelets of rats and dogs. The methods and the DGL inhibitor RHC 80267 are described in J. Biol. Chem. 257:14006, 1982. RHC 80267 at 100 uM (I_{50} = 4 uM) and indomethacin (40 uM) did not inhibit aggregation of GP platelets stimulated by bovine thrombin (0.5 u/ml). Aggregation of GP platelets with collagen (4 ug/ml) was inhibited by indomethacin (3 uM), but RHC 80267 at concentrations below 100 uM was not similarly inhibitory. Quinacrine, an indirect PLA_2 inhibitor, had an I_{50} of 15 uM against aggregation induced by collagen. Large differences exist in PLA_2/DGL ratios in platelets of common mammalian species. This could be true of other similarly compared cell types. Collagen does not appear to promote aggregation by a mechanism dependent upon DGL activity. RHC 80267 is a useful probe for investigation of the relative importance of PLA_2, PLC and DGL in the release of arachidonic acid from phospholipids.

Pharmacological Aspects of "Lipoclin," a New Hypolipidemic Agent

K. Suzuki, T. Irie, A. Nagata, S. Aono, K. Toki, and H. Nakatani

Sumitomo Chemical Co., Ltd., Pharmaceuticals Div., Osaka, Japan

"Lipoclin" is a new hypolipidemic agent having different pharmacological aspects from clofibrate. The hypolipidemic effect was studied in normal and in hyperlipidemic animals. "Lipoclin" effectively lowered serum levels of triglyceride and cholesterol, and the effect of this drug was 5 to 10 times more potent than that of clofibrate by weight basis. "Lipoclin" did not show hepatomegaly and peroxisome proliferation at dosage levels exerting significant hypolipidemic effect. Lithogenecity of this drug was not detected in rats and hamsters, whereas clofibrate showed a tendency to increase the lithogenic index.

Pharmacokinetic studies showed that most of the absorbed drug was eliminated into bile and, after enterohepatic circulation, excreted into feces as unchanged form. In the extensive toxicological studies, "Lipoclin" was shown to have very low toxicity and no carcinogenicity.

"Lipoclin" is a trade name, the property of Sumitomo Chemical Company, Ltd. (Code No. S-8527, clinofibrate[INN]).

Effect of Clinofibrate on Biliary Lipids in the Patients with Hyperlipidemia and with Biliary Diseases

Nozomu Takeuchi, Goro Kajiyama, and Takeo Asano

The Central Laboratory, Ehime University Hospital, Ehime-ken, Japan

Clinofibrate was given to 15 patients with hyperlipidemia and 10 patients with biliary diseases for 6-8 weeks at the daily dose of 600 mg, and its effect on biliary cholesterol, bile acid, phospholipids, and the lithogenic index was investigated. After clinofibrate treatment, 6 of the hyperlipidemic patients were given 1.5 g/day clofibrate for 6-8 weeks to compare the effect clofibrate with that of clinofibrate.

Since the molar percentage of biliary cholesterol and phospholipids to the total molar number of the three biliary lipid components decreased and that of bile acid increased during clinofibrate administration, the molar ratio of bile acid to cholesterol increased. Neither the lithogenic index calculated by the formula of Admirand and Small, nor that of Hegardt et al. was altered significantly by the treatment. There was no apparent relationship between the effect of the drug on the lithogenic index and any of the factors, such as initial lithogenic index, rate of decrease of serum lipid concentration or type of hyperlipidemia.

Although clofibrate had no significant effect on the maximum solubility of cholesterol in the bile, the molar percentage of biliary cholesterol was elevated and the lithogenic index increased, as compared with the control and clinofibrate period.

Enhancement of Experimental Atherogenesis in Hypercholesterolemic Rabbits by Dietary Omega-3 Polyunsaturated Fatty Acids

J. Thiery, M. Nauck, D. Niedmann, J. Glockmann, G. Rahlf, P. Schwartz, and D. Seidel

Abtl. Klinische Chemie, Zentrum Innere Medizin, Zentrum Pathologie and Zentrum Anatomie, Med. Univ.-Klinik, Goettingen, Germany

Platelet function as a possible factor in atherogenesis is influenced by the PGI_2/TXA_2 system. Dietary effects of polyunsaturated fatty acids of the omega-3 series on these prostaglandins have been postulated to explain the lower incidence of myocardial infarction and atherosclerosis in Eskimos (Dyerberg and Bang, 1979). An influence on experimental atherogenesis was studied in groups of rabbits (n = 8) fed a semisynthetic diet (I) supplemented with 1.5% cholesterol (II) and a purified fish oil concentrate (MAXEPA, 2 ml/d) (III) for 145 days.

Aortic atherosclerosis as measured by planimetry of sudanophilic lesions (%) amounted to 2.16 $\pm$ 2.7 (I), 43.61 $\pm$ 12.74 (II), and 73.31 $\pm$ 10.97 (III). Concomitantly, the biological half life span of ^{111}Indium-labeled platelets was significantly reduced to a similar extent in groups II and III.

Toxic effects of dietary omega-3 fatty acids might be responsible for an exceptional hepatosplenomegaly with steatosis and fibrosis of the liver in group III. Peroxides in serum, expressed as malondialdehyde equivalents, of 2.25 $\pm$ 0.6 μ mol/l (III) as compared to the basal values of 0.57 $\pm$ 0.18 mol/l persisting throughout the study in groups I and II may contribute to these alterations.

Contrary to our expectations, an enhancement rather than a prevention of atherosclerosis was found in hypercholesterolemic rabbits fed a concentrate rich in omega-3 polyunsaturated fatty acids.

Inhibition of Cholesterol Synthesis by Mevinolin Stimulates Low Density Lipoprotein Receptor Activity in Human Monocyte-Derived Macrophases

Maret G. Traber and Herbert J. Kayden

Dept. of Medicine, New York University School of Medicine, New York, New York

Mevinolin inhibited the incorporation of ^{14}C acetate into cholesterol by human monocyte-derived macrophages (HMD macrophases) when both mevinolin and ^{14}C acetate were added simultaneously to the culture medium. Longer incubation with mevinolin, 24 hours, led to a marked increase in the degradation of ^{125}I-low density lipoprotein (LDL) via the high affinity receptor for LDL by HMD macrophages. Furthermore, this increased LDL receptor activity in cells incubated for 24 hours with mevinolin and lipoprotein depleted serum (LPDS) led to a nearly 3-fold increase in the formation of cholesteryl esters when these cells were then incubated with LDL for 24 hours. Continuous exposure to mevinolin did not result in a constant increase in LDL receptor activity. Cells exposed to mevinolin for 24 hours on day 3 had increased LDL receptor activity, but exposure to mevinolin with 5% human serum (HS) from day 3 to 9 resulted in degradation of ^{125}I-LDL at the same rate as observed in cells incubated with 5% HS alone. Cholesterol synthesis from ^{14}C acetate was decreased in cells incubated for 24 hours in 5% HS + mevinolin compared with 5% HS alone, and in 10% LPDS + mevinolin compared with 10% LPDS alone; however, cells incubated with LPDS + mevinolin synthesized cholesterol at higher rates than did cells cultured in 5% HS alone. Continuous culture with 5% HS + mevinolin for 5 days resulted in cholesterol synthesis at control levels. These data show that following inhibition of cholesterol synthesis by mevinolin, HMD macrophages maintain cholesterol homeostasis by increasing LDL receptor activity to obtain cholesterol from LDL.

2-Tetradecylglycidyl-CoA, The Active Form of the Fatty Acid Oxidation Inhibitors, Methyl-2-Tetradecylglycidate (MeTDGA) and 2-Tetradecylglycidic Acid (TDGA)

G. F. Tutwiler and T. C. Kiorpes

McNeil Pharmaceutical, Spring House, Pennsylvania

TDGA and Me-TDGA, potent, specific inhibitors of long chain fatty acid oxidation, have frequently been used to delineate the inter-relationship of fatty acid oxidation, esterification and gluconeogenesis *in vivo* and *in vitro*. They are orally effective hypoglycemic and anti-ketogenic compounds. As these compounds are fatty acid analogs, it was of interest to follow selected aspects of their metabolic transformation *in vitro* in order to gain further insight into their mechanism of action. Both were converted to acyl-CoA derivatives by acyl-CoA synthetase with the enzyme showing a preference for (+)TDGA. The resulting TDGA-CoA was a substrate for glycerolipid synthesis as evinced by studies in hepatocytes using [C]TDGA but failed to undergo -oxidation. Instead, TDGA-CoA rapidly, irreversibly and stereospecifically (+ isomer) inhibited (Ki=300nM) mitochondrial carnitine:palmitoyl transferase (CPT). Only the outer CPT (A) was inhibited as revealed by digitonin separation of the inner and outer enzymes after *in vivo* Me-TDGA administration. *In vitro*, the intramitochondrial CPT-B converted TDGA-CoA to a carnitine ester, which indicated that this enzyme is not inhibitable. Our results clearly identify TDGA-CoA as the active form of these compounds and its inhibition of CPT-A as their site of action.

Natural Product Inhibitors of Cholesterol Absorption

George V. Vahouny

George Washington University, Dept. of Biochemistry, Washington, D.C.

We have recently surveyed a number of unrelated natural products for their direct effects on cholesterol absorption in the rat. These included various purified plant sterols, shellfish sterols, salmon oil, dietary fiber derivatives and a partially deacetylated product of chitin, chitosan. Effects on cholesterol (and fatty acid) absorption were determined by net recovery of administered lipid in the thoracic duct lymph, and was assessed by either acute administration of the agent, or following feeding of the agent for four weeks. Chitosan was the most effective of the agents tested and was equivalent to the effects of cholestyramine administration. Among the cholesterol analogues, sitosterol and stigmasterol were equally effective with lesser effects of shellfish sterols and no effect by fucosterol. Salmon oil, fed in equivalent amounts to either oleic acid or corn oil was also an effective inhibitor of sterol absorption. Among the dietary fibers, pectin, guar gum and alfalfa all exhibited effects on absorption of cholesterol, while bran and yeast cell wall polysaccharides were without significant effects.

Although the mechanisms of each class of biological agents on sterol absorption are different, further studies on these materials alone and in combination appears warranted.

Supported in part by USDA Grant 82-CR-CR-1-1001

Niphedipin (calcium-antagonist) does not Affect Serum Lipoproteins

G. Walldius

Dept. of Medicine, Karolinska Hospital and King Gustaf V Research Institute, Stockholm, Sweden

Background: In the long term treatment of angina pectoris (AP) and hypertension, it is important that haemodynamically active drugs do not affect serum lipoproteins undesirably. Increased conc of VLDL-triglycerides (TG) and decreased conc of HDL-cholestrol (chol) have been reported for some -blocking agents.

The aim of this study was to see if the calcium-antagonist niphedipin (N) affects lipoprotein conc.

Design: Nine males with stable AP (4 with hypertriglyceridaemia), mean age 58 years (43-69) were treated with N 30-40 mg/d for 14 weeks.

(SEE TABLE)

N did not affect any lipoprotein fraction significantly. We have previously reported that another ca-antagonist (verapamil) lowers total and LDL-chol.

Conclusion: We believe that calcium-antagonists have no undesirable effects on serum lipoprotein concentrations in long term treatment of AP and hypertension.

Results:

	Total		VLDL		LDL		HDL Tot.		HDL	HDL
	Chol	TG	Chol	TG	Chol	TG	Chol	TG	Chol	Chol
Before	7.2	2.2	0.9	1.6	5.0	0.4	1.2	0.2	0.4	0.8
After	6.9	2.4	0.9	1.7	4.6	0.5	1.2	0.2	0.5	0.8

Beclobrate, A New Lipid Lowering Agent - Results in Patients with Hypercholesterolaemia

A. Walther, H. Merki, R. Mordasini, W. Riesen, and H. P. Gurtner

Lipid Research Laboratory, Tiefenau-Hospital, and Cardiologic Unit (Inselspital) of the University of Berne, Switzerland

The efficacy and tolerance of Beclobrate, a new derivative of Clofibrate, was assessed in an open-study in 15 patients with primary hypercholesterolaemia. After a dietary pre-treatment period of at least three months, the trial was divided into four observation periods consisting of a four weeks' period of placebo-administration followed by two eight weeks' periods on Beclobrate one 25 mg capsule twice daily or one 50 mg capsule twice daily, respectively. This was followed by a further four-week placebo treatment period at the end of the study.

Cholesterol (CH) and Triglycerides (TG) were measured in whole serum and in the isolated lipoprotein fractions after ultracentrifugation. In addition, the apoproteins B (RID), A-I and A-II (EID) were determined as well as the usual safety parameters.

Total- and LDL-CH (about 20%) as well as apo-B (15%) and total- and VLDL-TG were significantly decreased. Both HDL-CH and the apoproteins A-I and A-II showed a significant increase. The lipid lowering effect as well as the influence on the HDL were dose related, the 100 mg daily dosage being more effective in lowering total CH- and LDL-CH as well as increasing the HDL. No side-effects were reported during Beclobrate administration, nor were any adverse changes noted in hematology and blood-chemistry studies.

Effect of Long Term Probucol Treatment on Serum Lipoproteins and Skin Xanthomas in Heterozygous Familial Hypercholesterolemia

Akira Watanabe, Hiroshi Mabuchi, Yasuyuki Sakai, Takeshi Sakai, Akira Yoshimura, Takanobu Wakasugi, Junji Koizumi, Susumu Miyamoto, and Ryoyu Takeda

Second Dept. of Internal Medicine, School of Medicine, Kanazawa University, Kanazawa, Japan

We studied the effects of probucol on serum lipoprotein lipids and skin xanthomas in 36 heterozygous patients with familial hypercholesterolemia (FH). Probucol was given at the dose of 1.0 g per day for 24 months. Serum cholesterol (TC) decreased from 334 ± 12 to 267 ± 12 (mean ± SE) mg/dl- a 17 per cent reduction ($p<0.001$). LDL-TC decreased by 19 per cent, from 256 ± 12 to 210 ± 14 mg/dl ($p<0.001$) and HDL-TC decreased by 29 per cent, from 41 ± 2 to 31 ± 2 mg/dl ($p<0.001$). VLDL-TC, VLDL-triglyceride (TG) and HDL-TG decreased significantly ($p<0.05$, $p<0.05$, $p<0.05$, respectively). Serum TG did not change significantly. LDL-TG showed a slightly upward trend and LDL-TC/LDL-TG ratio decreased significantly ($p<0.05$). The complete or partial regression of skin xanthomas was noticed in eight of 12 patients (66.7 per cent). The regression of xanthelasma palpebrarum was observed in five of seven patients (71.4 per cent) and tuberous xanthomas regressed in three of four patients (75 per cent).

These data suggest that probucol is an effective hypolipidemic agent in a heterozygus patient with FH.

Regression of Aortic Atherosclerosis Produced by Combined Therapy with Probucol and Cholestyramine

Robert W. Wissler and Dragoslava Vesselinovitch

Dept. of Pathology and Specialized Center of Research on Atherosclerosis, University of Chicago, Chicago, Illinois

Twenty adult male rhesus monkeys were all fed a high fat, high cholesterol ration for the first 13 months of this study. At this time, five of the animals were autopsied; their atherosclerotic lesions served as a reference for quantative morphometry. They were used for comparing the lesions resulting from treating the other 15 animals in groups of 5 with probucol (0.06g/kg body wt./day) alone, cholestyramine (0.57g/kg body wt./day) alone, or a combination of these two drugs, for a 12-month period, while the animals continued to receive the original atherogenic ration. The combined drug therapy led to remarkable lowering of the blood cholesterol from 931 to 217mg%, while the HDL cholesterol was higher than baseline and higher than the pretreatment level. The aortic atherosclerotic lesions of the treated groups all showed evidence of regression.

The most substantial regression was observed in the aortic lesions of the animals receiving the combined therapy with probucol and cholestyramine. Their microscopic lesions decreased on the average from a thickness of 0.26mm to 0.12mm and the total lipid observed in their lesions decreased from 0.42mm^2 to 0.19mm^2, while the total lesion areas observed in these standardized samples of the aorta decreased similarly as did the % of aortic medial involvement. The single therapy groups showed less regression, with the probucol treated animals demonstrating somewhat more lesion regression than the cholestyramine treated group.

Effects of Meprobamate (Equanil) on Plasma Lipids and Atherogenesis on Cockerels Fed an Atherogenic Diet

Harry Y. C. Wong, Ka-Kui S. Cheng, David T. Ng and Howard S. Kruth

Dept. of Physiol., Howard University College of Medicine, Washington, D.C., and Experimental Atherosclerosis, NHLBI, NIH, Bethesda, Maryland

Diazepam (Valium), a benzodiazepine, has been reported to lower plasma cholesterol and atherogenesis in roosters fed an (AD). Thus, we decided to study the effect of another tranquilizer, meprobamate (M), a carbamate derivative, on plasma lipids and aortic and coronary atheromatosis of cockerels fed an AD (2%) cholesterol + 5% cottonseed oil added to plain mash (PM). Total of 24 6-month old birds were divided into 4 groups: I. PM controls; II. PM+M; III. AD; and IV. AD+M.M (8.57 mg/kg) was administered twice daily _per os_ by a tube. After 10 weeks, following data were obtained: (1) hypercholesterolemia occurred in AD and AD+M, but there was no statistical difference in plasma lipids when AD was compared to AD+M ($p < 0.2$), nor PM to PM+M; (2) no gross lesion was observed in the thoracic (T) or abdominal (AB) aortas of PM controls, but 4 out of 6 PM+M had T lesions avg. grading of 1.0 (based on 0-4) and all had (AB) lesions (avg. 2.5). All AD had T and AB atheroma avg. 1.3 and 3.5; and in AD+M, lesions avg. 1.5 and 3.7, respectively; (3) histologic sections of aorta showed spontaneous lesions with lipid deposits in PM and PM+M groups. AD groups indicated infiltration of lipids into the aortas, and there were no differences between the groups. Examination of coronary arteries depicted some lesions in PM groups; AD groups had much more severe lesions than PM groups, but no difference was observed between AD groups.

Improving Effect of Panax Ginseng and Its Saponins on Hyperlipidemia in Rats and In Man

Masahiro Yamamoto, Yasushi Tamura and Akira Kumagai

Dept. of Internal Medicine, Nissei Hospital, Osaka; Second Dept. of Internal Medicine, Chiba University, Chiba and Toyama Med. Pharm. University, Toyama, Japan

Panax ginseng has been widely used in oriental countries for thousands of years for its tonic action. Chemical structure of ginseng saponins named ginsenosides were determined by Shibata et al. Biochemical and pharmacological actions of ginseng have been clarified recently (ex. Yamamoto et al. Arzneimittelforschung 27: 1169; 1404, 1977; 28: 2238, 1978).

It has been reported from our lab. that serum cholesterol (CH) and triglyceride (TG) were reduced with ginseng saponins in high CH diet-fed rats, plasma CH turnover after ^{14}C-CH injection was accelerated and that fecal sterol and bile acid excretion was increased with ginseng saponins.

In this paper, serum HDL-CH was increased, while CH, atherogenic index (AI), TG, NEFA as well as platelet adhesion were all decreased with oral administration of red ginseng powder manufactured by the Office of Monopoly, Republic of Korea, 1 g/kg/d., corresponding to 20-50 mg ginsenosides, in high CH diet-fed rats. Long-term administration of red ginseng powder 2.7 g/d. to patients with hyperlipidemia, significantly reduced CH, AI, TG, NEFA and lipoperoxide, while HDL-CH increased after 1 up to 24 months.

Prevention By Pantethine of HDL-C Reduction Induced by Probucol

T. Yasugi, G. Mizuno, H. Kishi, H. Izumida, T. Tochihara, U. Hara, T. Fujioka, and T. Shimizu

The Second Dept. of Medicine, Nihon University School of Medicine, Tokyo, Japan

It is well known that probucol induces marked reductions of serum cholesterol levels. However, a problem exists that HDL-C also decreases significantly on probucol administration. It might be well effective if reduction of HDL-C by probucol could be prevented by the utilization with other drugs together. So, in this study synergistic effects on serum lipids, lipoprotein and HDL apolipoproteins were studied by the administration of probucol and pantethine which activate lipolytic activity and biosynthesis of apoA-I and increase HDL-C.

Methods: Ten cases of heterozygote familiar hypercholesterolemis and combined hyperlipemia were subdivided into two groups. Then, 750 mg/day of probucol and 600 mg/day of pantethine were given for 8 weeks into the first group, and 1500 mg/day of probucol and 600 mg/day of pantethine to the other group.

Results: In the first group, serum cholesterol and LDL-C decreased significantly. However, HDL-C did not decrease at all. HDL apoA-I also did not change. On the contrary, in the second group, HDL-C, HDL and HDL apoA-I decreased significantly although serum cholesterol and LDL-C decreased more than those in the first group.

Conclusion: Synergistic administration of probucol and pantethine is effective to prevent the HDL-C reduction by probucol when dose of probucol is maintained under 750 g/day.

Three Way Comparative Double Blind Study of Probucol in Japan

T. Yasugi, H. Nakamura, C. Naito, F. Kuzuya, I. Fukui, A. Yamamoto, K. Ogino, H. Fukuzaki, K. Arakawa, and K. Oshima

Nihon University, Tokyo; Jikei University, Tokyo; Tokyo Teishin Hospital, Tokyo; Nagoya University, Nagoya; Kyoto Pref. Med. Univ., Kyoto; National Cardiovascular Center, Osaka; Kobe University, Kobe; and Fukuoka University, Fukuoka, Japan

To investigate the clinical usefulness of probucol in hyperlipidemia, probucol, 250 mg TID, was compared with nicomol, 400 mg TID, and dextran sulfate sodium 300 mg TID for 16 weeks in a three-way parallel double blind study.

Total 364 patients were included in the evaluations with 122 patients, 122 patients and 120 patients allocated to the probucol, nicomol and dextran sulfate sodium groups, respectively. All the lipid analyses were performed at one central laboratory. At 16 weeks, cholesterol reduction in the probucol group was 39 mg/dl (14%) compared to baseline. No consistent change of total serum cholesterol was observed in the nicomol and dextran sulfate sodium groups. The three drugs in this study decreased serum triglyceride to almost same extent. HDL-cholesterol decreased from baseline significantly with probucol at each four-week interval ($p<0.001$), whereas it was significantly elevated from baseline with nicomol at 4W, and with dextran sulfate sodium at 8W, 12W and 16W. The most commonly observed adverse reactions associated with nicomol were skin diseases.

Gastrointestinal disorders were the main adverse reactions associated with probucol and dextran sulfate sodium; however, these were not significantly different among the three drugs.

Judging from the results of effectiveness and safety, probucol is a useful drug in treatment of hyperlipidemia.

Effect of Streptococcus Faecium on the Serum Cholesterol and Triglyceride Level

Kazunaga Yazawa, Fumio Kuzuga, and Yasuo Kawai

Dept. of Clinical Biochemistry; Institute of Medical Science, Advance R&D Company, Kanagawa; Dept. of Geriatrics, School of Medicine, Nagoya University, Aichi; and Dept. of Microbiology, School of Medicine, Teikyo University, Tokyo, Japan

Effect of administration of *Streptococcus faecium* on the serum cholesterol and triglyceride levels was examined.

The oral administration (10^{10} viable cells/animal) of *Streptococcus faecium* lowered the serum levels of cholesterol and triglyceride by 20 to 40% and 15 to 60%, respectively, in both ex-germfree rats and mice.

The oral administration of the dead cells of *Streptococcus faecium* 10^{10}/day for 4 weeks lowered the serum cholesterol and triglyceride by 20 to 32% and 30 to 75%, respectively, in both conventional rats and mice.

When high cholesterol diet (1% cholesterol + 0.5% sodium cholate) was given, the serum cholesterol and triglyceride were lowered by 30% and 53%, respectively, by the streptococcal administration in conventional rats. And when fructose diet (60% fructose) was given, the serum cholesterol and triglyceride levels were lowered by 23.5% and 68%, respectively, by the streptococcal administration.

These effects were dose-dependent when 10^8 to 10^{11} dead cells of the streptococci/day/animal were administered for 4 weeks.

Then we obtained fractions from *Streptococcus faecium*: they are proteins and polysaccharides which lowered the serum cholesterol and triglyceride levels, respectively.

Beneficial Effects of Pantethine on Regression of Atherosclerosis

Yoji Yoshida, Masako Mitsumata, Toshio Fukuda, and Genju Ooneda

Dept. of Pathology, Yamanashi Medical College, Yamanashi; Dept. of Pathology, Gunma University Hospital, Maebashi; and Geriatrics Research Institute, Maebashi, Japan

Marked atherosclerotic lesions developed in the rabbit common carotid artery which had received a freeze-injury by liquid-N_2 and had been exposed to hyperlipidemia for 14 weeks.

First, effects of Pantethine (P) on development and regression of the lesions were investigated in vivo.

Animals placed on an atherogenic diet supplemented with 1% P. (w/w) for 14 weeks showed an average serum cholesterol level was 1,500 mg/dl being in contrast to 2,000 mg/dl in the controls without P. The areas of intimal thickening and the number of foam cells in the lesions reduced significantly as compared to those of the controls. The average areas of the intima in the center of the lesions were 739 x 10^3 in the experimentals and 1046 x $10^3\mu^2$ in the controls, respectively.

In the rabbits under regimen for atherosclerosis P. assumed to have beneficial effects on regress of the lesions.

Secondly, influence of P. on the rabbit aortic medial smooth muscle cells was studied in vitro. Acid cholesteryl esterase activity in cell homogenates showed increment of 140% at an hour to reach 226% p in maximum at 4 hours after addition of 100 μ MP into the culture media.

Acid phosphatase activity was also stimulated by P. Lysosomes increased in number in the cells under an electron microscope after the supplement.

Hypolipidemic Food Products: An Alternative to Pills and Powders

James H. Zavoral, Peter Hannan, Donna Fields, Ivan Frantz, and Madge Hanson

Dept. of Pediatrics, Hennepin County Medical Center, Minneapolis, Minnesota

Twenty-eight patients (17 adults, 11 children), 18 with familial hypercholesterolemia (FHC) and 10 normal family members (N) were fed four food products with Locust Bean Gum (LBG), 8-30 gm/day. Utilizing a cross-over design, identical food products with and without LBG were consumed by two groups of patients. Plasma cholesterol (C), low density lipoprotein cholesterol (LDL-C), high density lipoprotein cholesterol (HDL-C), very low density lipoprotein cholesterol (VLDL-C), and triglycerides (Tg) were measured at two-week intervals and compared to control feeding periods. In Group A, FHC C and LDL-C decreased by 10 and 11% ($p < .001$), N C and LDL-C decreased by 6 and 10% ($p < .001$). In Group B, FHC C and LDL-C decreased by 17 and 19%, N C and LDL-C decreased by 11 and 6% ($p < .001$). HDL-C and VLDL-C decreased in both groups compared to control diets but less dramatically. C and LDL-C decreased in FHC children and adults. N adults and children had a lessor decrease in lipids. Tg decreased in both groups slightly (N.S.). The LBG in food products was well accepted and without side effects. Food products offer a potential alternative to pills and powders for the hypolipidemic prevention of atherosclerosis in adults and children with FHC.

TO AGEING LIPIDOLOGISTS

"You are old, Father William," the young man said,
"And your hair has become very white;
And yet you incessantly stand on your head -
Do you think, at your age, it is right?"

"In my youth," Father William replied to his friend,
"I feared it might injure the brain
But now there are certainly drugs no end
Which will lower my lipids again."

"You are old," said the youth, "with receptors no more -
Your A1 and C3 are to blame,
Why bother to go looking for apos galore
And old fibrates to give a new name?"

"In my youth," said the sage, "there were lipids and proteins
And we thought there was nothing more subtle,
But now it is clear that we don't have the means
To know how they manage to couple."

"You are old," said the youth "and your mind is too weak
To discover another peptide,
Yet you will not give up, and measure each peak,
Although many are not bonafide."

"In my youth," said the Prof., "I thought that the heart
Was the source and giver of life
But now I know it's an irrelevant part
Interrupting laboratory strife."

"You are old," said the youth, "you cannot still wish
To be given by Nobel a prize
For lowering your lipids with enzymes of radish
And I doubt if it is really so wise."

"I have answered your questions and that is enough,
Of discussing the heart and such things,
Do you think I can listen all day to such stuff?
Be off, let me play with my chemical rings."

M. F. OLIVER

With apologies to Bill Holmes, Lewis Carroll, and Alice
(who lived in an alternative wonderland).

AUTHOR INDEX

SUBJECT INDEX

www.ingramcontent.com/pod-product-compliance
Lightning Source LLC
LaVergne TN
LVHW082023200926
848481LV00010B/2909
* 9 7 8 1 4 6 1 2 9 4 9 3 1 *